Mental Disorders in Primary Care

Jeanne Miranda
Ann A. Hohmann
C. Clifford Attkisson
David B. Larson

Editors

Mental Disorders in Primary Care

Jossey-Bass Publishers
San Francisco

Contributions by two of the editors, Ann A. Hohmann and David B. Larson, were made as part of their official duties as employees of the U.S. federal government.

Manufactured in the United States of America. Nearly all Jossey-Bass books and jackets are printed on recycled paper that contains at least 50 percent recycled waste, including 10 percent postconsumer waste. Many of our materials are also printed with vegetable-based ink; during the printing process these inks emit fewer volatile organic compounds (VOCs) than petroleum-based inks. VOCs contribute to the formation of smog.

Library of Congress Cataloging-in-Publication Data

Mental disorders in primary care / editors, Jeanne Miranda . . . [et al.]. — 1st ed.
p. cm.—(The Jossey-Bass health series) (The Jossey-Bass social and behavioral science series)
Includes bibliographical references and index.
ISBN 1-55542-660-3
1. Psychiatry. 2. Primary care (Medicine) I. Miranda, Jeanne, date. II. Series. III. Series: The Jossey-Bass social and behavioral science series.
RC454.4.M456 1994
616.89—dc20 94-6425
CIP

FIRST EDITION
HB Printing 10 9 8 7 6 5 4 3 2 1 *Code 9457*

A joint publication in
The Jossey-Bass Health Series and
The Jossey-Bass Social and Behavioral
Science Series

Contents

Preface

As this book goes to press, four work groups of primary care researchers and clinicians are completing a psychiatric diagnostic manual—the *Diagnostic and Statistical Manual of Mental Disorders-IV-Primary Care* (DSM-IV-PC)—that will help primary care practitioners to identify the mental disorders seen in primary care practices. This manual will be explicitly linked to the *Diagnostic and Statistical Manual of Mental Disorders-IV* (DSM-IV) that is also in preparation to be used in psychiatric settings. The work to produce the primary care version of the manual was supported by many organizations. These include the American Psychiatric Association (APA), the National Institute of Mental Health (NIMH), the American Academy of Pediatrics, the American College of Obstetrics and Gynecology, the Society of General Internal Medicine, and the American Academy of Family Physicians. This support demonstrates the cogency of the primary care research carried out in the last thirty years, particularly in the United Kingdom and the United States. In *Mental Disorders in Primary Care,* the prominent researchers in this field organize and present this important body of work.

Research has clearly shown that nearly half of all individuals seeking care for mental disorders go to primary care physicians rather than to psychiatrists or other mental health professionals. Unfortunately, few of the mental disorders are detected, diagnosed, or treated correctly by primary care physicians. No single volume has been available that summarizes the research literature on what is known about the recognition, treatment, and treatment outcomes for mental disorders in primary care. This book provides an organized presentation of that literature, with a historical perspective.

In addition to presenting what is known about mental disorders in primary care, a second and perhaps even more important goal of this book is to provide an agenda for mental health services research in primary care settings. In conceptualizing the book, we intended the authors, in the course of their reviews of the published research, to identify the major gaps in our general understanding of the presentation, identification, and treatment of mental disorders in primary care. Each chapter addresses the specific research issues that the field must confront in the next decade.

Audience for the Book

We have written this book for several groups. First, it will be valuable to those who are conducting, or plan to conduct, research on mental disorders in primary care settings. This book provides an overview of the current state of the field, as well as outlining areas for future research.

Mental Disorders in Primary Care has also been written for clinicians in the field. It clearly reviews the epidemiology, presentations, treatments for, and clinical sequelae of mental disorders in primary care. As such, the book should be useful to primary care physicians, consultation-liaison psychiatrists, health psychologists, and substance abuse counselors working with medical patients.

Those who pay for and regulate health care settings may find this book useful as well. It clearly spells out the impact of mental disorders on the medical system. In addition, strategies for evaluating interventions are delineated.

Finally, this book should contribute significantly to the education of medical students, psychiatrists, and mental health professionals. It fills an important gap, since no comprehensive study of mental disorders in primary care previously existed. This book should be useful in classroom settings, providing cogent information on a wide range of medical issues.

Overview of the Contents

Part One provides essential background material. In Chapter One, Jeanne Miranda, Ann A. Hohmann, and C. Clifford Attkisson sketch the epidemiological underpinnings of the field of mental disorders in primary care. We present data demonstrating the high prevalence of psychiatric disorders in primary care patients and document the pattern of service use by these patients. In Chapter Two, Barbara J. Burns provides a historical perspective on the development of this field. Barbara E. Havassy and Catherine J. Schmidt discuss substance abuse as it presents and impacts primary care medical settings in Chapter Three. Finally, in Chapter Four, Johan Ormel and Wim van den Brink define the problem by comparing outcomes of primary care patients with mental disorders to outcomes of similar patients without the mental disorders.

Part Two focuses on the co-occurrence of mental and medical disorders. Clearly medical disorders can cause mental disorders, mental disorders can complicate medical disorders, and other factors, such as stress, can cause both types of disorders. In Chapter Five, Jeanne Miranda, Patricia A. Arean, and Richard L. Rickman discuss the complex relationships between the two types of disorders in adults, while Nicholas Long, Barbara Starfield, and Kelly Kelleher discuss these relationships in children in Chapter Six.

Part Three covers presentation and recognition of mental disorders in primary care. W. Eugene Broadhead, in Chapter Seven, describes typical presentations of psychiatric disorders in primary care populations. Next, in Chapter Eight, Rolando Castillo, Howard Waitzkin, and Javier I. Escobar cover the atypical presentations of psychiatric distress often seen in immigrant and refugee populations. Daniel E. Ford evaluates what is known about physicians' roles and abilities in recognizing mental disorders in Chapter Nine. In Chapter Ten, Anne W. Riley and Lawrence S. Wissow discuss research on the ability of pediatricians to recognize emotional and behavioral problems and family violence in their patients. Finally, in Chapter Eleven, Linda Gask discusses important work on improving physicians' ability to detect mental disorders.

Part Four examines the current state of knowledge on treatment of mental disorders in primary care. In Chapter Twelve, Herbert C. Schulberg and Kathleen A. Pajer discuss the major issues in evaluating research on treatment of depression in primary care. Frank V. deGruy, in Chapter Thirteen, examines the treatment of anxiety in medical settings. In Chapter Fourteen, Kelly Kelleher and Vaughn I. Rickert review the relatively new area of management of pediatric mental disorders by primary care physicians. Finally, in Chapter Fifteen, Junius J. Gonzales and Grayson Norquist trace interventions in primary care that are conducted through consultation-liaison programs.

An important aspect of mental disorders in primary care is the consequences of the disorder for health services utilization. This is the topic of Part Five. In Chapter Sixteen, Philip J. Leaf presents an overview of the literature evaluating the impact of mental illness on medical services utilization. In addition, in Chapter Seventeen, Curtis J. Henke and Michael S. Pallak discuss economic analyses of treatment of mental disorders in primary care.

Part Six takes up the subject of methodology. In Chapter Eighteen, Michael Von Korff and Gregory E. Simon clearly outline the major methodologic issues confronting researchers in this area. They provide useful guidelines for getting answers to the most important questions in this field.

Acknowledgments

We would like to thank the chapter authors for their patience and for the time they devoted in helping us compile this book. Without their hard work and insightful syntheses of the literature, our vision of a state-of-the-art book on mental health issues in primary care would never have been realized. We also wish to thank Ed Klein for his very helpful contribution to the editorial work and Clifford Willis for his fine clerical services.

March 1994

Jeanne Miranda
San Francisco, California

Ann A. Hohmann
Baltimore, Maryland

C. Clifford Attkisson
Mill Valley, California

David B. Larson
Rockville, Maryland

The Editors

JEANNE MIRANDA is assistant professor in residence at the University of California, San Francisco (UCSF). She received her B.A. degree (1976) in psychology from Idaho State University and her Ph.D. degree (1986) in clinical psychology from the University of Kansas. She completed pre- and postdoctoral fellowships in clinical psychology at UCSF and a two-year, National Institute of Mental Health-sponsored clinical services research fellowship, also at UCSF.

Miranda is director of the depression clinic at San Francisco General Hospital, which treats depression in medical patients. In addition, she is director of the behavioral medicine program for the division of internal medicine at San Francisco General Hospital.

Miranda's research has focused on mental disorders in primary care patients, including treatment of depression in low-income and minority public care medical patients.

ANN A. HOHMANN is chief of the Special Populations and Research Methods Development Program in the Services Research Branch at the National Institute of Mental Health (NIMH). She received her B.A. degree (1978) from Pomona College and both her M.A. (1980) and Ph.D. (1983) degrees from Rutgers University, all in sociology. She received her M.P.H. degree (1987) from Harvard University.

Hohmann is currently responsible for the extramural research programs at NIMH related to mental health services for homeless, rural, and minority people and to research methods development. Her research since joining NIMH has focused on the prescription of psychotropic drugs and uses of formal and informal mental health services.

In 1992 Hohmann received an award from the director of NIMH for her contributions to the development of the NIMH program in clinical services research.

C. Clifford Attkisson is professor of medical psychology in the Department of Psychiatry at the University of California, San Francisco (UCSF), where he also serves as dean of the graduate division and associate vice chancellor for student academic affairs. He received his A.B. degree (1962) in psychology from the University of Richmond and his Ph.D. degree (1970) in psychology from the University of Tennessee. He completed psychoanalytic training at the San Francisco Psychoanalytic Institute in 1992 and is a member of the San Francisco Psychoanalytic Institute and Society.

Attkisson's teaching and research over the past twenty-three years have concentrated on program evaluation, information systems for human services, clinical services, and service systems research. His current research program is a study of innovative systems of care for children and adolescents who suffer from serious emotional disorders.

David B. Larson is president of the National Institute for Healthcare Research, located in Tyson's Corner, Virginia. During the last twelve years he has worked as senior researcher for the Department of Health and Human Services and the National Institute of Mental Health (NIMH). He is also an adjunct associate professor in the Department of Psychiatry at Duke University Medical Center.

Larson received his B.S. degree (1969) in humanities and technology from Drexel University and his M.D. degree (1973) from

Temple University Medical School. He completed his chief residency in psychiatry at Duke University Medical Center. He received his M.S.P.H. degree (1983) from the School of Public Health at the University of North Carolina.

Larson's research has focused on the impact of religious commitment on physical health, mental health, and social status; the method and use of analytic systematic reviews of research literature; the provision and delivery of mental health services in both the primary care and specialty mental health service sectors; and care issues concerning the prescription of psychotropic medications.

The Contributors

Patricia A. Arean has recently completed a National Institute of Mental Health–sponsored clinical services fellowship at the University of California, San Francisco. She received her Ph.D. degree (1991) in clinical psychology from Fairleigh Dickinson University. Her research focuses on depression in elderly medical patients.

W. Eugene Broadhead is associate professor of community and family medicine and chief of the research and education division, Duke University Medical Center. He received his M.D. degree (1981) from Duke University and his Ph.D. degree (1987) in epidemiology from the University of North Carolina School of Public Health. Broadhead serves on the editorial board of the *Archives of Family Medicine* and continues to practice family medicine part-time in the rural town of Yanceyville, North Carolina.

Barbara J. Burns holds academic appointments at Duke University as professor of medical psychology (Department of Psychiatry), associate research professor (Center for Health Policy Research and

Education), and senior fellow (Center for the Study of Aging and Human Development). She received her Ph.D. degree (1972) in counseling psychology from Boston College. Her major research interests are in the areas of child, adult, and elderly psychopathology and mental health services, with a focus on the quality and outcomes of care for populations with severe and persistent disorders.

Rolando Castillo is assistant clinical professor in psychosocial medicine in the Department of Medicine at the University of California, Irvine. He is also founder and executive director of the Consortium of Physicians from Latin America (COPHYLA), which operates widely in the state of California. Castillo received his Ph.D. degree (1992) in education from Claremont Graduate School of Education.

Frank V. deGruy is associate professor in the Department of Family Practice and Community Medicine at the University of South Alabama College of Medicine, where he is also director of research. He received his M.D. degree (1977) from the University of South Alabama and his M.S.F.M. degree (1982) from Case Western Reserve University, where he was a Robert Wood Johnson fellow from 1977–1980.

Javier I. Escobar is professor and interim chair of the Department of Psychiatry in the School of Medicine at the University of Connecticut. He is also a consultant to the World Health Organization and the National Institutes of Health and a member of the Food and Drug Administration Advisory Committee on Psychopharmacology. He received his M.D. degree (1967) from the University of Antioquia, Colombia.

Daniel E. Ford is assistant professor of medicine, epidemiology, and health policy and management in the Welch Center at Johns Hopkins Medical Institutions. He is a general internist conducting research on early symptoms of psychiatric disturbance in patients seen in primary care settings. He received his M.D. degree (1982) from the State University of New York at Buffalo and his M.P.H. degree (1986) from Johns Hopkins.

Linda Gask is senior lecturer in psychiatry at the University of Manchester in the United Kingdom and is also a consultant psychiatrist in Preston, Lancashire, in a community-based psychiatric service. She is an active member of the management committee of the Defeat Depression Campaign sponsored by the Royal College of Psychiatrists and the Royal College of General Practitioners. She received her M.D. degree (1979) from the University of Edinburgh and her Ph.D. degree (1992) in psychiatry from the University of Manchester.

Junius J. Gonzales is director of clinical programs and assistant professor in the Department of Psychiatry at Georgetown University Medical Center. He is also a member of the clinical economics research unit in the Department of Medicine and the university's Institute for Health Care Research and Policy. Gonzales received his M.D. degree (1986) from the University of Pennsylvania.

Barbara E. Havassy is adjunct professor of medical psychology in the Department of Psychiatry, School of Medicine, at the University of California, San Francisco, where she is codirector of the Clinical Services Research Postdoctoral Training Program (funded by the National Institute of Mental Health) and codirector of the Postdoctoral Training Program in Substance Abuse Treatment Research (funded by the National Institute of Drug Abuse). She received her Ph.D. degree (1969) in social psychology from the University of Colorado, Boulder. Havassy conducts services research in the fields of mental health and drug abuse.

Curtis J. Henke is an economist on the faculty of the Department of Medicine at the University of California, San Francisco. He also holds an adjunct faculty position in the Sacramento center of the School of Public Administration of the University of Southern California. He received his Ph.D. degree (1982) in economics from the University of California, Berkeley.

Kelly Kelleher is associate professor of pediatrics and psychiatry at Arkansas Children's Hospital and the University of Arkansas for Medical Sciences, where he is also the associate director of the Center for Applied Research and Evaluation and on the steering committee of the Centers for Mental Health Care Research. He received his M.D. degree (1984) from the Ohio State University and his M.P.H. degree (1988) from Johns Hopkins University.

Philip J. Leaf is professor in the Department of Mental Hygiene at the Johns Hopkins School of Public Health, with joint appointments in Health Policy Management and the Department of Psychiatry. He received his Ph.D. degree (1978) in sociology from the University of Wisconsin.

Nicholas Long is associate professor and director of pediatric psychology in the Department of Pediatrics at the University of Arkansas for Medical Sciences and Arkansas Children's Hospital. He received his Ph.D. degree (1985) in clinical child psychology from the University of Georgia. His primary research interests include parenting, the psychosocial adjustment of children to chronic medical conditions, common psychosocial problems in pediatric primary care, and the adjustment of children to divorce.

Grayson Norquist is deputy director of the Division of Epidemiology and Services Research and associate director for services research at the National Institute of Mental Health. He received his M.D. degree (1978) from the University of Mississippi and his M.S.P.H. degree (1989) from the School of Public Health at the University of California, Los Angeles (UCLA). Norquist completed his training in psychiatry at the UCLA Neuropsychiatric Institute, which was followed by an appointment as a Robert Wood Johnson Clinical Scholar at UCLA.

Johan Ormel is associate professor of psychiatric epidemiology (Department of Psychiatry) and of social epidemiology (Department of Health Sciences) at the University of Groningen in the Netherlands. He received his Ph.D. degree (1980) in medical sociology from the University of Groningen.

Kathleen A. Pajer is associate professor of psychiatry and director of psychiatry residency training at the Medical College of Pennsylvania, Allegheny campus. She received her M.D. degree (1982) from the University of South Alabama and her M.P.H. degree (1988) from Yale University.

Michael S. Pallak is partner in and vice president for research of Quality Behavior Health, Inc. He also serves as director of the organizational psychology program for the California School of Professional Psychology, Los Angeles campus, and is special assistant to the chancellor. He received his Ph.D. degree (1968) in social psychology from Yale University. He is the former chief executive officer of the American Psychological Association and former editor of the *American Psychologist,* of which he is currently an associate editor.

Vaughn I. Rickert is associate professor of pediatrics at the University of Arkansas for Medical Sciences and on staff at Arkansas Children's Hospital. He received his Psy.D. degree (1986) in clinical psychology from Central Michigan University after completing his internship at Johns Hopkins University School of Medicine. He is a fellow in the Society for Adolescent Medicine.

Richard L. Rickman is a postdoctoral fellow at the Center for AIDS Prevention Studies at the University of California, San Francisco (UCSF). He received his Ph.D. degree (1991) in clinical psychology from the University of Southern Florida and completed a clinical internship at UCSF, where he focused on mental health care delivery to medical outpatients. Rickman's current research examines the interpersonal aspects of condom use and other AIDS-relevant behavior among adolescents and young adults.

Anne W. Riley is assistant professor in the Department of Health Policy and Management at Johns Hopkins University. She received her Ph.D. degree (1986) in psychology from Virginia Polytechnic Institute and State University. Her current research focuses on the measurement of child and adolescent health status, the investigation of factors related to the type of treatment received by adolescents with mental health problems, and the role of pediatric providers in the management of children's emotional and behavioral problems.

Catherine J. Schmidt is assistant research sociologist at the University of California, San Francisco, and research analyst at Family Caregiver Alliance in San Francisco. She received her Ph.D. degree (1980) in sociology from the State University of New York at Stony Brook.

Herbert C. Schulberg is professor of psychiatry, psychology, and medicine at the University of Pittsburgh and director of the primary care consultation program at Western Psychiatric Institute and Clinic. He received his Ph.D. degree (1960) in clinical psychology from Columbia University.

Gregory E. Simon is assistant scientific investigator at the Center for Health Studies, Group Health Cooperative of Puget Sound, and research assistant professor in the Department of Psychiatry and Behavioral Sciences at the University of Washington. He received his M.D. degree (1982) from the University of North Carolina and his M.P.H. degree (1990) from the University of Washington.

Barbara Starfield is professor and head of the Division of Health Policy at the Johns Hopkins University School of Public Health, with a joint appointment in the Department of Pediatrics at the medical school. She received her M.D. degree (1959) from the State University of New York (Health Sciences Center in Brooklyn) and her M.P.H. degree (1963) from Johns Hopkins University. She is a fellow of the American Academy of Pediatrics and a member of the Institute of Medicine.

Wim van den Brink is professor of clinical epidemiology and addiction at the University of Amsterdam, where he is also associate professor of psychiatry. In addition, he is program director of the clinical epidemiology program of the Amsterdam Institute for Addiction Research. He received his M.D. degree (1981) from the Free University of Amsterdam and his Ph.D. degree (1989) in psychiatry from the University of Groningen in the Netherlands.

Michael Von Korff is associate director of research at the Center for Health Studies, Group Health Cooperative of Puget Sound. He received his Sc.D. degree (1978) in health operations research from the School of Hygiene and Public Health, Johns Hopkins University, where he also received postdoctoral fellowship training (1979–1980) in mental disorder epidemiology.

Howard Waitzkin is professor of medicine and social sciences and attending physician in internal medicine at the University of California, Irvine. He received his M.D. degree (1972) and his Ph.D. degree (1972) in sociology from Harvard University. His current research focuses on psychosocial issues in primary care and health policy issues such as access to health care and proposals for a national health program. He has authored *The Second Sickness: Contradictions of Capitalist Health Care* (1983) and *The Politics of Medical Encounters: How Patients and Doctors Deal with Social Problems* (1991).

Lawrence S. Wissow is associate professor of pediatrics at the Johns Hopkins University School of Medicine. He received his M.D. degree (1979) from Duke University and his M.P.H. degree (1984) from Johns Hopkins University. He has a long-standing interest in the detection and treatment of family violence and is the author of *Child Advocacy for the Clinician* (1990).

Mental Disorders in Primary Care

Part One

Mental Disorders in Primary Care: The Scope of the Problem

Jeanne Miranda
Ann A. Hohmann
C. Clifford Attkisson

1

Epidemiology of Mental Disorders in Primary Care

Most individuals who suffer from mental disorders are seen by primary care physicians rather than psychiatrists or other mental health professionals. This surprising fact became known as a result of data from the Epidemiologic Catchment Area (ECA) study (Regier, Goldberg, & Taube, 1978). The ECA study was the first attempt to evaluate the incidence and prevalence of psychiatric disorders in the United States as a whole. The development of the Diagnostic Interview Schedule (DIS)—an instrument that allows lay interviewers to determine psychiatric diagnoses reliably (Robins, Helzer, Croughan, & Ratcliff, 1981)—made this large-scale study possible. The DIS was used to interview 20,291 adults in the community as well as in institutions in five areas of the United States. One year later, 78 percent of these adults were reinterviewed during the second wave of data collection. In addition, the use of mental health and medical services by those with and without a psychiatric diagnosis was evaluated. As a result of the data from this comprehensive study, the widespread use of medical services for mental health purposes became known.

In this chapter, we present ECA and other epidemiological data that serve as the underpinnings of the field of mental disorders in primary care. The prevalence of mental and addictive disorders in adults and children as seen in primary care settings will be discussed. In addition, we will review current knowledge of service use by those with mental and addictive disorders.

Epidemiology of Mental Disorders in Primary Care

Recent analyses of both waves of the ECA data have provided important information about the rates of mental disorders in the community, as well as clarifying the relationship between presence of a psychiatric disorder and use of medical services (Regier et al., 1993). First, in the United States as a whole, mental and addictive disorders have a six-month prevalence rate of 16 percent. However, for primary care patients who use medical services frequently (at least once in six months), mental and addictive disorders have a six-month prevalence rate of 21.7 percent (Kessler, Cleary, & Burke, 1987). The high prevalence of mental disorders in primary care patients has been confirmed in studies of primary care patient populations. For example, using the same diagnostic instrument as in the ECA studies, the one-month prevalence of mental and addictive disorders in primary care patients in an inner-city group practice was 25 percent (Von Korff et al., 1987). Thus, mental and addictive disorders are more frequent in primary care settings than in the community as a whole.

Overall, 14.7 percent of adults receive mental health services during a year. In contrast, 28.5 percent of those who have a diagnosable psychiatric disorder seek mental health or addictive service care. Many patients use the general medical sector for mental health services. Of those with a diagnosable psychiatric disorder who seek care, 40 to 50 percent seek care from the general medical sector. Sociodemographic factors influence the probability of seeking mental health services from primary care physicians rather than mental health professionals. In particular, nonwhites and lower-income individuals are less likely to seek mental health treatment from any source than are more affluent white persons. For example, the Los Angeles ECA studies found that Mexican Americans with a recently diagnosed mental disorder were only half as likely as non-Hispanic whites (11 versus 22 percent, respectively) to have seen a mental health professional. Thus, many patients with psychiatric disorders fail to seek treatment.

Given that less than 30 percent of persons with mental or addictive disorders seek mental health services, a logical next question is what percentage of persons who have, but do not seek treatment for, mental or addictive disorders visit a general medical physician so that treatment or referral could be made if the disorder were detected. Over 78 percent of those with mental or addictive disorders receive health care services (Regier et al., 1978). Thus, the vast majority of those who fail to seek treatment for mental or addictive disorders are seen in the general health sector and could receive treatment if the disorders were detected.

A problem arises when studying overall rates of mental and addictive disorders in primary care. Specifically, many studies include diagnoses for common and minor disorders such as minor phobias. These disorders have dramatically different consequences than more severe disorders such as depression or panic disorder. For this reason, we turn next to the prevalence and medical utilization consequences of severe disorders, including depression, anxiety, somatization, psychotic disorders, and alcohol and other substance abuse disorders. In a separate section, we will consider childhood mental disorders as seen in pediatric primary care settings.

Depression

Depression is the most prevalent major mental disorder, in both the community and in primary care medical settings. According to estimates from the ECA date, approximately 5 percent of the population suffers a depressive episode in any one year.

Numerous studies have investigated the prevalence of depression in primary care patients. Eight studies have been conducted in the United States, using the same diagnostic instrument as the ECA study. In seven of these studies (Burnham, Wells, Rogers, & Potts, 1989; Coulehan, Schulberg, Block, Janosky, & Arena, 1990; Hoppe, Leon, & Realini, 1989; Kessler et al., 1987; Schulberg et al., 1985; Von Korff et al., 1987; Zich, Attkisson, & Greenfield, 1990), approximately 4.1 to 8.6 percent of patients met criteria for major depression—rates somewhat higher than the population as a whole. In the eighth study (Pérez-Stable, Miranda, Muñoz, & Ying, 1990), an inner-city sample of predominantly low-income and minority patients, approximately 16 percent had major depression. Two studies in the United States used the Schedule for Affective Disorders (SADS) (Endicott & Spitzer, 1978). One found a 5.6 percent rate of major depression (Hoeper, Nycz, Cleary, Regier, & Goldberg, 1979) and the other—a study of rural patients—found 2.2 percent major depression and 6.4 percent masked major depression or depression presenting with predominantly physical complaints (Barrett, Barrett, Oxman, & Gerber, 1988). International studies find similar rates. A study in Great Britain found a 4.8 percent rate of major depression in medical patients (Blacker & Clare, 1988), and a study in the Netherlands found 5.6 percent cases of depression (Ormel, van den Brink, & Koeter, 1990). These studies confirm that depression is extremely prevalent in medical patients, with rates comparable to that of hypertension—the most common medical disorder.

Several studies have evaluated the course of depression in primary care patients. In two studies, researchers followed depressed patients for six months and estimated that between 29 percent (Schulberg, McClelland, & Gooding, 1987) and 36 percent (Kessler, Cleary, & Burke, 1985) continued to meet criteria for depression. In two studies, depressed patients were followed for a year. Using clinical interviews, 25 percent were judged to have chronic depression and 22 percent improved depression (Mann, Jenkins, & Belsey, 1981). Using the Center for Epidemiological Studies Depression (CESD) scale, a measure of depressive symptomatology, 50 percent remained symptomatic (Hankin & Locke, 1982). In a study of geriatric outpatients, 52 percent were found to remain depressed thirty-three months later (Kukull, Koepsell, & Inui, 1986). In sum, these studies suggest that depression is persistent among primary care patients.

Data from the ECA study provide information regarding use of services by individuals with diagnoses of depression. Among those with major depression, 49 percent seek professional care during a year's time; 27.8 percent seek this care from mental health specialists and 25.3 percent from physicians in the general medical sector (Regier et al., 1993). Clearly, nearly half of all persons who are depressed and seek care do so from their primary care physicians.

Anxiety

Although anxiety in general is very common, the more serious and debilitating anxiety disorders—panic disorder and obsessive-compulsive disorder—are less common in the community. Approximately 1.3 percent of the population in the general community has panic disorder in any one year; 2.1 percent has obsessive-compulsive disorder (Regier et al., 1988, 1993).

A few studies have examined the prevalence of anxiety disorders among primary care patients. Two studies (Schulberg et al., 1985; Von Korff et al., 1987) found that just less than 2 percent of patients in general medical settings met criteria for panic disorder and that 1 percent had obsessive-compulsive disorder. These rates are similar to those found in the community in general.

Two studies evaluated the less debilitating diagnosis of generalized anxiety disorder in medical patients. There are no community-based data for this disorder, and so no community comparisons can be made. Between 3 and 4.6 percent of general medical patients met criteria for generalized anxiety disorder (Barrett, Oxman, & Gerber, 1987; Von Korff et al., 1987). Only one study followed general medical patients with anxiety over time. It found that only 2 percent with general anxiety continued to meet criteria six months later (Kessler, Cleary, & Burke, 1985). Although generalized anxiety disorders are relatively common in primary care patients, they appear to be transient.

In general, persons with anxiety disorders are as likely to seek treatment in general medical clinics as in specialty mental health settings: 29.7 percent of those with panic disorders are treated in general medical settings and 33.6 percent in mental health specialty settings. Similarly, 18.3 percent of those with obsessive-compulsive disorders are seen by general medical practitioners and 25.3 percent by mental health specialists (Regier et al., 1993).

Somatization

Somatization disorder is rare in the general population; approximately 0.2 percent of the population meet criteria for this disorder sometime during their lifetime (Regier et al., 1988, 1993; Swartz, Landerman, George, Blazer, & Escobar, 1990). However, because these patients experience their suffering as physical illness, they are also frequent users of general medicine for nonmental health treatment. As a result, they are overrepresented in primary care clinic populations. For example, deGruy, Columbia, and Dickinson (1987) found that 5 percent of patients in an academic family practice setting met criteria for somatization disorder (compared with 0.2 percent in the general population).

Of those with somatization disorder, approximately 70 percent seek mental health treatment. Of those somatizers who seek mental health services, 49.4 percent seek the services from the general medical sector. However, many (42.5 percent) also seek care from mental health specialists (Regier et al., 1993).

Although DSM-III-R Somatization Disorder is generally rare, people with unexplained somatic complaints but who do not have enough of these symptoms to meet diagnostic criteria for somatization disorder are highly prevalent. Escobar, Burnam, Karno, Forsythe, and Golding (1987) estimate that 4.4 percent of the general population in Los Angeles are somatizers under an abridged definition (having symptoms of somatization disorder but fewer than are required for diagnosis), whereas in Puerto Rico, 18 to 20 percent meet this criterion (Escobar, Rubio-Stipec, Canino, & Karno, 1989). In a low-income, predominantly minority sample of inner-city medical patients, nearly 25 percent meet this abridged criterion (Miranda, Pérez-Stable, Muñoz, Hargreaves, & Henke, 1991). Although use of services for those with somatic symptomatology has not been well studied, one investigation suggests that these patients overuse medical services when they experience life stress (Miranda et al., 1991).

Psychotic Disorders

The psychotic disorders are among the most severe and debilitating mental disorders. Approximately 3 percent of the general population experience schizophrenia or bipolar disorder during any one-year period (Regier et al., 1993). Surprisingly, studies in primary care settings find few patients with these disorders. Less than 1 percent of primary care patients meet criteria for schizophrenia or bipolar disorder (Von Korff et al., 1987; Schulberg et al., 1985).

Despite these small numbers in primary care populations, many patients with psychotic disorders seek mental health care from general medical practitioners. For example, approximately 29 percent of patients who meet diagnostic criteria for schizophrenia are treated by physicians in the general medical sector; 14 percent are seen exclusively in the general medical system. Those with bipolar disorder are equally likely to be seen in general medical or mental health specialty settings, with approximately 33 percent seen in each.

Alcohol and Other Substance Abuse

According to the ECA study, nearly 9.5 percent of the general population meets criteria for substance abuse disorder during any year. In surveys of medical patients, substantial numbers have current substance abuse disorders. Von Korff et al., (1987) found 5.0 percent of their medical patients to meet criteria for alcoholism. Similarly, Schulberg et al. (1985) found that 8.2 percent met criteria for alcoholism; 7.1 percent abuse drugs.

Nearly 10 percent of those who abuse substances seek care from medical personnel, whereas 11.2 percent use specialty mental health and addictive services. As with psychiatric illness, substance abuse is common in the general medical sector, and general physicians are frequently sought out to treat these disorders.

Mental Disorders in Children and Adolescents

Although mental disorders in pediatric settings have been less well studied than in adult settings, the existing data suggest that, as with adults, children with mental disorders are overrepresented in pediatric practices and that few are seen by mental health specialists. Estimates of the number of children with mental disorders vary widely, depending on the informant (that is, parents versus pediatrician) and the diagnostic criteria used (Gould, Wunsh-Hitzig, & Dohrenwend, 1980). The best estimates suggest that at least 10 percent of school-aged children have one or more significant mental health problems (Achenbach & Edelbrock, 1981).

As with adults, children with mental health problems are overrepresented in primary care pediatric samples. For example, Costello et al. (1988) gave a random sample of children attending pediatric clinics the Child Behavior Checklist or CBCL (Achenbach & Edelbrock, 1983). National age- and gender-stratified norms are available for this questionnaire, with 10 percent of children scoring in the clinically significant range. In Costello's pediatric sample, 24.7 percent (195 of 789) scored above the clinical cutoff.

Few of the children with mental disorders seen in pediatric practices are treated by mental health specialists. In a recent study of children with mental disorders seen by pediatricians, only 16 percent were referred to specialty services; 40 percent received intervention by the pediatrician, 31 percent had no active intervention, and 13 percent had disorders where treatment was not indicated (Horwitz, Leaf, Leventhal, Forsyth, & Speechley, 1992). Similarly, Lavigne et al. (1993) found that 51.7 percent of children with an emotional/behavioral problem in a pediatric practice had not received counseling, medication, or a mental health referral. Not surprisingly, children whose problems were rated moderate to severe were twice as likely to be referred as children with mild problems.

Mental Health Services Research in Primary Care

Psychiatric morbidity influences use of ambulatory medical services. Generally, psychiatric distress is a predictor of high medical care utilization; patients with psychiatric distress use more services than do their less distressed counterparts (for example, see Follette & Cummings, 1967; Mechanic, Cleary, & Greenley, 1982; Myers & Weissman, 1980; Shapiro et al., 1984). However, much of this increased use of services may be for medical rather than psychiatric complaints. In addition, medical patients often reduce their level of utilization of general health services following mental health treatment (National Institute of Mental Health, 1986).

Mental health services provided in health care settings differ from those in mental health settings. For instance, patients who are seen for mental health or addiction problems are seen less frequently in medical as compared to mental health settings. That is, if they are seen in medical rather than mental or addictive disorder specialty settings, they make fewer visits per year for mental health services (Narrow, Regier, Rae, Manderscheid, & Locke, 1993). Unfortunately, few data are available on the differential effectiveness of these treatments.

Conclusion

Epidemiological research has consistently found that people with mental disorders are overrepresented in primary care medical patient populations. In addition, almost half of those with mental disorders who seek treatment do so from primary care physicians rather than mental health specialists. Many who do not seek services for their mental disorders are seen by primary care physicians and could be treated if the disorder was detected. Patients with mental disorders tend to use more medical services than do those without mental disorders. These epidemiological data clearly point to the need for further research on detection and treatment of mental disorders in primary care patients.

References

Achenbach, T. M., & Edelbrock, C. S. (1981). Behavioral problems and competencies reported by parents of normal and disturbed children aged 4 through 16. *Monograph of Social Research on Child Development, 46,* 1.

Achenbach, T. M., & Edelbrock, C. S. (1983). *Manual for the child behavior checklist.* Burlington: University of Vermont.

Barrett, J., Oxman, T., & Gerber, P. (1987). Prevalence of depression and its correlates in a general medical practice. *Journal of Affective Disorders, 12,* 167–174.

Barrett, J. E., Barrett, J. A., Oxman, T. E., & Gerber, P. D. (1988). The prevalence of psychiatric disorders in a primary care practice. *Archives of General Psychiatry, 45,* 1100–1106.

Blacker, C.V.R., & Clare, A. W. (1988). The prevalence and treatment of depression in general practice. *Psychopharmacology, 95,* 514–517.

Burnham, A., Wells, K., Rogers, W., & Potts, M. (1989, May). *Prev-*

alence of depression in general medical and mental health outpatient practices in three health care systems. Paper presented at the annual meeting of the American Psychiatric Association, San Francisco.

Costello, E. J., Edelbrock, C., Costello, A. J., Dulcan, M. K., Burns, B. J., & Brent, D. (1988). Psychopathology in pediatric primary care: The new hidden morbidity. *Pediatrics, 82,* 415–424.

Coulehan, J. L., Schulberg, H. C., Block, M. R., Janosky, J. E., & Arena, V. C. (1990). Medical comorbidity of major depressive disorder in a primary medical practice. *Journal of General Internal Medicine, 150,* 2363–2367.

deGruy, F., Columbia, L., & Dickinson, P. (1987). Somatization disorder in a family practice. *Journal of Family Practice, 25,* 45–51.

Endicott, J., & Spitzer, R. L. (1978). A diagnostic interview: The schedule for affective disorders and schizophrenia. *Archives of General Psychiatry, 35,* 837–844.

Escobar, J. I., Burnam, A., Karno, M., Forsythe, A., & Golding, J. M. (1987). Somatization in the community. *Archives of General Psychiatry, 44,* 713–718.

Escobar, J. I., Rubio-Stipec, M., Canino, G., & Karno, M. (1989). Somatic symptoms index (SSI): A new abridged somatization construct. *Journal of Nervous and Mental Disease, 177,* 140–146.

Follette, W., & Cummings, N. A. (1967). Psychiatric services and utilization in a prepaid health plan setting. *Medical Care, 5,* 24–35.

Gould, M. S., Wunsch-Hitzig, R., & Dohrenwend, B. P. (1980). Formulation of hypotheses about prevalence, treatment, and prognostic significance of psychiatric disorders in children in the United States. In B. P. Dohrenwend, M. S. Gould, & B. Link (Eds.), *Mental illness in the United States: Epidemiological estimates* (pp. 9–44). New York: Praeger.

Hankin, J. R., & Locke, B. Z. (1982). The persistence of depressive symptomatology among prepaid group practice enrollees: An exploratory study. *American Journal of Public Health, 72,* 1000–1007.

Hoeper, E. W., Nycz, G. R., Cleary, P. D., Regier, D. A., & Goldberg, I. D. (1979). Estimated prevalence of RD mental disorder in primary medical care. *International Journal of Mental Health, 8,* 6–15.

Hoppe, S. K., Leon, R. L., & Realini, J. P. (1989). Depression and anxiety among Mexican Americans in a family health center. *Social Psychiatry and Epidemiology, 24,* 63–68.

Horwitz, S. M., Leaf, P. J., Leventhal, J. M., Forsyth, B., & Speechley, K. N. (1992). Identification and management of psychosocial and developmental problems in community-based, primary care pediatric practices. *Pediatrics, 89,* 480–485.

Kessler, L., Cleary, P., & Burke, J. (1985). Psychiatric disorders in primary care. *Archives of General Psychiatry, 42,* 583–587.

Kessler, L., Cleary, P., & Burke, J. (1987). Psychiatric diagnoses of medical service users: Evidence from the Epidemiologic Catchment Area Program. *American Journal of Public Health, 77,* 18–24.

Kukull, W. A., Koepsell, T., & Inui, T. S. (1986). Depression and physical illness among general medical clinic patients. *Journal of Affective Disorders, 10,* 153–162.

Lavigne, J. V., Binns, H. J., Christoffel, K. K., Rosenbaum, D., Arend, R., Smith, K., Hayford, J. R., McGuire, P. A., & Pediatric Practice Research Group. (1993). Behavioral and emotional problems among preschool children in pediatric primary care: Prevalence and pediatricians' recognition. *Pediatrics, 91,* 649–655.

Mann, A., Jenkins, R., & Belsey, E. (1981). The twelve-month outcome of patients with neurotic illness in general practice. *Psychosomatic Medicine, 11,* 535–550.

Mechanic, D., Cleary, P. D., & Greenley, J. R. (1982). Distress syndrome, illness behavior, access to care, and medical utilization in a defined population. *Medical Care, 20,* 361–372.

Miranda, J., Pérez-Stable, E. J., Muñoz, R. F., Hargreaves, W., & Henke, C. J. (1991). Somatization, psychiatric disorder, and stress in utilization of ambulatory medical services. *Health Psychology, 10*(1), 46–51.

Myers, J., & Weissman, M. (1980). Recognition of depression. *American Journal of Psychiatry, 141,* 1081–1084.

Narrow, W. E., Regier, D. A., Rae, D. S., Manderscheid, R. W., & Locke, B. Z. (1993). Use of services by persons with mental and addictive disorders: Findings from the National Institute of Mental Health Epidemiologic Catchment Area Program. *Archives of General Psychiatry, 50,* 95–107.

National Institute of Mental Health. (1986). *Mental health impact on medical care cost and utilization under Medicare and Medicaid—a study design.* Bethesda, MD: Author.

Ormel, J., van den Brink, W., & Koeter, M.W.J. (1990). Recognition, management, and outcome of psychological disorders in primary care: A naturalistic follow up study. *Psychosomatic Medicine, 20,* 909–923.

Pérez-Stable, E., Miranda, J., Muñoz, R., & Ying, Y. (1990). Depression in medical outpatients: Underrecognition and misdiagnosis. *Archives of Internal Medicine, 150,* 1083–1088.

Regier, D. A., Boyd, J. H., Burke, J. D., Rae, D. S., Myers, J. K., Kramer, M., Robins, L. N., George, L. K., Karno, M., & Locke, B. Z. (1988). One-month prevalence of mental disorders in the United States: Based on five Epidemiologic Catchment Area sites. *Archives of General Psychiatry, 45,* 977–986.

Regier, D. A., Goldberg, I. D., & Taube, C. A. (1978). The de facto US mental health services system: A public health perspective. *Archives of General Psychiatry, 35,* 685–693.

Regier, D. A., Narrow, W. E., Rae, D. S., Manderscheid, R. W., Locke, B. Z., & Goodwin, F. K. (1993). The de facto US mental and addictive disorders service system: Epidemiologic Catchment Area prospective 1-year prevalence rates of disorders and services. *Archives of General Psychiatry, 50,* 85–94.

Robins, L., Helzer, J., Croughan, J., & Ratcliff, K. (1981). National Institute of Mental Health Diagnostic Interview Schedule: Its history, characteristics, and validity. *Archives of General Psychiatry, 41,* 949–958.

Schulberg, H., McClelland, M., & Gooding, W. (1987). Six month outcome for medical patients with major depressive disorders. *Journal of General Internal Medicine, 4,* 312–317.

Schulberg, H. C., Saul, M., McClelland, M., Ganguli, M., Christy, W., & Frank, R. (1985). Assessing depression in primary medical and psychiatric practice. *Archives of General Psychiatry, 42,* 1164–1170.

Shapiro, S., Skinner, E. A., Kessler, L. G., Von Korff, M., German, P. S., Tischler, G. L., Leaf, P. J., Benham, L., Cottler, L., &

Regier, D. A. (1984). Utilization of health and mental health services: Three Epidemiological Catchment Area sites. *Archives of General Psychiatry, 41,* 971-978.

Swartz, M., Landerman, R., George, L., Blazer, D., & Escobar, J. (1990). Somatization disorder. In L. N. Robins & D. Regier, (Eds.), *Psychiatric disorders in America.* New York: Free Press.

Von Korff, M., Shapiro, S., Burke, J. D., Teitelbaum, M., Skinner, E. A., German, P., Turner, R. W., Klein, L., & Burns, B. (1987). Anxiety and depression in a primary care clinic: Comparison of Diagnostic Interview Schedule, General Health Questionnaire, and practitioner assessments. *Archives of General Psychiatry, 44,* 152-156.

Zich, J. M., Attkisson, C. C., & Greenfield, T. K. (1990). Screening for depression in primary care clinics: The CES-D and the BDI. *International Journal of Psychiatry and Medicine, 20,* 259-277.

2

Barbara J. Burns

Historical Considerations of Mental Disorders in Primary Care

Primary care mental health services research focuses on the nature, recognition, classification, and treatment of people with mental disorders in primary care settings. The ultimate goal of the research is to improve mental health services in the general health sector. The major foci of the research over the past twenty years in the United States include:

- Documenting the extent of illness and types of mental disorder in general medical populations
- Describing and assessing the mental health practices of health professionals and patterns of service use by the population
- Modifying mental health practices of general medical professionals and assessing client and system level outcomes
- Evaluating the impact of organizational structures and financing mechanisms on health and mental health service use and client outcomes

Note: The author would like to acknowledge Junius Gonzales, M.D.—current chief of the NIMH Primary Care Research Program—for a program update. This chapter was supported in part by NIMH grant MH45750.

Throughout the development of primary care mental health research in the United States, the National Institute of Mental Health (NIMH) has provided the leadership and support for its growth as a field. A series of articles that span more than a decade have documented the scientific development of the field (Burns, Regier, Goldberg, & Kessler, 1979; Hankin & Oktay, 1979; Burns & Burke, 1985; Wilkinson, 1985; Burns, Taube, & Regier, 1986; Kamerow, Pincus, & MacDonald, 1986; Taube & Burns, 1988; Schulberg & Burns, 1988; Morlock, 1989; Schulberg, 1991). This chapter uses the preceding review documents to show the progression of thematic developments in primary care mental health research and provides a context for understanding its emergence in the United States. Because of NIMH's central role in the development and progression of research in this area and the author's direct involvement at NIMH in the field's emergence, this history is written from that perspective.*

Early Influences

Creation of the Primary Care Research Program was influenced by a combination of U.S. health policy developments, international research and directives, and NIMH data collection efforts related to primary care.

Policy Context

The Primary Care Research Program at NIMH emerged out of a period of rapid growth of the mental health system in this country. During the 1960s and the early 1970s, there was optimism in the United States about the potential to provide specialist mental health services to the entire population. This optimism stemmed from several factors: (1) enactment of the Community Mental Health

*The author brings a perspective developed through direct involvement in this history, both in a primary care research setting before coming to NIMH (a neighborhood health center with mental health services in Boston) and as an integral part of the NIMH staff involved in primary care mental health services research (1978–1987).

Centers Act in 1963, promising a shift away from care in large psychiatric hospitals to services in the community; (2) a dramatic rise in the number of psychiatrists, psychologists, psychiatric social workers, and psychiatric nurses due, in part, to NIMH support for their training; and (3) the addition of psychiatric benefits to health insurance plans, with states mandating at least minimal inpatient and outpatient coverage. Health policy developments during this period were even more dramatic and added to the sense of optimism. Medicaid and Medicare—which increased access to health care for low-income persons, the elderly, and the disabled—were passed in the early 1960s, and President Kennedy promised national health insurance by 1970.

By the early 1970s, revolutionary developments in health and mental health services looked much less probable. Gains in the provision of services were threatened by serious economic problems and more conservative governments. Efforts to reduce the cost of health care became evident in prospective payment and managed care, a deemphasis on specialist medical care, and mandates to strengthen primary care medicine. Within the mental health sector, the hopes of the 1960s were diminished as progress slowed in the 1970s. Only 50 percent of the community mental health centers (CMHCs) proposed were ever established, and funds for them were impounded during the Nixon administration. Ultimately, the increasing numbers of deinstitutionalized patients on the streets, in nursing homes, or in jails made it clear that CMHCs were not meeting the needs of those suffering from mental illness, particularly those with severe mental disorders. Support for clinical training of mental health professionals was cut drastically, despite predictions of shortages in psychiatry (Graduate Medical Education National Advisory Committee, 1981). Further, gains in psychiatric benefits in insurance plans were showing signs of erosion. These developments made the primary care sector of the health care system an increasingly likely source of care for individuals with severe mental disorders.

International Perspective

The Primary Care Research Program was influenced substantially by an international perspective on the place of primary care in the delivery of mental health services. Outside the United States, in both developed and developing countries, an expectation that mental health specialists would assume responsibility for most mental illness did not evolve as it did in this country. In fact, a World Health Organization work group stated in 1973 that "the primary care team is the cornerstone of psychiatry" (World Health Organization, 1973). Access to specialist care in most of the world is restricted by mechanisms such as gatekeepers, explicit or implicit rationing, and professional shortages.

The difference in how mental health services are actually provided in the United States and elsewhere has led to differences in perspectives about the nature and role of primary care. The international perspective about the critical role of primary care in the delivery of mental health services helped shape the NIMH Primary Care Research Program. Critical to the formation of the NIMH program was Shepherd's work in the General Practice Research Unit in London.

Epidemiological research directed by Shepherd, beginning in the 1950s, established that the great majority of patients with mental disorders make no contact with specialty mental health service providers and that the care of these patients falls primarily to the general practitioner (Shepherd, Cooper, Brown, & Kalton, 1966). The early and ongoing consultation by Shepherd and other investigators from his unit was critical to the development of the NIMH program.

NIMH Data Context

Data gathered by NIMH in the 1960s and 1970s also influenced the focus of the Primary Care Research Program. The NIMH National Reporting Program (NRP) was established to survey use of specialty mental health clinics and public and private psychiatric hospitals. The NRP expanded in the late 1960s to include surveys of the new CMHCs and to collect the first data on mental health services in the general health sector—that is, on psychiatric units in general hospitals. This latter step represented an initial recognition that a national picture of mental health service use would be incomplete without information on mental health service use in the general health sector.

Several researchers within NIMH in the Division of Biometry and Epidemiology perceived the need to extend the picture beyond the hospital to primary care services in the community. They developed a combined estimate of mental health services provided by psychiatrists and primary care physicians in one large county in New York. In the three types of primary care settings surveyed, the annual prevalence of mental disorder ranged from 5.4 to 20.2 percent, while only 1.6 to 5.2 percent of persons in the preceding groups were found on the psychiatric case register in Monroe County, New York (Rosen, Locke, Goldberg, & Babigian, 1972; Goldberg, Babigian, Locke, & Rosen, 1978). These findings, which documented a critical gap (3.8 to 15 percent) between having a mental disorder and receiving psychiatric care, helped direct attention to a potentially significant mental health role for primary health care providers. These findings supported Shepherd's research in London and made it clear that a mental health role for primary care providers was not solely attributable to gatekeeping in the British National Health Service but was probably more universal.

NIMH Research Agenda

Health policy developments in the United States, international research and directives, and NIMH data collection efforts related to primary care highlighted the need for a primary care research program within NIMH, but the focus for such a program was lacking. Darrel A. Regier was recruited to NIMH in 1975 by Irving Goldberg, chief of the Biometry Branch, for the express purpose of providing this focus.

Establishing the Research Agenda

To establish the NIMH agenda, Regier began by analyzing national surveys of health and mental health service use and case register data to estimate the proportion of the population with mental disorders who received mental health services. He found that only 20 percent of persons with mental illnesses were receiving any care from mental health specialists; 60 percent were receiving care only from primary care physicians, and another 20 percent went entirely without treatment. Later published as the "de facto" paper (Regier, Goldberg, & Taube, 1978), the above finding solidified the need for further investigation and was used by the President's Commission on Mental Health (1978) to reinforce this need. By 1977, with the support of Herbert Pardes, then NIMH director, the research program was formally organized to address the following questions:

1. What is the prevalence of mental disorders identified in the U.S. primary health care sector?
2. What are the validity and reliability of psychiatric diagnoses made by primary health care providers?
3. What mental health treatment services are primary health care providers currently offering?
4. What is the outcome or effectiveness of mental health services provided in the primary health care sector?
5. What is the optimal division of responsibility between the primary care sector and the specialty mental health sector in the treatment of patients with mental disorders?
6. What kind of mental health training programs will enable primary health providers to deal most effectively with their patients requiring mental health services?
7. What is the effect of different organizational and financing structures of primary health and mental health specialty services on the utilization and cost of both mental health services and other health services for patients with mental disorders?
8. What is the overall cost of mental health services provided in the primary health care sector?
9. What is the effect of different organizational and financing structures on health and mental health?

This set of carefully considered research directions set the stage for an initial sequence of studies and a long-term research agenda. Despite gains in many areas, this agenda remains relevant in the 1990s.

Initial steps to launch the program included a comprehensive literature review and a national conference. NIMH commissioned a state-of-the-art review (Hankin & Oktay, 1979), which provided the background for future research and for the 1979 conference, "Mental Health Services in Primary Care Settings." At this conference, investigators and key government officials—including the Secretary of the Department of Health and Human Services, Julius Richmond—met to assess the mental health service needs of the population and the policy interests of the government. The outcome of this meeting was a more specific set of research recommendations, which called for epidemiologic, clinically oriented, institutionally oriented, and health systems studies in primary care.

Pivotal Research Under Contract

Since the creation of the Primary Care Research Program predated the grants mechanism for mental health services research (initiated in 1979), and since few investigators would have been prepared to respond to a request for proposals, request for applications, or program announcement on this topic, the early research was directed by NIMH Primary Care Research Program staff and conducted under contract.

This was an exciting five-year period (1978–1983) for NIMH staff recruited to initiate the program. In essence, an intramural research program enabled staff investigators to design studies that were then conducted under contract in the field. The challenge was to translate the primary care research questions into relevant and feasible studies. Contracts were awarded on a competitive basis; analysis and subsequent publications were often joint efforts between NIMH staff and university-based investigators.

The early research contracts focused on the prevalence of mental disorder in primary care patients, the differences between clinical practices of mental health specialists and generalists, and patterns of health service use by patients receiving mental health services. Selected contract research on these topics is briefly described below.

- *Four Settings Studies.* In two fee-for-service (Bunker Hill Health Center of the Massachusetts General Hospital and the Marshfield Wisconsin Medical Plan) and two health maintenance organizations (Columbia, Maryland and Marshfield, Wisconsin), rates of mental health specialist and generalist care were examined and contrasted (Regier, Goldberg, et al., 1982; Hankin et al., 1982).

- *Prevalence of Mental Illness in Adults.* The rates of various types of mental disorder were examined for the first time using research diagnostic criteria in medical users of the Marshfield Medical Plan (Hoeper, Nycz, Cleary, Regier, & Goldberg, 1979).
- *Pre-Post Psychiatric Utilization.* To further examine the offset issue (that is, reduction of medical service use following mental health treatment), which had shown promising findings in preliminary studies (Jones & Vischi, 1979), use of medical services was examined for several years before and after the use of mental health services in two patient populations: Bunker Hill Health Center and the Columbia Medical Plan (Borus et al., 1985; Hankin, Kessler, Goldberg, Steinwachs, & Starfield, 1983).
- *Monroe County Pediatrician Study.* Through a survey of pediatricians, the prevalence of emotional and behavioral problems among children in their practices was estimated (Goldberg, Roghmann, McInerny, & Burke, 1984).
- *Pittsburgh Child HMO Study.* Using a standardized psychiatric interview, the Diagnostic Interview Schedule for Children (DIS-C), rates of emotional disturbance in children were contrasted with pediatrician awareness of these conditions. Use of mental health services was also examined (Costello, Costello, et al., 1988; Costello, Burns, et al., 1988).

Several research contracts focused on issues associated with altering mental health practices among primary care physicians.

- *Family Physician Training at the Medical University of South Carolina.* The relationship between improved interviewing skills (for example, using more open-ended questions) and detection of emotional distress based on General Health Questionnaire Scores was examined in family medicine residents (Goldberg, Steele, Smith, & Spivey, 1980).
- *Screening for Mental Disorder.* An attempt to replicate a British study by Johnstone and Goldberg (1976) to increase the detec-

tion of psychological distress in primary care patients in Marshfield, Wisconsin did not yield findings similar to the British study (Hoeper, Nycz, Kessler, Burke, & Pierce, 1984).

- *Secondary Prevention of Mental Disorder.* A further test of the usefulness of providing mental health screening information to general internists at a Johns Hopkins clinic produced slightly more promising findings for screening among select groups (Shapiro et al., 1987).

Other research contracts moved the program into quite different directions: classification of psychosocial problems and organizational linkages.

- *Psychosocial Classification in Primary Care.* The World Health Organization, as part of its primary care focus, was seeking to improve primary care recognition of mental health problems with a classification system to identify symptoms and social problems that were prediagnostic; a classification was developed and tested briefly (Regier, Burke, et al., 1982).
- *Linkages Between Community Health Centers and Community Mental Health Centers.* The placement of mental health liaison workers in health centers to consult, triage, and refer patients to community mental health centers was evaluated (Goldman, Burns, & Burke, 1980; Burns, Burke, & Ozarin, 1983).

Building the Field

By the early 1980s, funds for contracts became increasingly less available. Concurrently, primary care research grant applications began coming in at the rate of one to three per year, starting in 1980. NIMH primary care staff activities shifted away from directing the research to identifying potential investigators and providing consultation on grant-supported research and delineating special initiatives. The intramural role became more one of interpreting national patterns of service need and use based on national surveys, such as the National Ambulatory Medical Care Survey, the National Medical Care Utilization and Expenditure Survey, and the Epidemiologic Catchment Area study.

Identifying Investigators

Identifying a pool of investigators was an incremental process. Initially, young investigators in psychiatry were attracted through a special initiative to encourage research on consultation-liaison psychiatry (Larson et al., 1987). More established mental health investigators were slower to recognize primary care research as an important and viable area in the early years of the program. The other group that was critical, but difficult to attract into this field, was primary care practitioners. Not only was there a national shortage of these health providers to deliver primary health care, but the number of primary care practitioners with any research training or experience was extremely small; the number of those who also had an interest in mental health was probably less than five. To respond to this need, a decision was made to recruit primary care physicians applying for the Public Health Service's Epidemiology Fellowship Program into NIMH. The Primary Care Research Program was fortunate to be able to recruit three over time: a family physician, a general internist, and a pediatrician. All were able to provide leadership within their professional organizations, encouraging primary care colleagues to consider mental health–related research.

New Initiatives

Although the broad topics encompassing primary care mental health services research had been announced to the field (see Table 2.1), to truly promote growth of the field a number of further steps were essential. Expanding specific research issues, highlighting high-priority topics, and identifying new issues all served to stimulate emerging areas of work. Small research conferences and commissioned reviews published by NIMH (see Table 2.2) were mechanisms employed both to generate ideas and to further build a network of investigators.

As the list of conferences in Table 2.2 shows, the Primary Care Research Program has put an emphasis on children and adolescents, treatment of depression, and issues related to classification in primary care settings. The concern with children and depressive disorders is also reflected in NIMH's current primary care

Table 2.1. NIMH Interests in Primary Care Mental Health Research.

Epidemiological

- Incidence and prevalence of mental disorders and psychosocial problems in primary care and the course of these disorders: duration, recurrence, and remission
- Relationships between co-occurring medical and psychiatric conditions
- Differences in presentation of mental disorders across the life span (for example, is depression different in the elderly?)

Clinical Practice

- Relationships between the prevalence of mental disorders and the extent and adequacy of recognition, diagnosis, and treatment (particularly use of psychotropic medications)
- Barriers to providing mental health care: attitudes, training, time, medical decision making, reimbursement, and effect of medical role models
- Examination of approaches to improve clinical practice: usefulness of screening measures, physician and patient education, mental health consultation, availability of referral sources, value of computer-assisted diagnosis, design of clinical protocols for management of mental disorder in primary care, and special approaches for children, the elderly, and low-income populations
- Differences between the mental health role of health professionals and mental health professionals

Service System

- Effect of type of health organization (for example, fee-for-service versus prepaid health plan) on the mental health care provided
- Effect of integrating mental health specialists into health organizations on the mental health care provided
- Effect of the gatekeeper role on referral to mental health specialists
- Effect of different reimbursement approaches on the use of mental health services, choice of setting, and cost of care

Methodological

- Classification of mental disorder and psychosocial conditions in primary care, with attention to identifying syndromes not previously classified
- Validation of screening measures for mental disorder
- The adequacy of outcome measures for diagnosis, functioning, disability, symptoms, social support, and stressors over repeated administrations
- Correspondence between patient and provider report of mental health conditions and treatment provided
- Classification of mental health treatments used in primary care

Source: Parron & Solomon, 1980.

Table 2.2. NIMH Primary Care Mental Health Services Workshops and Conferences.

1985	Consultation-Liaison Research, Rockville, Maryland
1987	Decision Analysis in Mental Health, Harvard University, Boston
1987	Psychosocial Screening in Pediatrics, NIH, Bethesda, Maryland
1987	Research on Mental Disorders in General Health Settings, Seattle, Washington
1987	Screening for Depression (Attkisson & Zich, 1990), Tiburon, California
1988	The Treatment of Mental Disorders in General Health Settings: A Research Conference, Western Psychiatric Institute, Pittsburgh, Pennsylvania
1989	Mental Health Services for Children and Adolescents in Primary Care Settings: A Research Conference, Yale University, New Haven, Connecticut
1990	Fourth NIMH International Research Conference on the Classification, Recognition, and Treatment of Mental Disorders in General Medical Settings: A Research Conference, Rockville, Maryland
1991	Fifth NIMH International Research Conference on the Classification, Recognition, and Treatment of Mental Disorders in General Medical Settings: A Research Conference, Rockville, Maryland
1992	Co-occurring Physical and Mental Disorders in Children and Adolescents: A Research Workshop, Washington, D.C.
1992	Sixth NIMH International Conference on Primary Care Mental Health Research, Tysons Corner, Virginia
1992	Technical Assistance Workshop on Rural Primary Care Mental Health Research, Tysons Corner, Virginia

research grant portfolio. The reemergence of classification issues, which were part of the early program efforts with the World Health Organization in 1979, is related to joint efforts by NIMH and the American Psychiatric Association to produce a *Diagnostic and Statistical Manual for Primary Care* (DSM-IV-PC), in conjunction with the publication of DSM-IV in 1994.

Two other significant themes are apparent among current Primary Care Research Program grants: a broadening of the research focus and an increasing use of clinical trials to generate client outcome data.

The research focus of the Primary Care Research Program now includes mental illness in all general health care settings, including primary care, secondary care in general hospitals, and tertiary care in nursing homes and rehabilitation facilities. Initial work in this area began earlier in the program's history with analyses of national survey data, especially surveys from the National Center for Health Statistics of short-stay hospitals (Allen, Burns, & Cook, 1983) and the 1985 National Nursing Home Survey (for example, Burns et al., 1985).

The need for an increasing emphasis on clinical trials was supported by Wilkinson's (1985) review of the primary care mental health research literature. Of the 612 published scientific papers, government reports, and books on the topic that he surveyed—which were the work of 800 authors and coauthors—only ten studies (less than 2 percent) assessed outcomes at the client level. Since this 1985 review, a few intervention studies using primary care practitioners and measuring client outcome have appeared in the literature (Smith, Monson, & Ray, 1986; Magruder-Habib, Zung, & Feussner, 1990).

Assuming that the U.S. economy will not adequately support treatment for mental illness by specialists, and also that most people will continue to expect primary care physicians to be qualified to treat mental illness, it is increasingly important to be able to determine whether treatments mental health specialists use can be transferred to primary care physicians (Schulberg, 1991). These treatments should be as effective for primary care patients as for patients of psychiatrists. A current trial of antidepressant drugs and supportive psychotherapy in a primary care setting is an example of this type of research. Research on treatment effectiveness and on improving provider practices will play a key role in the future.

Conclusion

In a research program that currently supports over twenty-five grants, developments can be expected in multiple areas. Some will involve revisiting old themes in new ways; for example, currently funded NIMH grants include those with a focus on consultation-liaison services in child psychiatry. Others address new and important issues in primary care, such as services to individuals with co-occurring substance abuse disorders and severe and persistent mental illness.

While there is ample room to investigate a broad range of

topics, it will be particularly important to focus on the recognition, diagnosis, and treatment of mental illness in primary health care and on recent findings showing significant disability among depressed primary care patients (Wells et al., 1989; Broadhead, Blazer, George, & Tse, 1990). The greatest benefits of research on mental disorders in primary care are likely to come from highly focused research on the clinical outcomes of specific interventions for carefully selected mental disorders. With the knowledge from these interventions, the next critical step will be to train primary care providers to implement effective clinical interventions. Comparing the data from the "de facto" and other papers that focus on the recognition and treatment of mental disorders in primary care with data on the current state of practice will be essential. When that point is reached, we would hope to see improved recognition and treatment of mental illness in primary care patients.

References

Allen, G. S., Burns, B. J., & Cook, W. A. (1983). The provision of mental health services in the health care sector: United States. In C. A. Taube & S. A. Barrett (Eds.), *Mental health, United States, 1983* (DHHS Publication No. ADM 83-1275). Rockville, MD: National Institute of Mental Health.

Attkisson, C. C., & Zich, J. M. (Eds.). (1990). *Depression in primary care: Screening and detection.* London: Routledge, Chapman, and Hall.

Borus, J. F., Olendzki, M. C., Kessler, L., Burns, B. J., Brandt, U. C., Broverman, C. A., & Henderson, P. R. (1985). The offset effect of mental health treatment on ambulatory medical care utilization and charges. *Archives of General Psychiatry, 42,* 573–580.

Broadhead, W. E., Blazer, D. G., George, L. K., & Tse, C. K. (1990). Depression, disability days, and days lost from work in a prospective epidemiological survey. *Journal of the American Medical Association, 264,* 2524–2528.

Burns, B. J., & Burke, J. D. (1985). Improving mental health practices in primary care: Findings from recent research. *Public Health Reports, 100,* 294–300.

Burns, B. J., Burke, J. D., & Ozarin, L. D. (1983). Linking health and mental health services in rural areas. *International Journal of Mental Health, 12,* 130–143.

Burns, B. J., Larson, D. B., Goldstrom, I. D., Johnson, W. E., Taube, C. A., Miller, N. E., & Mathis, E. S. (1985). Mental disorder among nursing home patients: Preliminary findings from the National Nursing Home Survey Pretest. Paper presented at the World Psychiatric Association meeting, Edinburgh, Scotland.

Burns, B. J., Regier, D. A., Goldberg, I. D., & Kessler, L. G. (1979). Future directions in primary care/mental health research. *International Journal of Mental Health, 8,* 130–140.

Burns, B. J., Taube, C. A., & Regier, D. A. (1986). A view from abroad: Building primary care/mental health research in the USA. In M. Shepherd, G. Wilkinson, & P. Williams (Eds.), *Mental Illness in Primary Care Settings* (pp. 180–194). London: Tavistock.

Costello, E. J., Burns, B. J., Costello, A. J., Edelbrock, C., Dulcan, M., & Brent, D. (1988). Services utilization and psychiatric diagnosis in pediatric primary care: The role of the gatekeeper. *Pediatrics, 82,* 435–441.

Costello, E. J., Costello, A. J., Edelbrock, C., Burns, B. J., Dulcan, M. K., & Brent, D. (1988). DSM-III disorders in pediatric primary care: Prevalence and risk factors. *Archives of General Psychiatry, 45,* 1100–1106.

Goldberg, I. D., Babigian, H. M., Locke, B. Z., & Rosen, B. M. (1978). Role of non-psychiatrist physicians in the delivery of mental health services: Implications from three studies. *Public Health Reports, 93,* 240–254.

Goldberg, I. D., Roghmann, K. J., McInerny, I. K., & Burke, J. D. (1984). Mental health problems among children seen in pediatric practice: Prevalence and management. *Pediatrics, 73,* 278–293.

Goldberg, D. P., Steele, J. J., Smith, C., & Spivey, L. (1980). Training family doctors to recognise psychiatric illness with increased accuracy. *Lancet, 2,* 521–523.

Goldman, H. H., Burns, B. J., & Burke, J. D. (1980). Integrating primary health care and mental health services: A preliminary report. *Public Health Reports, 96,* 535–539.

Graduate Medical Education National Advisory Committee. (1981).

Final report to the Secretary, United States Department of Health and Human Services (Vol. 1) (Publication No. HRA-81-651). Washington, DC: U.S. Government Printing Office.

Hankin, J. R., Kessler, L. G., Goldberg, I. D., Steinwachs, D. M., & Starfield, B. H. (1983). A longitudinal study of offset in the use of non-psychiatric services following specialized mental health care. *Medical Care, 21,* 1099–1109.

Hankin, J. R., & Oktay, J. S. (1979). *Mental disorder and primary medical care: An analytical review of the literature* (DHHS Publication No. ADM 78-661). Washington, DC: U.S. Government Printing Office.

Hankin, J. R., Steinwachs, D. M., Regier, D. A., Burns, B. J., Goldberg, I. D., & Hoeper, E. W. (1982). Use of general medical care services by persons with mental disorders. *Archives of General Psychiatry, 39,* 225–231.

Hoeper, E. W., Nycz, G. R., Cleary, P. D., Regier, D. A., & Goldberg, I. D. (1979). Estimated prevalence of RDC mental disorder in primary medical care. *International Journal of Mental Health, 8,* 615.

Hoeper, E. W., Nycz, G. R., Kessler, L. G., Burke, J. D., & Pierce, W. E. (1984). The usefulness of screening for mental illness. *Lancet, 8367,* 33–35.

Johnstone, A., & Goldberg, D. P. (1976). Psychiatric screening in general practice. *Lancet,* 7960, 605–608.

Jones, K. R., & Vischi, T. R. (1979). Impact of alcohol, drug abuse, and mental health treatment on medical care utilization: A review of the research literature. *Medical Care, 17* (Suppl.), 12.

Kamerow, D. B., Pincus, H. A., & MacDonald, D. I. (1986). Alcohol abuse, other drug abuse, and mental disorders in medical practice: Prevalence, costs, recognition, and treatment. *Journal of the American Medical Association, 255,* 2054–2057.

Larson, D. B., Kessler, L. G., Burns, B. J., Pincus, H. A., Houpt, H. A., Fiester, S., & Chaitkin, L. (1987). The research development workshop: The case of NIMH and c-I psychiatry. *Hospital and Community Psychiatry, 38,* 1106–1109.

Magruder-Habib, K. M., Zung, W. W. K., & Feussner, J. R. (1990). Improving physicians' recognition and treatment of depression in general medical care: Results of a randomized clinical trial. *Medical Care, 28,* 239–250.

Morlock, L. L. (1989). Recognition and treatment of mental health problems in the general health care sector. In C. A. Taube, D. Mechanic, & A. A. Hohmann (Eds.), *The future of mental health services research.* Washington, DC: U.S. Government Printing Office.

Parron, D. L., & Solomon, F. (Eds.). (1980). *Mental health services in primary care settings: Report of a conference, April 2–3, 1979* (DHHS Publication No. ADM 80-995). Washington, DC: U.S. Government Printing Office.

President's Commission on Mental Health. (1978). *Report to the President* (Vol. 1). Washington, DC: U.S. Government Printing Office.

Regier, D. A., Burke, J. D., Burns, B. J., Clare, A., Bultinat, W., Lipkin, M., Spitzer, R., Williams, J., & Wood, M. (1982). *Proposed classification of health problems* (pp. 153–184). In M. Lipkin & K. Kupka (Eds.), Psychosocial factors affecting health. New York: Praeger.

Regier, D. A., Goldberg, I. D., Burns, B. J., Hankin, J. R., Hoeper, E. W., & Nycz, G. R. (1982). Specialist/generalist division of responsibility for patients with mental disorders. *Archives of General Psychiatry, 39,* 219–224.

Regier, D. A., Goldberg, I. D., & Taube, C. A. (1978). The de facto US mental health services system. *Archives of General Psychiatry, 35,* 685–693.

Rosen, B. M., Locke, B. Z., Goldberg, I. D., & Babigian, H. M. (1972). Identification of emotional disturbance in patients seen in general medical clinics. *Hospital and Community Psychiatry, 23,* 364–370.

Schulberg, H. C. (1991). Mental disorders in the primary care setting: Research priorities for the 1990s. *General Hospital Psychiatry, 13,* 156–164.

Schulberg, H. C., & Burns, B. J. (1988). Mental disorder in primary care: Epidemiologic diagnostic and treatment research directions. *General Hospital Psychiatry,* 10, 79–87.

Shapiro, S., German, P. S., Skinner, E. A., Von Korff, M., Turner, R. W., Klein, L. E., Teitelbaum, M. L., Kramer, M., Burke, J. D.,

& Burns, B. J. (1987). An experiment to change detection and management of mental morbidity in primary care. *Medical Care, 25,* 327–339.

Shepherd, M., Cooper, B., Brown, A. C., & Kalton, G. W. (1966). *Psychiatric illness in general practice.* London: Oxford University Press.

Smith, G. R., Monson, R. A., & Ray, D. C. (1986). Psychiatric consultation in somatization disorder: A randomized controlled study. *New England Journal of Medicine, 314,* 1407–1413.

Taube, C. A., & Burns, B. J. (1988). Mental health services system research: The National Institute of Mental Health program. *Health Services Research, 22,* 837–855.

Wells, K. B., Stewart, A., Hay, R. D., Burnam, M. A., Rogers, W., Daniels, M., Berry, S., Greenfield, S., & Ware, J. (1989). The functioning and well-being of depressed patients. *Journal of the American Medical Association, 262,* 914–919.

Wilkinson, G. (1985). Mental health practices in primary care settings: An annotated bibliography, 1977–85. London: Tavistock.

World Health Organization. (1973). *Report of a working group.* Copenhagen: Author.

Barbara E. Havassy
Catherine J. Schmidt

3

Alcohol and Other Drug Abuse Disorders in Primary Medical Settings: Current and Future Research

The aim of this chapter is to highlight the central issues in the treatment of alcohol and other drug abusers in primary medical care settings. The literature in this area manifests several themes. The first theme concerns the extent to which alcohol and other drug abusers present for treatment in primary care settings. Recent literature documents high rates of alcohol and drug abusers in these settings. The second theme concerns the issues surrounding detection and recognition of alcohol and other drug abuse (AODA) problems. The literature indicates widespread failure to detect these problems and multiple barriers to their recognition in medical settings. A third distinct theme concerns techniques of screening for AODA problems in medical settings. We reviewed empirically based research findings for each of these themes and have suggested areas for future research. We did not include studies in our review that addressed (1) the contribution of alcohol and other drugs to medical emergency room visits and utilization of trauma centers or (2) detection and treatment of AODA in perinatal and obstetric care contexts. Although these topics merit attention, they are too specialized for the focus of this chapter.

Before proceeding with a review of completed work and research recommendations, we note a few caveats. The literature reveals serious gaps in knowledge and distinct biases. It is characterized by an inadequate empirical foundation and by descriptive rather than hypothesis-testing investigations. The work is overwhelmingly clinical, and didactic medical texts focusing primarily on techniques for recognition of alcoholism are overrepresented. Furthermore, attention to alcoholism overshadows that of other drugs: problems concerning drug abusers in primary medical care settings have not received sufficient attention.

Estimates of the Prevalence of Alcoholism and Other Drug Abuse Disorders

The consensus is that many medical patients seen in primary care settings suffer from AODA disorders and that these disorders are undetected and underdiagnosed to a large extent. Although data on drug users are sparse, data from a wide variety of sources on alcoholics indicate that they frequent medical rather than specialty settings for their problems. Data from the NIMH Epidemiologic Catchment Area (ECA) study indicate that over 50 percent of persons with AODA disorders received all of their care in the general medical sector and that only about 10 percent saw a mental health specialist (Shapiro et al., 1984). Data from the National Ambulatory Medical Care Survey (Shurman, Kramer, & Mitchell, 1985) indicate that 47.5 percent of all office visits that had a primary or secondary diagnosis of AODA occurred in the offices of nonpsychiatrist physicians; 87 percent of these were in the primary care sector.

Findings such as these have led to a significant amount of work on estimating prevalence of AODA problems in primary care settings. We reviewed a number of these studies and emphasized those published after 1980. We found few studies of the prevalence of substance abuse problems in medical care settings. Of the seventeen studies we reviewed, only four included any mention of drug abuse disorders. We include only one of these; the other did not yield findings that could serve as prevalence rates.

Any examination of prevalence estimates across studies is complicated due to variability in the screening measures, cutoff points, and time frames employed. The most frequently used standardized diagnostic and/or screening measures are alcohol and substance abuse sections of the NIMH Diagnostic Interview Schedule (DIS) (Robins, Helzer, Croughan, & Ratcliff, 1981); the Michigan Alcoholism Screening Test (MAST) (Selzer, 1971); one of two shortened versions of the MAST, the brief MAST (Porkorny, Miller, & Kaplan, 1972) or the SMAST (Selzer, Vinokur, & vanRooijen, 1975); and the CAGE (Mayfield, McLeod, & Hall, 1974). Of these, only the DIS was developed to be used in deriving estimates of prevalence in large samples; the remainder were developed as clinical tools to quickly screen for possible AODA.

The MAST and SMAST are composed of twenty-five and thirteen easily answered yes-no questions, respectively. These simple questionnaires have been frequently used as the "gold standard" against which other screening techniques have been evaluated (for example, Cyr & Wartman, 1988), and a great deal of research has been accumulated on them. Descriptive and psychometric information about them can be found in several publications (examples include Selzer, 1971; Porkorny et al., 1972; Skinner & Sheu, 1982; Zung, 1984). Recent research on the MAST and SMAST assesses the sensitivity and specificity of these screening tools, frequently in comparison to laboratory tests and to clinical judgment.

The CAGE is comprised of four clinical interview questions to assist in making a diagnosis of alcoholism (Ewing, 1984). The four questions ask about whether the patient has ever done the following: thought about *C*utting down on drinking, been *A*nnoyed by criticism (of drinking), had *G*uilty feelings about drinking, and had morning "*E*ye-openers." The convention is to identify alcoholism by two or more affirmative responses (Mayfield et al., 1974). Work by King (1986), conducted in London, yielded sensitivity of 84 percent and specificity of 95 percent using the standard cutoff of two affirmative CAGE responses.

Buchsbaum and colleagues at the Medical College of Virginia (Buchsbaum, Buchanan, Lawton, & Schnoll, 1991) examined alcohol consumption and disorders in 468 randomly selected adult attendees of the general medical clinic. Of these, 459 agreed to participate in the study and received the alcohol section of the DIS. This group was composed primarily of women (66 percent), African

Americans (80 percent), persons who did not complete high school (73 percent), and persons who were unemployed (72 percent). Those who met criteria for an alcohol abuse or dependence disorder who experienced symptoms in the year prior to testing were designated as meeting criteria for a current disorder, and those whose most recent symptom occurred before one year prior to testing were designated as meeting criteria for a past disorder. A total of 31 percent met criteria for a DSM-III diagnosis of past or current alcohol abuse/dependence: 12 percent met criteria for a current disorder, and 19 percent met criteria for a past disorder. Most of these patients met criteria for dependence rather than abuse. Twenty-four percent met criteria for current or past dependence: 10 percent for current dependence and 14 percent for past dependence. The lifetime prevalence of alcohol use disorders was significantly higher in men than women ($p < .0005$). Current disorder was more prevalent in younger than older subjects ($p < .0005$). Race had no effect on prevalence rates.

Cleary et al. (1988) administered the DIS to a sample of outpatients seeking care at a hospital-based primary care practice. The rate of alcohol abuse and dependence obtained, with current and past disorders combined, was lower than in the Buchsbaum et al. (1991) study: only 20 percent met DSM-III criteria for past or current alcohol abuse or dependence compared to the Buchsbaum et al. rate of 31 percent. The rates for "past" alcohol disorders obtained in the two studies were somewhat similar: 14.6 percent in the Cleary et al. study and 19 percent in the Buchsbaum et al. study. The lower rate obtained by the Cleary group is apparently attributable to many fewer patients who met criteria for current disorder (5.4 percent) than in the Buchsbaum et al. sample (19 percent). Unfortunately, there was a great deal of attrition from the identified sample before administration of the DIS, which may have influenced prevalence rates. That is, of the 591 adult patients assessed for study participation, only 41 percent were administered the DIS: 30 percent were not contacted due to scheduling and logistic problems, 18 percent refused participation, and 11 percent were excluded for not speaking English or because preexisting conditions made DIS administration problematic.

Coulehan, Zettler-Segal, Block, McClelland, and Schulberg

(1987) used the DIS to study AODA problems in new adult outpatients of two academic family health centers and one academic internal medicine clinic. Only 294 of the 1,040 eligible patients received the DIS, so the rates are highly biased. In addition, women and younger patients were significantly overrepresented. The time frame for experiencing symptoms was the preceding six months. A total of 14 percent (42 patients) met criteria for alcohol or other substance abuse. Of the 42, 45 percent abused only alcohol, 31 percent abused alcohol and other drugs, and 24 percent abused only other drugs. Alcohol abuse was diagnosed in 10.9 percent of the sample. Drugs of abuse were as follows: alcohol, 76 percent; barbiturates and benzodiazepines, 29 percent; amphetamines, 26 percent; and opiates, 19 percent.

Several studies using the MAST and SMAST obtained virtually identical rates of alcoholism. Cyr and Wartman (1988) administered the MAST to a sample of 232 new patients in an ambulatory medical care unit in an urban teaching hospital. The sample was predominantly Caucasian (59 percent), female (63 percent), and currently unemployed (53 percent). Using a MAST cutoff of five points, 47 patients (20 percent) were classified as alcoholic. Leckman, Umland, and Blay (1984) conducted a study at a university family practice center in New Mexico and obtained a similar alcoholism prevalence rate of 19 percent, using a cutoff score of five points. The sample consisted of 147 adults: 72 percent were women, 58 percent were unemployed, and 19 percent were either Hispanic or African-American. Woodall (1988) administered the SMAST to patients in an urban family practice center. Among 276 patients in the sample, 138 reported drinking and were asked to complete the SMAST. The SMAST identified 16 percent of these (22 patients) as alcoholics using a cutoff score of three or more points. Chart audits identified 3 additional alcoholics who scored below three on the SMAST, bringing the total identified alcoholics to 18 percent of the 138 patients who reported any drinking.

Using the CAGE, Moore and Malitz (1986) obtained higher prevalence rates in a sample of 95 patients of residents of the internal medicine group practice at Johns Hopkins Hospital. The sample was predominantly African-American (87 percent) and female (63 percent). Only 16 percent were employed, 54 percent were retired or unemployed, and employment data were missing on 30 percent. Using a CAGE score of two points, 36 percent of the 87 respondents were classified as probable alcoholics; of these, 52 percent were women and 97 percent were African-American.

A subsequent comprehensive diagnostic study (Moore et al., 1989) targeted all new adult admissions to the inpatient services of the Johns Hopkins Hospital. A total of 2,002 patients—all of the new admissions except for elective surgery, short-stay, and detoxification admissions—were screened using the CAGE, the SMAST, and several quantity-frequency alcohol consumption questions. Those who provided at least two affirmative responses on the CAGE or who scored at least five points on the SMAST were considered alcoholic. The rates of alcoholism varied by clinical department, from a low of 12 percent in obstetrics and gynecology to a high of 43 percent in ear, nose, and throat surgery. Intermediate rates included the following: urology surgery, 14 percent; neurosurgery, 16 percent; neurology, 19 percent; general surgery, 21 percent; medicine and cardiac surgery, each 24 percent; orthopedic surgery, 28 percent; and psychiatry, 30 percent.

A similar investigation of alcoholism rates assessed surgical as well as general medical settings in a suburban community hospital outside Chicago (Sherin, Piotrowski, Panek, & Doot, 1982). This study resulted in lower, albeit substantial, alcoholism rates in comparison with Moore et al. (1989). They found the following rates: orthopedics, 16 percent; surgery, 15 percent; medicine, 9 percent; obstetrics, 9 percent; and gynecology, 5 percent. The overall prevalence rate was 11 percent.

The estimated prevalence rates of these studies indicate that approximately one in five patients in primary medical settings is a probable alcoholic. The extremes of the range are 5 and 43 percent. Magruder-Habib, Durand, and Frey (1991) report a generally similar range of rates in their review of prevalence studies conducted with medical patients in inpatient and outpatient settings and published primarily in the 1980s. In these studies, rates from inpatient settings varied from a low of 13–15 percent (Moore et al., 1989, and Nolan, 1965—university hospital service) to a high of 60–61 percent (McCusker, Cherubin, & Zimberg, 1971—general hospital; Aderhold, 1980—VA). Rates obtained in outpatient settings varied from a low of 4–5 percent (Powers & Spickard, 1984—general medical clinic; Nicol & Ford, 1986—general practice, women; and Hurt, Morse, & Swenson, 1980—Mayo Medical Clinic) to a high of 31–33 percent (Magruder-Habib, Fraker, & Peterson, 1983—VA; Nicol & Ford, 1986—general practice, men).

Problems of Detection and Recognition in Primary Care Settings

Despite the substantial prevalence of AODA problems among primary medical care patients, many physicians do not recognize or correctly diagnose these problems. In this section, we summarized recent studies that demonstrate the extent of the failure to recognize AODA problems and studies that address the causes of failed detection.

Failure to Detect and Recognize AODA

Numerous studies substantiate the low rates of detection of AODA in primary practice (for example, Coulehan et al., 1987; Fisher, Mason, Keeley, & Fisher, 1975; Moore et al., 1989). These studies indicate that, in general, physicians fail to detect between 50 and 95 percent of persons with AODA problems.

In Woodall's (1988) study of family practice residents, cited earlier, residents detected fewer than half of the alcoholic patients. In a sample of 276 outpatients, 218 were surveyed for alcoholism using the SMAST and by conducting chart audits. Chart audits were conducted by the investigator. The investigator apparently examined whether a diagnosis of alcoholism had been given, whether residents recorded asking the patient questions about alcohol use, and whether residents appeared to have examined chart notes from previous visits. Residents detected only 12 of the 25 alcoholics identified by the SMAST and/or chart audit. Moreover, of these 12, 9 had been identified in earlier chart entries as being alcoholic. The failure of these residents to ask patients appropriate questions may partially account for their failure to recognize alcoholism. According to charts, residents asked questions concerning drinking of only 28 of 51 patients (55 percent) who presented for physical examinations and of only 6 of 157 patients (4 percent) who presented for follow-up or episodic care.

In the Moore and Malitz (1986) survey of 95 internal medicine patients at the Johns Hopkins Hospital, patients completed the CAGE and a questionnaire on alcohol consumption. Of 31 who scored at least two on the CAGE, residents diagnosed only 14 (45 percent) as alcoholics. Of 20 patients with a score of at least three, residents detected 11 (55 percent).

A study of 56 randomly chosen general practitioners conducted in England (Reid, Webb, Hennrikus, Fahey, & Samson-Fisher, 1986) investigated the accuracy of detecting patients with a high alcohol intake. A total of 2,081 patients were recruited from these physicians' waiting rooms and were asked quantity-frequency questions about their drinking habits. Based on their answers to these questions, patients were classified (according to Australian Medical Association criteria) as high-risk drinkers or not (men: 60 g or more of alcohol per day; women: 40 g or more). Then physicians were asked to classify their patients' levels of alcohol intake (light, moderate, high), according to their own criteria. Only 27.5 percent of patients who were classified as "high-risk" drinkers using the Australian criteria were identified as moderate or heavy drinkers by their physicians. Only 45.2 percent of patients who described themselves as drinking four or more drinks per day were classified by physicians as "moderate to heavy" drinkers.

In the Coulehan et al. (1987) study cited earlier, 14 percent of the 294 adult primary care patients received diagnoses of alcohol or other substance abuse disorders, per the DIS. Primary care physicians correctly identified only 40 percent of these patients. Clinically identified patients were older, more likely to be married, and more often used multiple drugs. In addition, they more frequently had antisocial personality disorders. Patients not clinically recognized often were depressed. Logistic regression analysis indicated that the factors most strongly associated with clinical recognition of AODA problems were the presence of antisocial personality, the absence of a coexisting depressive disorder, and better social functioning scores.

In a study of mental health services in primary health care settings (Hoeper, Nycz, & Cleary, 1979), it was noted that only about

10 percent of those meeting research diagnostic criteria for substance abuse or mental disorder were recognized by primary care physicians, even when any indication of potential recognition (chart notation or a psychotropic drug prescription, for example) was counted. Emergency room physicians recognized fewer than half of the patients identified as alcoholics by the brief MAST (Solomon, Vanga, Morgan, & Joseph, 1980).

The best AODA detection rates were found in the Cleary et al. (1988) study of 242 outpatients of 19 senior medical residents in a hospital-based, primary care setting. Residents' judgments about their patients were compared to results of DIS administration. Residents noted serious alcohol problems in 77 percent of their patients who met DSM-III criteria for current alcohol abuse or dependence (within the past year). In contrast, they correctly identified only 35 percent of patients diagnosed with lifetime but not current alcohol disorders and only identified 36 percent of patients with less serious alcohol problems ("problem drinkers").

Barriers to Detection and Recognition

Lack of physician training is thought to be a major contributor to missed diagnoses of AODA problems. Many researchers criticize the paltry amount of training about alcoholism, drug abuse, and addiction provided in medical schools. Generally, 1 percent of didactic hours are devoted to alcoholism and drug abuse (Kamerow et al., 1986; Delbanco & Barnes, 1987), and only 3 percent of medical students receive a course on alcoholism (Spickard, 1986). In a recent survey of general practitioners (Roche, Guray, & Saunders, 1991), respondents stated that their medical training had not prepared them to respond to patients with drug and alcohol problems and that they had little understanding of these problems until encountering them in practice. Conversely, several articles (for example, Chappel & Schnoll, 1977) describe apparently successful attempts to remedy this lack, and some medical school curricula are including more didactic work and clinical experience (Lewis, Niven, Czechowicz, & Trumble, 1987; Roche et al., 1991).

The following factors contribute to underdetection of AODA

problems: (1) characteristics of physicians, (2) characteristics of alcohol and drug abusers, and (3) the nature of AODA problems.

Characteristics of Physicians. Many studies report physicians' hostile and negative stereotypes and attitudes toward chemically dependent persons. These attitudes include the belief that those with AODA problems are difficult and demanding, as well as attitudes that alcoholics and drug abusers are "morally" lacking. Among the 1,106 nursing, medical, social work, and counseling students in the Wechsler and Rohman study (1982), 20 percent felt that alcoholics had little remorse about their drinking habits, 46 percent felt that alcoholics were not honest about their drinking, and 32 percent believed that alcoholics had no one to blame for their problems but themselves. Of the sample, 61 percent endorsed the statement that alcoholics were "very demanding, difficult, and uncooperative patients," and 48 percent felt that alcoholics were "harder to relate to than people whose problems were not self-inflicted." The latter statement was endorsed by 55 percent of nursing students and 58 percent of medical students. Abed and Neira-Muñoz (1990) and Glanz (1986) found that 72 percent and 76 percent, respectively, of primary care practitioners in their samples considered drug addicts as particularly difficult or uncooperative. Addicts were characterized as patients who often disagreed with their doctor's judgment about the underlying cause of symptoms, failed to comply with advice, and frequently missed appointments. A survey of a 5 percent random sample of general practitioners in England and Wales (Glanz, 1986) indicated that respondents generally regarded opiate abusers as especially difficult to manage, beyond their competence to treat, and less acceptable as patients than others in need of care.

Roche et al. (1991) conducted a qualitative study of attitudes and experiences of forty-four general practitioners in seven focus groups in Sydney and in rural New South Wales, Australia. These physicians were more sympathetic to patients with alcohol and minor tranquilizer problems; opiate users were least favored, and most of the physicians expressed hostility toward them. Hospitalized substance abusers were stereotyped as usually "end-stage cases" in detox wards and as "nasty, dangerous people who waste the precious time and limited and expensive hi-tech resources of the hospital." One senior specialist was quoted as referring to an alcoholic as an "ex-member of the human race."

Physicians' negative attitudes have two critical consequences. First, these attitudes appear to be related to an unwillingness to work with patients with AODA problems and/or to a tendency to disregard issues of alcohol and drug use. Anderson (1985) and Clement (1986) both found that doctors with negative attitudes about working with drinkers undertook less work related to alcohol problems in their practice. Attitudes in both studies were measured by the Alcohol and Alcohol Problems Perception Questionnaire (AAPPQ, fourth version) (Cartwright, 1980). Anderson found that those with scores in the highest sixth of the range (most positive attitudes) performed more alcohol problem tasks than those in the lowest sixth. For example, 60 percent of high scorers initiated discussions about alcohol at least once a week, compared with 30 percent of low scorers. Further, 83 percent of high scorers discussed alcohol with more than three-quarters of patients who presented with gastritis, compared with 59 percent of low scorers. Clement (1986) found that both perception of role adequacy (working knowledge of alcohol and alcohol-related problems and knowing how to counsel drinkers over the long term) and role support (could find help in dealing with a drinker) were positively correlated with the proportion of patients with alcohol problems with whom the physicians reported working.

Another consequence of negative attitudes to those with AODA is that physicians often fail to consider alcohol and drug abuse problems in patients who are socially acceptable (employed, relatively healthy, and so on)—that is, those who do not conform to their negative stereotypes (for example, Schuckit, 1987). Schuckit noted that many physicians and other health professionals develop negative stereotypes during training in large urban areas where they were exposed to skid-row alcoholics and street drug users. Iber (1991) also noted that physicians' experience with skid-row alcoholics during training establishes the attitude that abusing persons are often dirty and unkempt, riddled with communicable diseases, and infrequently rehabilitated. Influenced by these experiences, many physicians fail to notice that the "typical" abuser in primary practice is not a skid-row alcoholic or street drug user (Schuckit, 1987).

According to Schuckit (1985), more than 90 percent of alcoholics and drug users in primary practice settings are employed and reasonably healthy. According to Iber (1991), the derelict alcoholic or drug addict makes up less than 3 percent of all alcoholics and 5 percent of all other drug abusers.

Some physicians may be better than others at recognizing substance abuse problems. Many physicians feel that management of addiction to illicit drugs is beyond their competence (see for example, Glanz, 1986; Abed & Neira-Muñoz, 1990). In a 1982 AMA poll (Kennedy, 1985), 71 percent of physicians stated they felt either incompetent or ambivalent about treating alcoholism. Roche et al. (1991) reported that doctors appeared more confident in dealing with the medical aspects of alcohol problems than in their ability to influence patients' alcohol consumption. In a survey of primary care physicians (Wechsler, Levine, Idelson, Rohman, & Taylor, 1983), only 3 percent reported that they felt "very successful" in helping their patients with alcohol and 5 percent with other drug abuse problems.

Linn and Yager (1989), in a survey of internists, family physicians, and psychiatrists, found ADOA disorder recognition to be correlated positively with volume of outpatients and inpatients seen, younger age, more work in primary rather than specialty patient care, less academic work, stronger belief in the efficacy of treating alcoholism, and greater religiosity. Both Abed and Neira-Muñoz (1990) and Glanz (1986) found that younger general practitioners had a more positive attitude toward drug addicts and were more prepared to take an active part in their management. In the Glanz study, recently graduated general practitioners were somewhat more favorable in their views than longer-practicing physicians: 40 percent of general practitioners who began practice in the 1970s and 1980s agreed that they were as willing to treat opiate users as other patients, compared to 25 percent of general practitioners who began practice before 1970. Those physicians in Linn and Yager's study with a greater breadth of experience in treating alcoholism were significantly more likely to believe in what they were doing and to feel that such treatment was efficacious.

Gottlieb, Mullen, and McAlister (1987) studied physicians' self-efficacy, outcome expectations, and practices regarding smoking, alcohol and over-the-counter drug problems, and illicit drug use in a random sample of 442 primary care physicians. Multivariate discriminant analysis showed that year of graduation, specialty, self-efficacy, and outcome expectation for patient compliance were predictive of many practice behaviors. More recently trained physicians, internists, and family practice specialists were more likely to practice in the substance abuse areas. Internists were most likely to take substance abuse histories. Higher levels of self-efficacy and outcome expectations were positively related to history taking and counseling and negatively related to outside referral.

Not all studies obtained differences in recognition related to age and specialty of practitioner. For example, Brown, Carter, and Gordon (1987) studied diagnostic practices by using computer-simulated patients with symptoms of alcohol abuse. They found that physicians' diagnoses and the patterns of questions asked in order to formulate diagnoses were not associated with age, gender, specialty, duration of training, or reported personal impact of alcoholism.

Characteristics of Alcohol and Drug Abusers. Another impediment to the discovery of AODA problems in primary medical care settings is patients' attitudes. Patients often are wary of bringing up emotional, alcohol, or drug problems, believing that they are not "legitimate" topics to discuss with a general practitioner (Kamerow et al., 1986). Furthermore, in much of the clinical literature, patients' denial of the AODA problem is seen as a major obstacle to recognition: "It is not uncommon for an alcoholic to sit in a physician's office, noticeably intoxicated in the middle of the day, with a swollen red nose and advanced cirrhosis, and still seriously claim to be a social drinker" (Spickard, 1986). According to Barnes (1987), an understanding, systematic approach to denial may help the newly diagnosed patient begin to engage in treatment, although he or she may require multiple confrontations over time before accepting the need for treatment. Thom and Téllez (1986) note that patients, particularly women, are often reluctant to mention drinking for fear of physicians' negative judgments. Unfortunately, despite the acceptance of the notion that patients' denial is an obstacle to detection and to appropriate care, there is virtually no empirical research in this area about denial.

The Nature of AODA Problems. Even under the best of circumstances, AODA problems may be difficult to detect. For example, individual responses to drinking are highly variable, and there are no hard-and-fast rules to determine exactly when alcohol consumption becomes a problem (Thom & Téllez, 1986). Furthermore, AODA problems can be manifested psychosocially as well as biomedically. Psychosocial symptoms tend to be more difficult for physicians, since they have less training in this area. Although some patients present symptoms in both domains, others' symptoms appear only in one area. Often only the later-stage alcoholics present clear-cut biomedical sequelae. Primary care physicians in the Brown et al. (1987) study used a computerized, simulated encounter with an alcoholic patient and diagnosed the psychosocial problem, alcoholism, with much less accuracy and certainty than two biomedical problems, peptic ulcer and gastritis. Of ninety-five physicians, only 32 percent diagnosed alcoholism with maximal certainty. One-third misinterpreted symptoms of alcoholism and erroneously made other psychiatric diagnoses, chiefly anxiety or depression. More than 40 percent did not make any psychosocial diagnosis. Brown et at. (1987) also noted that physicians often are not aware of the extent to which alcoholism and its psychosocial consequences can mimic or elicit symptoms of anxiety or depression.

Making diagnoses of AODA problems is often perceived as difficult and time consuming. Physicians often feel insufficiently compensated for time spent evaluating and counseling. Abusers are widely perceived to require more services and to provide less likelihood of reimbursement (Iber, 1991). Many physicians respond to these issues by referring quickly and by assuming little responsibility (Delbanco & Barnes, 1987).

Diagnoses of alcoholism and/or drug abuse often carry negative implications for patients and physicians alike. For physicians, it may mean continued attention to a condition with serious medical, psychological, and social sequelae and one where success is difficult to measure. Or it may mean responsibility for making an effective referral (Barnes, 1987). It could also mean losing patients diagnosed as having an AODA problem. Thom and Téllez (1986) point out that offering the diagnosis of alcoholism and/or substance abuse could end the relationship: "I have had patients who have changed doctors. They have gone off our list because we have insisted that they did have a drinking problem." Thus, the fear of losing patients may cause physicians to delay or not present a substance abuse diagnosis.

Screening for Alcoholism and Drug Use in Medical Settings

The prevalence of alcoholism and related medical problems, as well as the failure to recognize these conditions, has led to efforts to improve detection of alcoholism. There has been no equivalent research emphasis concerning identification and diagnosis of substance use disorders in medical settings. Only two of the articles we reviewed attempted to screen for drug use problems.

The development of routine procedures to screen for alcoholism follows at least three major avenues: clinical screening interviews/questionnaires (discussed earlier), laboratory tests, and protocols for clinical examination.

Laboratory Tests and the Identification of Alcoholism

A significant amount of work has addressed identification of laboratory measures that could function as reliable biological markers for alcoholism. Since many heavy drinkers deny their drinking and alcohol-related problems in response to questionnaires, laboratory tests have the potential for more accurate identification of problem drinkers. Among the markers receiving the most attention in the literature are the following: (1) serum g-glutamyl transpepidase (GGTP), (2) mean corpuscular volume (MCV), (3) blood alcohol level (BAL), and (4) high-density lipoproteins (HDL).

Two studies that examined laboratory tests as markers were those by Robinson, Monk, and Bailey (1979) and Cushman, Jacobson, Barboriak, and Anderson (1984). Neither reported promising results. Robinson and colleagues found no significant correlation between self-reported alcohol consumption and serum GGTP level in 260 apparently healthy men coming to a medical center for a routine health examination. Subjects who reported the highest levels of alcohol intake had the widest range of serum GGTP values. There was no definite trend of serum GGTP values increasing with alcohol consumption. Cushman et al. (1984) examined a panel of seven blood tests considered to be markers for alcohol abuse in 543 male and female "relatively healthy alcoholics" entering an ambulatory alcohol treatment program. These markers were MCV, glutamine oxaloacetic transaminase (SGOT), GGTP, alkaline phosphatase (AP), bilirubin (B), HDL, and BAL. Used individually, the markers were found to be unsatisfactory; their sensitivity was unacceptably low. When combined, the sensitivities improved. The most sensitive individual marker for both genders was GGTP (49 percent), followed by MCV (41 percent). The combination of SGOT, GGTP, and MCV was the most useful; this combination yielded a sensitivity of 72 percent for men and 61 percent for women. Both groups of authors concluded that the sensitivity of these tests alone or in combination leaves much to be desired in healthy alcoholics.

Comparisons Among Screening Questionnaires, Laboratory Tests, and Clinical Examinations

By far the most revealing and useful studies of improving detection of alcoholism are those that compare brief interviews, laboratory tests, and clinical examination protocols.

Screening Interviews Compared to Laboratory Tests. Each of the following studies examines the sensitivities and specificities of screening interviews and laboratory tests alone and combined. Although the particular screening interviews and laboratory tests studied are sometimes different, these studies have a great deal in common. Each of these studies found that when used alone, the screening interviews had better sensitivity and specificity than any single biological test; however, when combined, a screening interview plus laboratory test was always better than either measure alone. Mayfield and Johnston (1980) completed one of the most comprehensive studies of this type. It resulted in a complementary combination of screening techniques that balanced the advantages and limitations of biological markers and questionnaires. The sample was 126 male inpatients drawn from all services of a general hospital (the first 100 subjects were selected at random at admission; the procedure for selecting the other 26 was not specified). Subjects received a breathalyzer at admission to obtain BAL values, a drinking practices and consumption interview, the CAGE, the MAST, the SMAST, and the Alcoholic Stages Index Subscales (ASIS) (Mulford, 1977). MCV and GGTP tests were conducted. Subjects were classified as alcoholic based on the interview, a review of the complete medical record, and the MCV and BAL values. Then sensitivity and specificity were calculated for each indicator alone, and each biological test was paired with each questionnaire. The biological markers had greater specificity but less sensitivity than the questionnaires. The positive and negative predictive values as well as the efficiency (proportion of patients tested who were correctly assigned) was lower for the biological tests than for the questionnaires. The best of all of the measures was the MAST, with sensitivity at 86 percent, specificity at 81 percent, and efficiency at 83 percent. The SMAST was second, with sensitivity at 80 percent, specificity at 77 percent, and efficiency at 79 percent. The test with the worst performance (although with the best specificity) was the BAL, with sensitivity at 13 percent, specificity at 97 percent, and efficiency at 58 percent. The authors examined the combinations of each questionnaire with each laboratory test. All of the combinations resulted in a better sensitivity than either test alone at the cost of decreased specificity, except for the combination of the MAST with BAL. The combination of the MAST with BAL was the most favorable, producing a sensitivity of 90 percent, specificity of 81 percent, and efficiency of 86 percent. The next best combination was MAST with MCV, yielding 96 percent sensitivity, 69 percent specificity, and 82 percent efficiency.

Bernadt, Mumford, Taylor, Smith, and Murray (1982) and Bernadt, Mumford, and Murray (1984) compared the brief MAST, the CAGE, and the Reich test (Reich et al., 1975) to eight laboratory tests, among them MCV, GGTP, HDL, and AP. (The Reich test is a brief eight-item interview with a branching structure, resulting in a binary classification, alcoholic or nonalcoholic. Most respondents are classified by the first few questions. This test is cited infrequently in the literature.) The sample consisted of 198 consecutive male admissions and 187 women, every second admission, to two English psychiatric hospitals. Criteria for alcoholism were (1) self-reported "excessive drinking"—consuming more than sixteen "drinks" per day during the year before admission (that is, > 160 mg ethanol/day)—or (2) a primary or secondary diagnosis of alcoholism by the time of discharge. Correlations between self-reported amount of alcohol consumed per day and the laboratory tests were low. Sensitivity and specificity of each of the five best laboratory tests were calculated against the excessive drinking indicator and the alcoholism diagnosis indicator. With both, the sensitivity of MCV, GGTP, and three other tests was quite low (0–36 percent), although the specificity ranges were acceptable (83–99 percent). In contrast, the sensitivities and specificities of the three questionnaires were good, ranging from 85 to 98 percent and from 76 to 89 percent, respectively. The optimum screening combination was the Reich questionnaire and glutamate dehydrogenase (GDH) laboratory test (Bernadt et al., 1984). The sensitivity was 100 percent, the specificity was 84 percent, the positive predictive value was 59 percent, and the negative predictive value was 100 percent using either excessive drinking or diagnosis of alcoholism as a criterion.

History of trauma is widely thought to signal the presence of alcohol abuse. To assess the diagnostic value of trauma, Skinner, Holt, Schuller, Roy, and Israel (1984) derived a scale from five short questions embedded in a medical history and compared it to three laboratory tests: GGTP, MCV, and HDL. There were 197 subjects: 68 subjects in outpatient alcoholism treatment, 68 matched social drinkers, and 61 family practice patients. Outpatients in alcoholism treatment reported significantly more traumatic injuries ($p < .01$) and had a mean scale score two points higher than the social drinkers ($p < .0001$). The trauma questionnaire correctly identified 68 percent of the alcohol abusers. In contrast, the best laboratory test—MCV—identified only 49 percent of the alcohol abusers. The trauma scale also performed better than MCV in the family practice patients. It detected 67 percent of excessive drinkers and had a specificity of 70 percent. GGTP was the best laboratory test for this group, with a sensitivity of 33 percent. Overall, the laboratory tests had much lower sensitivities (0–33 percent) but better specificities (87–94 percent). Because the trauma scale yielded more acceptable sensitivities and the laboratory tests better specificities, the authors combined them and found that diagnostic accuracy increased. The combination yielded a sensitivity of 81 percent and a specificity of 94 percent in distinguishing alcoholic outpatients from social drinkers and a sensitivity of 86 percent and specificity of 83 percent in detecting excessive drinking in family practice patients. The efficiency of the combinations was 88 percent among alcohol abusers and 84 percent among family practice patients.

Comparisons of Screening Questionnaires, Laboratory Tests, and Clinical Judgment. Skinner, Holt, Sheu, and Israel (1986) compared clinical information from a physical examination that focused on signs of excessive drinking, a self-administered medical history questionnaire, and an extensive battery of twenty-two laboratory tests. Subjects were 131 outpatients with documented alcohol problems, 131 social drinkers matched to the outpatients on age and gender, and 52 patients from a family practice. The laboratory tests included the following: GGTP, BAL, HDL, and MCV. The alcohol problem group and social drinkers were different in terms of alcohol consumption and alcohol-related consequences as measured by the MAST and a quantity-frequency consumption index. Excessive drinkers from among the social drinkers and the family practice group were excluded from the sample. Clinical signs had an overall accuracy of 85–91 percent in distinguishing the alcoholics from social drinkers and from family practice patients. Items from the medical history had a range of 84–88 percent accuracy, while laboratory tests had a range of 71–83 percent in correctly differentiating the alcoholics from the social drinkers. Further analyses revealed that seventeen clinical signs and thirteen medical history items (but none of the laboratory tests) formed a highly diagnostic instrument. If four or more clinical signs were found or four or more medical history items were ascribed to, the probability of alcohol abuse exceeded 0.90.

Cleary et al. (1988) compared results from the SMAST, several laboratory tests, and physicians' examinations to DIS diagnoses. Physicians correctly identified 77 percent of patients who met

DSM-III criteria for alcohol abuse or dependence in the past year and 35 percent of those who met lifetime criteria. The SMAST did better than the physicians: it correctly identified all of the patients who met criteria in the past year and 82 percent of those who met lifetime criteria. None of the laboratory tests performed as well as the SMAST or physician judgments, although all tests varied according to cutoffs used; the more stringent the criteria, the lower the sensitivity and the higher the specificity.

Skinner, Holt, Allen, and Haakonson (1980) conducted an examination of the Munich Alcoholism Test (MALT), which incorporates data from a physical examination and laboratory tests (Part A) with self-report items such as those found on the MAST (Part B). The authors administered the MALT to a sample of 106 males from the Canadian Forces referred for a suspected alcohol problem. The subjects had a median age of twenty-six years and were healthy. According to MALT scoring conventions, 92.5 percent of subjects were classified as definite alcoholics, 5.6 percent as suspected alcoholics, and 1.9 percent as not alcoholic. Although the total MALT score was significantly positively correlated with both the Part A (medical) scores ($r = .74$, $p < .01$) and the Part B (self-report) scores ($r = .80$, $p < .01$), scores on the two sections were not related ($r = .18$). The authors suggest that the lack of correlation is due to the relative independence of the two parts and that self-report of the extent of alcohol problems was independent of the results of the physical examination. However, when the authors examined the psychometric properties of Parts A and B, they found that Part A was not internally consistent; the items correlated only minimally with each other and with the composite score. In contrast, Part B items formed a homogeneous scale with acceptable levels of internal consistency. This complex set of relationships both within and between each part of the MALT indicates that more developmental work is required in each domain—particularly the medical domain—before attempting to combine the two.

Screening for Drug Use Problems in Medical Settings

We found virtually no literature on screening for drug abusers in primary medical settings. Two studies concern screening techniques; however, both were conducted in drug treatment settings. The first (Calsyn, Saxon, & Daisy, 1991) examined the validity of the Millon Clinical Multiaxial Inventory (MCMI) Drug Abuse Scale as measured by the percent of known drug abusers obtaining scores above the established cutoff points. The MCMI is a self-report measure of psychopathology and personality and contains a drug abuse scale. The MCMI was not intended as a screening measure and is problematic to employ in this fashion. Calsyn, Saxon, & Daisy (1991) administered the MCMI to 110 consecutively admitted male veterans entering substance abuse treatment, 73 primary opiate addicts, and 37 primary cocaine addicts. This study found the MCMI to have low sensitivity: only 26 percent of this sample of opiate and cocaine addicts in treatment obtained scores that indicated "prominence" of a drug abuse syndrome; 23 percent obtained scores indicating the presence of "syndrome symptomatology." This scale did not identify the remaining 51 percent, all of whom openly admitted to illicit drug use and to drug use problems. Calsyn et al. note that Marsh, Stile, Stoughton, and Trout-Landen (1988) obtained similar results. In the latter study, the MCMI identified only 49 percent of 159 opiate addicts in methadone maintenance as drug abusers.

Lavelle, Hammersley, and Forsyth (1991) compared the Drug Misuse Scale—a thirty-seven-item subscale empirically derived from the Minnesota Multiphasic Personality Inventory (MMPI)—to a scale similarly derived by MacAndrew (1965) to identify alcoholics. The MacAndrew Scale also distinguishes between drug abusers and those who do not use drugs, but not between alcoholics and drug abusers. Lavelle et al. administered the Drug Misuse Scale and the MacAndrew Scale to men and women in alcohol and drug treatment programs and to a control group. The Drug Misuse Scale correctly identified 80 percent of the drug treatment group, 30 percent of the alcohol treatment group, and 92 percent of the control group. The Drug Misuse Scale distinguished drug abusers from alcoholics, unlike the MacAndrew Scale. Nevertheless, since the Drug Misuse Scale identified only 30 percent of the alcoholics, the MacAndrew Scale appears more appropriate for suspected alcoholism. Based on these findings, the Drug Misuse scale holds promise as a screening technique for drug abuse in clinical settings.

In summary, the amassed data clearly indicate the superiority of brief screening questionnaires over laboratory tests and clinical examinations for identifying AODA problems. If laboratory tests are available, the data indicate that these in combination with a screening questionnaire provide the most accurate means of identifying patients with alcohol and drug use problems.

Conclusion

The comprehensive work on prevalence of alcoholism rates and alcohol-related problems in primary care settings is complemented by the work on detection of alcohol problems. The progress in these two areas serves to highlight what has not yet been accomplished. First, the lack of studies about the presentation of drug abuse/dependence in medical settings is especially apparent. Investigations of the prevalence of drug abuse and dependence in primary medical patients are needed. In addition to providing estimates of the prevalence of drug use disorders, we need to identify: (1) the drugs abused by patients seen in these settings, (2) the medical conditions associated with abuse of these drugs, (3) the putative reasons that drug-involved persons are seeking care at primary care settings, and (4) psychosocial factors that describe these patients. Such studies should yield important information about the barriers to diagnosis and treatment of drug problems and to the screening for these problems.

Second, research is needed on treatment interventions that can be initiated or accomplished in the context of providing care in primary medical settings. Empirical research that addresses relative efficacies of different interventions in medical settings is lacking. If we assume that health care providers can be trained to obtain information that identifies problems, we still need efficacious ways of attending to the problem. Researchers should be encouraged to conduct studies that explore productive ways of initiating treatment and referrals in the primary care relationship. Research on the characteristics of patients who seek out specialty care for AODA problems, as well as on the frequency and precursors of these attempts, should contribute to the design of research on primary medical care intervention and referral strategies.

Third, aside from treatment interventions, service delivery

issues related to these patient groups also warrant more attention—specifically, better identification of risk groups. Despite increased sophistication in conducting prevalence studies, little information has emerged concerning the characteristics of identified alcoholics that might assist in developing appropriate services. For example, our review of prevalence studies indicated that although researchers intended to sample randomly or representatively, many of the samples were ultimately samples of convenience, in which women, African Americans, and unemployed persons predominated. The next steps should include research that develops models predictive of those at greatest risk for a primary or secondary AODA diagnosis among primary care patients. Once we have a better idea of which primary care patients are at greatest risk for having AODA problems, more insightful and effective interventions and service systems can be developed.

Fourth, recent research on screening strategies is impressive, yet it too highlights the need for better methods. Studies reveal that laboratory tests are far from satisfactory as markers for alcoholism. Most of this research assesses the value of different biological markers, using medically accepted normal ranges as cutoff values. Future research, however, should consider the cutoff points used, rather than discarding tests that are not good markers when using conventional cutoff points. Experimentation with different cutoff values may be productive.

Fifth, improving methods for making and communicating a diagnosis of alcohol or drug abuse should parallel research on screening techniques. Schulberg, McClelland, Coulehan, Block, and Werner (1986) studied identification of psychiatric disorders in general medical practice and noted that many physicians do not use screening tools or their results when available, although the reasons are unknown. To address this problem, Schulberg et al. (1986) recommended research on medical decision making and problem-solving processes. Such research could improve medical training. We concur with these recommendations and argue that these inquiries should address alcohol and substance abuse as well as psychiatric disorders.

In summary, the prevalence of AODA problems in primary care settings indicates that patients find such settings and health care providers acceptable sources of help for these problems. Research in the areas described should result in more effective responses to patients.

References

Abed, R. T., & Neira-Muñoz, E. (1990). A survey of general practitioners' opinions and attitudes to drug addicts and addiction. *British Journal of Addiction, 85,* 131–136.

Aderhold, R. M. (1980). Determinants of alcoholism diagnosis and treatment. *Proceedings of the Annual Meeting of the Robert Wood Johnson Foundation for Clinical Scholars.* Princeton, NJ: Robert Wood Johnson Foundation.

Anderson, P. (1985). Managing alcohol problems in general practice. *British Medical Journal, 290,* 1873–1875.

Barnes, H. N. (1987). Presenting the diagnosis: Working with denial. In H. N. Barnes, M. D. Aronson, & T. L. Delbanco (Eds.), *Alcoholism: A guide for the primary care physician* (pp. 59–65). New York: Springer-Verlag.

Bernadt, M. W., Mumford, J., & Murray, R. M. (1984). A discriminant-function analysis of screening tests for excessive drinking and alcoholism. *Journal of Studies on Alcohol, 45*(1), 81–86.

Bernadt, M. W., Mumford, J., Taylor, C., Smith, B., & Murray, R. M. (1982). Comparison of questionnaire and laboratory tests in the detection of excessive drinking and alcoholism. *Lancet, 1,* 325–328.

Brown, R. L., Carter, W. B., & Gordon, M. J. (1987). Diagnosis of alcoholism in a simulated patient encounter by primary care physicians. *Journal of Family Practice, 25*(3), 259–264.

Buchsbaum, D. G., Buchanan, R. G., Lawton, M. J., & Schnoll, S. H. (1991). Alcohol consumption patterns in a primary care population. *Alcohol & Alcoholism, 26*(2), 215–220.

Calsyn, D. A., Saxon, A. J., & Daisy, F. (1991). Validity of the MCMI drug abuse scale varies as a function of drug choice, race, and axis II subtypes. *American Journal of Drug and Alcohol Abuse, 17*(2), 153–159.

Cartwright, A. K. J. (1980). The attitudes of helping agents towards the alcoholic client: The influence of experience, support, training and self-esteem. *British Journal of Addiction, 75,* 413–431.

Chappel, J. N., & Schnoll, S. H. (1977). Physician attitudes: Effect on the treatment of chemically dependent patients. *Journal of the American Medical Association, 237,* 2318–2319.

Cleary, P. D., Miller, M., Bush, B. T., Warburg, M. M., Delbanco, T. L., & Aronson, M. D. (1988). Prevalence and recognition of alcohol abuse in a primary care population. *American Journal of Medicine, 85,* 466–471.

Clement, S. (1986). The identification of alcohol-related problems by general practitioners. *British Journal of Addiction, 81,* 257–264.

Coulehan, J. L., Zettler-Segal, M., Block, M., McClelland, M., & Schulberg, H. C. (1987). Recognition of alcoholism and substance abuse in primary care patients. *Archives of Internal Medicine, 147,* 349–352.

Cushman, P., Jacobson, G., Barboriak, J. J., & Anderson, A. J. (1984). Biochemical markers for alcoholism: Sensitivity problems. *Alcoholism: Clinical and Experimental Research, 8*(3), 253–257.

Cyr, M. G., & Wartman, S. A. (1988). The effectiveness of routine screening questions in the detection of alcoholism. *Journal of the American Medical Association, 259*(1), 51–54.

Delbanco, T. L., & Barnes, H. N. (1987). The epidemiology of alcohol abuse and the response of physicians. In H. N. Barnes, M. D. Aronson, & T. L. Delbanco (Eds.), *Alcoholism: A guide for the primary care physician* (pp. 3–8). New York: Springer-Verlag.

Fisher, J. C., Mason, R. L., Keeley, K. A., & Fisher, J. V. (1975). Physicians and alcoholics: The effect of medical training on attitudes toward alcoholics. *Journal of Studies on Alcohol, 36*(7), 949–955.

Glanz, A. (1986). Findings of a national survey of the role of general practioners in the treatment of opiate misuse: Views on treatment. *British Medical Journal, 293,* 543–545.

Gottlieb, N. H., Mullen, P. D., & McAlister, A. L. (1987). Patients' substance abuse and the primary care physician: Patterns of practice. *Addictive Behaviors, 12,* 23–32.

Hoeper, E. W., Nycz, G., & Cleary, P. D. (1979). *The quality of mental health services in an organized primary health care setting: Final report* (NIMH Contract No. 278-77-0071 (DB)). Rockville, MD: National Institute of Mental Health.

Hurt, R. D., Morse, R. M., & Swenson, W. B. (1980). Diagnosis of Alcoholism with a self-administered screening test: Results of 1002 patients receiving general examinations. *Mayo Clinical Proceedings, 55,* 365–370.

Iber, F. L. (Ed.). (1991). *Alcohol and drug abuse as encountered in office practice.* Boca Raton, Fla.: CRC Press.

Kamerow, D. B., Pincus, H. A., & MacDonald, D. I. (1986). Alcohol abuse, other drug abuse, and mental disorders in medical practice: Prevalence, costs, recognition, and treatment. *Journal of the American Medical Association, 255,* 2054–2057.

Kennedy, W. (1985). Chemical dependency: A treatable disease. *Ohio State Medical Journal, 71,* 77–79.

King, M. (1986). Brief communication: At risk drinking among general practice attenders: Validation of the CAGE questionnaire. *Psychological Medicine, 16,* 213–217.

Lavelle, T., Hammersley, R., & Forsyth, A. (1991). A short scale for predicting drug misuse using selected items from the MMPI. *British Journal of Addiction, 86,* 49–55.

Leckman, A. L., Umland, B. E., & Blay, M. (1984). Prevalence of alcoholism in a family practice center. *Journal of Family Practice, 18*(6), 867–870.

Lewis, D. C., Niven, R. G., Czechowicz, D., & Trumble, J. G. (1987). A review of medical education in alcohol and other drug abuse. *Journal of the American Medical Association, 257*(21), 2945–2948.

Linn, L. S., & Yager, J. (1989). Health care delivery: Factors associated with physician recognition and treatment of alcoholism. *Western Journal of Medicine, 150*(4), 468–472.

MacAndrew, C. (1965). The differentiation of male alcohol outpatients by means of the MMPI. *Quarterly Journal of Studies on Alcohol, 26,* 238–246.

McCusker, J., Cherubin, C. E., & Zimberg, S. (1971). Prevalence of alcoholism in a general hospital population. *New York State Journal of Medicine, 71,* 751–754.

Magruder-Habib, K., Durand, A. M., & Frey, K. A. (1991). Alcohol abuse and alcoholism in primary health care settings. *Journal of Family Practice, 32*(4), 406–413.

Magruder-Habib, K. M., Fraker, G. C., & Peterson, C. L. (1983). Correspondence of clinicians' judgments with the Michigan Alcoholism Screening Test in determining alcoholism in Veterans Administration outpatients. *Journal of Studies on Alcohol, 44,* 872–884.

Marsh, D. T., Stile, S. A., Stoughton, N. L., & Trout-Landen, B. L. (1988). Psychopathology of opiate addiction: Comparative data from the MMPI and MCMI. *American Journal of Drug and Alcohol Abuse, 14,* 17–27.

Mayfield, D. G., & Johnston, R. G. M. (1980). Screening techniques and prevalence estimation in alcoholism. In W. E. Fann, I. Karacan, A. D. Porkorny, & R. L. Williams (Eds.), *Phenomenology and treatment of alcoholism* (pp. 33–44). New York: SP Medical & Scientific Books.

Mayfield, D. G., McLeod, G., & Hall, P. (1974). The CAGE questionnaire: Validation of a new alcoholism screening instrument. *American Journal of Psychiatry, 131,* 1121–1123.

Moore, R. D., Bone, L. R., Geller, G., Mamon, J. A., Stokes, E. J., & Levine, D. M. (1989). Prevalence, detection, and treatment of alcoholism in hospitalized patients. *Journal of the American Medical Association, 261*(3), 403–407.

Moore, R. D., & Malitz, F. E. (1986). Underdiagnosis of alcoholism by residents in an ambulatory medical practice. *Journal of Medical Education, 61,* 46–52.

Mulford, H. A. (1977). Stages in the alcoholic process: Toward a cumulative nonsequential index. *Journal of Studies on Alcohol, 38,* 563–583.

Nicol, E. F., & Ford, M. J. (1986). Use of the Michigan Alcoholism Screening Test in general practice. *Journal of the Royal College of General Practitioners, 36,* 409–410.

Nolan, J. P. (1965). Alcohol as a factor in the illness of university service patients. *American Journal of Medical Science, 249,* 135–142.

Porkorny, A. D., Miller, B. A., & Kaplan, H. B. (1972). The brief MAST: A shortened version of the Michigan Alcoholism Screening Test. *American Journal of Psychiatry, 129,* 118–121.

Powers, J. S., & Spickard, A. (1984). Michigan Alcoholism Screening Test to diagnose early alcoholism in general practice. *South Medical Journal, 77,* 852–856.

Reich, T., Robins, L. N., Woodruff, R. A., Taibleson, M., Rich, C., & Cunningham, L. (1975). Computer-assisted derivation of a screening interview for alcoholism. *Archives of General Psychiatry, 32,* 847–852.

Reid, A. L. A., Webb, G. R., Hennrikus, D., Fahey, P. P., & Samson-Fisher, R. W. (1986). Detection of patients with high alcohol intake by general practitioners. *British Medical Journal, 293,* 735–737.

Robins, L. N., Helzer, J. E., Croughan, J., & Ratcliff, K. (1981). National Institute of Mental Health Diagnostic Interview Schedule: Its history, characteristics, and validity. *Archives of General Psychiatry, 38,* 381–389.

Robinson, D., Monk, C., & Bailey, A. (1979). The relationship between serum gamma-glutamyl transpeptidase level and reported alcohol consumption in healthy men. *Journal of Studies on Alcohol, 40*(9), 896–901.

Roche, A. M., Guray, C., & Saunders, J. B. (1991). General practitioners' experiences of patients with drug and alcohol problems. *British Journal of Addiction, 86,* 263–275.

Schuckit, M. A. (1985). Overview: Epidemiology of alcoholism. In M. A. Schuckitt (Ed.), *Alcohol patterns and problems* (pp. 1–42). New Brunswick, NJ: Rutgers University Press.

Schuckit, M. A. (1987). Why don't we diagnose alcoholism in our patients? *Journal of Family Practice, 25*(3), 225–226.

Schulberg, H. C., McClelland, M., Coulehan, J. L., Block, M., & Werner, G. (1986). Psychiatric decision making in family practice: Future research directions. *General Hospital Psychiatry, 8,* 1–6.

Selzer, M. L. (1971). The Michigan Alcoholism Screening Test: The quest for a new diagnostic instrument. *American Journal of Psychiatry, 127,* 89–94.

Selzer, M. L., Vinokur A., & vanRooijen L. (1975). A self-administered Short Michigan Alcoholism Screening Test (SMAST). *Journal of Studies on Alcohol, 36,* 117–126.

Shapiro, S., Skinner, E. A., Kessler, L. G., Von Korff, M., German,

P. S., Tischler, G. L., Leaf, P. J., Benham, L., Cottler, L., & Regier, D. A. (1984). Utilization of health and mental health services: Three epidemiologic catchment area sites. *Archives of General Psychiatry, 41,* 971–978.

Sherin, K. M., Piotrowski, Z. H., Panek, S. M., & Doot, M. C. (1982). Screening for alcoholism in a community hospital. *Journal of Family Practice, 15*(6), 1091–1095.

Shurman, R. A., Kramer, P. D., & Mitchell, J. B. (1985). The hidden mental health network: Treatment of mental illness by nonpsychiatrist physicians. *Archives of General Psychiatry, 42*(1), 89–94.

Skinner, H. A., Holt, S., Allen, B. A., & Haakonson, N. H. (1980). Correlation between medical and behavioral data in the assessment of alcoholism. *Alcoholism: Clinical and Experimental Research, 4*(4), 371–377.

Skinner, H. A., Holt, S., Schuller, R., Roy, J., & Israel, Y. (1984). Identification of alcohol abuse using laboratory tests and a history of trauma. *Annals of Internal Medicine, 101,* 847–851.

Skinner, H. A., Holt, S., Sheu, W. J., & Israel, Y. (1986). Clinical versus laboratory detection of alcohol abuse: The alcohol clinical index. *British Medical Journal, 292,* 1703–1708.

Skinner, H. A., & Sheu, W. J. (1982). Reliability of alcohol use indices: The lifetime drinking history and the MAST. *Journal of Studies in Alcoholism, 43,* 1157–1170.

Solomon, J., Vanga, N., Morgan, J. P., & Joseph, P. (1980). Emergency-room physicians' recognition of alcohol misuse. *Journal of Studies on Alcohol, 41*(5), 583–586.

Spickard, A., Jr. (1986). Alcoholism: The missed diagnosis. *Southern Medical Journal, 79*(12), 1489–1492.

Thom, B., & Téllez, C. (1986). A difficult business: Detecting and managing alcohol problems in general practice. *British Journal of Addiction, 81,* 405–418.

Wechsler, H., Levine, S., Idelson, R. K., Rohman, M., & Taylor, J. O. (1983). The physician's role in health promotion—survey of primary-care practitioners. *New England Journal of Medicine, 308*(2), 97–100.

Wechsler, H., & Rohman, M. (1982). Future caregivers' views on alcoholism treatment: A poor prognosis. *Journal of Studies on Alcohol, 43*(9), 939–955.

Woodall, H. E. (1988). Alcoholics remaining anonymous: Resident diagnosis of alcoholism in a family practice center. *Journal of Family Practice, 26*(3), 293–296.

Zung, B. J. (1984). Reliability and validity of the short MAST among psychiatric inpatients. *Journal of Clinical Psychology, 40,* 347–350.

Johan Ormel
Wim van den Brink

4

Outcome of Common Psychiatric Disorders and Symptoms in Primary Care

Anxiety and depressive disorders are common in primary care (Barrett, Barrett, Oxman, & Gerber, 1988; Blacker & Clare, 1987; Goldberg & Bridges, 1987; Ormel et al., 1990; Regier, Burke, Manderscheid, & Burns, 1985; Shepherd, Cooper, Brown, & Kalton, 1966; Von Korff et al., 1987). In addition, recent epidemiologic studies in community, primary care, and outpatient settings have documented a moderate but clinically significant association of psychiatric symptom severity with disability (impaired physical and role function as well as increased number of disability days) (Berkman et al., 1986; Broadhead, Blazer, George, & Tse, 1990; Craig & Van Natta, 1983; Dohrenwend, Dohrenwend, Link, & Levav, 1983; Hecht, Von Zers-

Note: This research was supported by the Medical Foundation of the Dutch Organization for Scientific Research (NWO), grants 900-556-002 and 900-556-050, and the Prevention Fund, grant 28-1209. Part of the analysis and writing was done at the Center for Health Studies of the Health Cooperative and the Department of Psychiatry and Behavioral Sciences of the University of Washington, Seattle. Parts of this chapter are based on a study also reported on in Ormel et al. (in press).

sen, & Wittchen, 1990; Von Korff, Ormel, Katon, & Lin, 1992; Wells et al., 1989; Wohlfarth, van den Brink, Ormel, Koeter, & Oldehinkel, 1993). This combination of psychiatric symptoms and associated disability may have considerable impact on personal well-being, social relationships, and public health cost and economic consequences (Broadhead et al., 1990; Stoudemire, Frank, Hedemark, Kamlet, & Blazer, 1986; Wells et al., 1989). The extent of the problem, however, is highly dependent on the (long-term) outcome of these disorders. If these psychiatric illnesses and the associated disability are self-limiting or transient, public health intervention is less necessary. But if many are not, a substantial public health problem exists. To date, few cross-sectional (Casey, Tyrer, & Platt, 1985) and longitudinal (Von Korff et al., 1992) studies have been published that address psychopathology and social disability simultaneously in primary care settings. Therefore, it seems expedient to further examine the medium- and long-term outcome of common psychiatric and associated social disability in primary care.

Major diagnostic classification systems like DSM-III do not adequately incorporate the minor anxiety and depressive disorders and nonspecific psychiatric symptoms that are frequently presented in primary care. In addition, these classification systems have a hierarchical structure that hampers research on anxiety-depression comorbidity. Patients who have psychiatric symptoms but do not meet the diagnostic criteria for major disorders may present with a series of somatic complaints, nonspecific distress complaints, and mixed specific symptoms of anxiety and depression. Nonspecific distress includes symptom patterns without a clear depressive or anxiety component. General practitioners (GPs) often recognize and treat these patients, although they rarely make a formal diagnosis. How significant these minor disorders and nonspecific symptoms are in terms of associated disability and outcome is less well known compared to the "diagnosable" disorders (Broadhead et al., 1990; Von Korff et al., 1992). Therefore, we explicitly include these minor disorders and nonspecific symptoms.

In sum, this chapter addresses the medium- and long-term outcome of common psychiatric disorders and symptoms and the associated disability as well as evaluating how symptom severity and disability level track each other over time—that is, their longitudinal relationship. We focus on social, or role, disability, which refers to a (temporary) deficiency in the ability to perform activities and behaviors that are expected in the context of well-defined social roles (Wiersma, DeJong, & Ormel, 1988; Weissmann, 1975). Deficiency in role functioning is inferred from behavioral deviations from norms and expectations of the relevant reference group, usually the local community. This conceptualization of social disability clearly follows the World Health Organization definition of disability as "any restriction or lack of ability to perform an activity in the manner or within the range considered normal for a human being" (World Health Organization, 1980, p. 28).

Conceptual and Methodologic Issues

A number of conceptual and methodologic issues merit discussion.

Long-Term Outcome

For the two major mental disorders that are most common—depression and anxiety—long-term outcomes have primarily been examined among psychiatric in- and outpatients. For depressive disorders in general, these studies have documented that at one-year follow-up, approximately 20 to 35 percent of patients still meet the diagnostic criteria and that another 25 percent, on average, relapse (Bronisch, Wittchen, Krieg, Rupp, & Von Zerssen, 1985; Ceroni, Nevi, & Pezolli, 1984; Keller et al., 1984). However, it is unclear whether these findings can be extrapolated to primary care settings because of subject selection bias. Since only a minority of patients with common mental disorders are referred to specialist settings in Western countries (Giel, Koeter, & Ormel, 1990; Shapiro et al., 1984), this constitutes a major obstacle for extrapolation. The reverse problem complicates extrapolation from longitudinal community studies to primary care settings, since many factors determine consultation of medical professionals, including clinical severity, disability, and sociocultural variables (Mechanic, 1978). As a matter of fact, both help seeking and referral are influenced by diagnosis, symptom severity, and social disability (Dohrenwend et al., 1983; Giel et al., 1990; Mechanic, 1978). Furthermore, the nature of psychopathology in primary care is different with increased prevalences of mixed depression and anxiety and minor disorders, and processes of stigmatization are largely absent among primary care patients with psychiatric symptoms (Link, 1982).

In general, community studies report somewhat better outcomes than patient-based studies (Murphy, Olivier, Sobol, Monson, & Leighton, 1986; Sargeant, Bruce, Florio, & Weissman, 1990). In the one-year follow-up of subjects with major depression identified in the baseline of the Epidemiologic Catchment Area (ECA) study, 20 percent were found to meet diagnostic criteria for major depression again (Sargeant et al., 1990). This estimate is intermediate between the rates of chronicity and the sum of chronicity and relapse, since it does not include patients who relapsed and remitted again. In general, community studies, as well as studies among psychiatric outpatients, suggest that depressive disorders and nonspecific distress have more favorable long-term outcomes than anxiety disorders (Angst, 1990; Wittchen & Von Zerssen, 1987).

Large variations in outcome have also been observed in primary care populations, both between patients and studies (Cooper, Fry, & Kalton, 1969; Hankin & Locke, 1982; Kessler, Cleary, & Burke, 1985; Mann, Jenkins, & Belsey, 1981; Parker, Holmes, & Manicavasagar, 1986; Schulberg, McClelland, & Gooding, 1987). For instance, one-fifth to one-half of patients with depression were found to be still depressed at the various follow-up times.

Methodologic Considerations

Findings on course and outcome are difficult to interpret because of various limitations. These limitations concern unrepresentative primary care settings (physicians), patient sampling limited to conspicuous cases, measurement instruments limited to self-report measures, and nonstandardized measurement procedures and diagnostic allocation. Other problems include short enrollment periods, resulting in oversampling of high utilizers of primary health care and in seasonal bias; high nonresponse rates; differences in diagnostic classification systems; and short follow-up periods of less than one year. Two further issues—lack of control for recency of onset and rarely combining a categorical and dimensional approach—need some discussion.

Controlling for recency of onset may be especially important for the following reasons. Outcome studies typically enroll consecutive patients who meet a priori selected severity and diagnostic criteria. These samples include cases covering the full spectrum of recency of onset, ranging from very recent to very remote. This means that selected cases include patients at different phases in the natural history of the disorder—that is, at different points in the course of their illness trajectory, such as symptom formation, flare-up, remission, complication, and so on. The time at which people visit their general physician frequently represents different time points in the natural history of their individual disorders, although first onsets and flare-ups are powerful predictors of visits. Since degrees of psychopathology and disability are associated with time since onset of symptoms, distinguishing recent-onset cases from more remote should facilitate interpretation.

Outcome studies using standardized interviews that allow diagnostic classification have typically adopted the categorical approach. Outcome is expressed as the proportion of baseline cases that do not meet diagnostic-level criteria at follow-up. This approach may blur reality, since it does not indicate the extent of improvement. In the end, people may have recovered fully and become asymptomatic, or they may have only partly recovered and may still suffer subclinical/subthreshold disorders and persistent symptoms without meeting diagnostic criteria.

The Present Study

The three-wave study described below addresses the medium- (one-year) and long-term (three-year) outcome of psychopathology and associated disability in primary care patients with common psychiatric disorders or nonspecific symptoms. We used well-validated and reliable measures of psychopathology and social disability based on standardized, semistructured personal interviews—the Present State Examination (PSE) (Wing, Cooper, & Sartorius, 1974) and the Groningen Social Disability Schedule (GSDS) (Wiersma et al., 1988). We will stratify analysis by recency of onset and contrast depressive illness, anxiety disorders, comorbidity of depression and anxiety, and nonspecific distress.

We will show that although most cases of depression, anxiety, and anxiety-depression comorbidity are no longer cases at follow-up, many do not regain symptom levels found among normals. This holds more strongly for minor disorders and anxiety than for depression. Improvement in social function is clearly related to improvement in psychopathology. In general, recent cases improved more fully than cases with onsets more than one year prior to index visit. Some of the findings have been published or submitted elsewhere (van den Brink, Leenstra, Ormel, & van de Willige, 1991; Ormel et al., 1990; Ormel & Wohlfarth, 1991; Wilmink, 1989).

Methods

The study was carried out in the province of Groningen, the Netherlands, during the late 1980s. The relevant methods of the study are described here. A full description of methods is provided elsewhere (Ormel et al., 1990; Wilmink, 1989).

Subjects

Sampling of primary care patients occurred in three stages. At stage 1, a representative sample of twenty-five GPs was drawn from the total population of GPs in the city of Groningen and some surrounding towns (with a total population of 275,000).

At stage 2, each GP handed out the thirty-item General Health Questionnaire (GHQ) (Goldberg, 1979; Koeter & Ormel, 1991) to all patients aged sixteen to sixty-five who came for consultation on any of ten prespecified days (index consult; $N = 2237$). Patients were asked to fill out the GHQ at home and return it by mail. Nonrespondents (11 percent) did not differ from respondents ($N = 1994$) in age and presence of a mental health problem as assessed by the GP. Males were slightly more likely to be nonrespondents than females (13 versus 9 percent). Using the conventional GHQ-30 cutoff of five, 863 patients (43 percent) were classified as GHQ+ cases. During the index consult, the GPs indicated on the study form whether the patient's complaints and symptoms were likely to be a manifestation of a mental health problem (GP+ cases; N = 556, 28 percent). The GPs also indicated whether a similar diagnosis had been made during the twelve months prior to the index visit (patients who were less than twelve months on the physician's panel had already been excluded). If this was the case, the patient was denoted an "old" patient (N = 544, 27 percent). Patients who had *no* mental health problem diagnosed in the preceding year were denoted "new" patients (N = 1450, 73 percent).

At stage 3, we cross-classified both "old" and "new" patients according to their GP (GP+/GP-) and GHQ (GHQ+/GHQ-) status. Since we were particularly interested in the long-term outcome of incident cases, the study sampled "new" cases (not necessarily recent-onset cases) with much higher probability than "old" cases. From the four "new" groups, we sampled as follows: all 206 GP+ patients, 62 from the GHQ-/GP- patients, and 91 from the GHQ+/GP- patients. From the four groups of "old" patients, we sampled only from the GHQ+/GP+ group (42 patients). Thus, this nonproportional stratified sampling procedure resulted in 296 subjects (26 percent nonresponse). Due to missing values, most baseline (T1) analyses are based on 285 subjects.

Patients were followed up approximately thirteen (T2) and forty-two (T3) months after the index consult visit. The "new" GHQ-/GP- patients were not examined at T2 and have been excluded from the longitudinal analyses. Attrition at T2 was minimal, but it was substantial at T3. Total attrition amounted to 20 percent but was unrelated to psychiatric status at baseline. The longitudinal three-wave analyses are based on 143 complete cases. The difference between these 143 and the 296 from the baseline analyses is due to exclusion of the patients without elevated psychiatric symptoms at baseline. (PSE-TOT < 3; N = 91), attrition at follow-up (N = 44), and missing data on one or more variables (N = 18).

Measures

Usually within one week of the index visit, well-trained clinical psychologists and physicians administered the PSE and the GSDS. The time frame of both instruments was the past four weeks. The same interviewers partly administered the PSE and GSDS at T2 and T3.

The PSE is a standardized semistructured *psychiatric interview* developed for use in psychiatric in- and outpatient settings but also frequently used in primary care studies. To rate a symptom present in the PSE, four conditions typically have to be met: the symptom is experienced as (1) unpleasant, (2) not under voluntary control, and (3) out of proportion (for example, grief); in some cases, (4) the symptom must have been present for a substantial period of time in the past four weeks. Interviewer-observer reliability of the PSE was generally good, with kappas for individual items ranging from .50 to .81 (Wilmink, 1989). We used the PSE data to construct PSE-TOT and PSE-ID. PSE-TOT is a simple symptom total that takes into account the total number and severity of PSE symptoms. PSE-ID is a weighted-sum score that also takes into account specificity of the symptoms and indicates the probability of the presence of a specific psychiatric diagnosis.

Recency of onset refers to the time of onset of psychiatric symptoms present at the index visit. Time of onset was established by the interviewer during a short semistructured interview. If symptoms had different times of onset, priority was given to the symptoms that had brought the patient to the index visit. Time of onset was classified as recent onset (onset less than twelve months prior to the index visit) or chronic. The latter category was further divided into with and without recent exacerbation.

The GSDS is a standardized semistructured interview that measures level of *role dysfunction*. It provides substantially more information on the specific nature of social role impairment than self-report disability schedules. Within the framework of the GSDS, disability refers to a deficiency in the ability to perform activities and manifest behaviors, as these are expected in the context of well-defined social roles. The deficiency is inferred from deviations from norms and expectations as these prevail within the context of the relevant reference group. Scores on each role range from 0 (no disability), through 1 (some but significant disability), to 2 (marked or severe disability). In this chapter, we focus on four roles (self-care, family role, social role, and occupational role) and their total score (range 0–8). Self-care encompasses how well people take care of and present themselves to others in everyday encounters. Family role function is evaluated in terms of participation in and preservation of the family or household as an independent unit. Social role entails the quantity and quality of contacts with other than family members and professional colleagues. Occupational role concerns daily activities at work (gainful employment, volunteer work, housekeeping), activities directed at securing a job (study, job searching), and structuring of daily activities in the case of retirement. Interviewer-observer reliability has been shown to be good in a variety of populations, with weighted kappas for different social roles ranging from .63 to .93 (Wiersma et al., 1988). Analyses showed that the four roles constitute a one-dimensional hierarchical scale (Loevinger's H-coefficient $>$ .50).

Diagnostic Classification

Psychiatric diagnoses were made according to the Bedford College Criteria, which are more useful than DSM-III criteria for differentiating common psychiatric disorders in primary care patients (Finlay-Jones et at., 1980). *Depression* is defined as depressed mood *and* four or more of the following ten symptoms: hopelessness, suicidal ideas or actions, weight loss, early waking, delayed sleep, poor concentration, neglect due to brooding, loss of interest, self-depreciation, and anergia. *Anxiety* is either (1) free-floating autonomic anxiety more than 50 percent of the time *or* more than five panic attacks, or (2) free-floating autonomic anxiety less than 50 percent of the time *and* one to four panic attacks, or (3) situational autonomic anxiety *and* marked generalization of avoidance. *Minor psychiatric disorder* includes *minor depression* (depressed mood *and* at least one of the ten symptoms listed for depression) and *minor anxiety,* which is defined as either (1) free-floating autonomic anxiety less than 50 percent of the time, or (2) less than five panic attacks, or (3) situational autonomic anxiety *and* avoidance whenever possible. To these four Bedford College diagnoses, we added the category of *nonspecific distress (or symptoms),* consisting of subjects with nonspecific psychiatric symptoms such as worrying, tension pains, muscular tension, tiredness, restlessness, hypochondriasis, irritability, and poor concentration. This category was assigned to all patients with PSE-TOT greater than or equal to 3 and no anxiety or depression as defined above. The diagnoses of depression and anxiety are not mutually exclusive, allowing for *comorbidity* of these disorders.

Results

The results are presented in three sections. We first summarize data collected at baseline, then turn to data collected during medium and long-term follow-up, and finally explore the correlation between psychopathology and social disability—specifically whether symptom improvement is associated with improved functioning.

Baseline Data

Baseline data included sociodemographic characteristics, levels of social and occupational role functioning, and the degree of disability by diagnostic category.

Sociodemographic Characteristics. Table 4.1 depicts the sociodemographic characteristics of the patients with three or more psychiatric symptoms broken down by recency of onset and of the controls;

Table 4.1. Demographic Characteristics of Patients with Psychiatric Disorders or Symptoms and Controls by Recency of Onset (Unweighted Baseline Data, *N* = 285).

			Educational Attainment		
Patient Group	*Women (%)*	*Mean Age*	*Low*[a]	*High*[b]	*(N)*[c]
Cases: recent onset[d]	63.5	34.0	14.5	43.5	63
Cases: onset > 1 year[d]	71.0	39.0	21.1	28.1	131
"Controls"[e]	53.8	37.7	22.2	34.4	91

[a] Graduated from elementary school only.

[b] Graduated from high school (Dutch VWO and HAVO).

[c] The table total does not add up to 296 because of missing values on the recency variable.

[d] T1 PSE-TOT 3 or more.

[e] T1 PSE-TOT less than 3.

the latter had less than three PSE symptoms at the index visit. Higher proportions of women are found in the caseness (diagnostic-level) groups relative to the controls, which is consistent with the reports of others (for example, Marks, Goldberg, & Hillier, 1979). No association between mean age and educational attainment, and caseness status was observed. Cases with a recent onset were somewhat more likely to be male, younger, and better educated than cases with an onset more than one year prior to the index visit.

Levels of Social and Occupational Role Functioning. Table 4.2 presents the percentage of patients with at least a minor impairment for each role, for recent-onset cases, cases with an onset more than one year prior to the index visit, and the controls. For reasons of comparison, data from psychiatric outpatients have been included. Cases differed strongly from controls in terms of disability. Most disability was in the domains of social and occupational role functioning; self-care and family (or household) roles were almost invariably intact. No marked differences were observed between recent-onset and chronic cases, except that occupational function

Table 4.2. Psychiatric Morbidity (PSE) and Social Disability (GSDS) (Baseline Data, Unweighted).

			Percent with at Least Minor Impairment in			
Primary Care Patient Group	*Mean PSE-TOT Score*	*Mean GSDS Score*	*Self-Care*	*Family Role*	*Social Role*	*Occupational Role*
Cases: recent onset[a]	12.0	1.57	6.3	12.7	49.2	50.8
Cases: onset > 1 year[a]	11.6	1.23	6.9	11.5	46.6	38.9
"Controls"[b]	0.7	0.43	3.3	3.3	21.1	11.1
Psychiatric outpatients (N = 40)[c]	15.5	1.51	13.0	18.1	70.2	59.1

[a]PSE-TOT 3 or more.
[b]PSE-TOT less than 3.
[c]Consecutive series of forty intakes at the psychiatric outpatient clinic of the nonuniversity hospital in the city of Groningen.

was more impaired among recent-onset cases. Compared to psychiatric outpatients, the primary care cases have lower levels of disability. The proportion of controls with at least minor impairment in social role suggests that interviewers may have applied too high a standard for this role.

Degree of Disability by Diagnostic Category. Table 4.3 presents mean disability scores by diagnostic category. While depressive illness showed higher disability than anxiety and minor disorders, the latter two showed higher disability levels than the nonspecific distress group. Similar trends were observed for the individual roles. The findings suggest that depression in particular, with or without anxiety, is associated with disability. However, the estimates for the patients with anxiety and anxiety-depression comorbidity are based on only ten cases each.

Medium- and Long-Term Outcomes

In the follow-up data collection period, we focused on the association between recency of onset and (1) outcome psychopathology and (2) outcome disability.

Outcome Psychopathology. Table 4.4 presents follow-up data on psychopathology broken down by recency of onset for patients with

Table 4.3. Mean Disability Scores by Study Diagnosis (Baseline Data, Unweighted).

	Nonspecific Distress[a]	*Minor Disorder*[b]	*Anxiety*[c]	*Depression*[d]	*Comorbidity*[e]
Cases: recent onset	1.18	1.35	0.67	2.60	1.67
Cases: onset > 1 year	0.79	1.00	1.29	2.18	2.67
Total (*N*)	63	81	10	38	10

[a] PSE-TOT equal to or greater than 3 and no specific diagnosis.
[b] Minor anxiety and/or minor depression; largely cases with minor anxiety.
[c] Anxiety with or without minor depression.
[d] Depression with or without (minor) anxiety.
[e] Comorbidity of depression and anxiety.

Table 4.4. Medium- and Long-Term Outcome of Psychiatric Disorders and Symptoms (Unweighted Data).

	Baseline (T1)	*One-Year Follow-up (T2)*	*Three-Year Follow-up (T3)*
Recent onset (*N* = 53)			
Mean PSE-TOT	12.2	4.8	3.1
% PSE-TOT ≥ 3	100.0	50.1	30.2
% PSE-TOT ≥ 10	64.2	13.2	9.4
% Anxiety and/or depression	35.8	1.9	5.7
Onset > 1 year prior to T1 (*N* = 104)			
Mean PSE-TOT	11.6	8.3	5.4
% PSE-TOT ≥ 3	100.0	81.7	59.6
% PSE-TOT ≥ 10	47.1	33.7	18.2
% Anxiety and/or depression	29.8	12.5	5.8

Note: Patients with incomplete data and T1 PSE-TOT less than 3 were excluded.

a psychiatric disorder or symptoms at baseline and complete follow-up data. There was substantial improvement as defined by mean symptom level (PSE-TOT), proportion of highly distressed persons (PSE-TOT ≥ 10), and proportion of subjects with a disorder. Among recent-onset cases, the improvement was more pronounced. Most of the improvement occurred in the first year of the follow-up period. However, although most cases significantly improve, many do not become symptom free, as shown by the proportion of patients with still at least three PSE symptoms at T1 and T2. This holds true in particular among patients with an onset dating back more than a year from index consult.

Table 4.5 shows data about the extent of partial recovery broken down by initial severity. Four outcome categories were distinguished: (1) less than three PSE symptoms, (2) nonspecific distress, (3) minor anxiety and/or minor depression, and (4) anxiety and/or depression. Most baseline cases improve substantially but do not fully recover. For instance, only 23 percent of the patients with

Table 4.5. Many Improve but Few Recover Fully: Outcome Status at Follow-up by Severity at Index Consult (Unweighted Data).

Baseline Severity (Diagnostic Status T1)	*Outcome Status at First Follow-up (T2)*				
	0–2 (%)[a]	*NS (%)*	*MINOR (%)*	*MAJOR (%)*	*Total (100%)*
Nonspecific symptoms (NS)	50	39	9	1	54
Minor disorder (MINOR)	16	21	58	6	73
Anxiety and/or depression (MAJOR)	23	27	32	18	

Baseline Severity (Diagnostic Status T1)	*Outcome Status at Second Follow-up (T3)*				
	0–2 (%)[a]	*NS (%)*	*MINOR (%)*	*MAJOR (%)*	*Total (100%)*
Nonspecific symptoms (NS)	73	23	4	0	
Minor disorder (MINOR)	36	22	39	3	64
Anxiety and/or depression (MAJOR)	36	24	26	14	50

Note: Patients with incomplete data and T1 PSE-TOT less than 3 were excluded.

[a]PSE-TOT less than 3.

depression and/or anxiety at index consult had less than three PSE-symptoms at T2 and only 36 percent at T3, more than three years after the index visit. Very similar findings are observed when using PSE total score and PSE Index of Definition as indicators of severity at index consult and follow-up. From the ninety-seven patients with PSE-TOT scores of 10+ at T1, the distribution at T2 was as follows: 0–1 symptoms, 16 percent; 2–4 symptoms, 20 percent; 5–9 symptoms, 26 percent; and 10+ symptoms, 38 percent. At T3, these proportions were as follows: 0–1 symptoms, 34 percent; 2–4 symptoms, 19 percent; 5–9 symptoms, 24 percent; and 10+ symptoms, 23 percent.

Outcome Disability. Table 4.6 shows data on the medium- and long-term outcome of disability broken down by recency of onset for

Table 4.6. Medium- and Long-Term Outcome of Disability (Unweighted Data).

	Baseline (T1)	*One-Year Follow-up (T2)*	*Three-Year Follow-up (T3)*
Recent onset (*N* = 47)			
Mean GSDS score	1.55	0.36	0.43
% Self-care ≥ 1	6.4	0.0	2.1
% Family role ≥ 1	17.0	8.5	2.1
% Social role ≥ 1	44.7	21.3	29.8
% Occupational role ≥ 1	46.8	2.1	6.4
Onset > 1 year prior to index consult (*N* = 95)			
Mean GSDS score	1.35	0.98	0.72
% Self-care ≥ 1	8.4	6.3	3.1
% Family role ≥ 1	14.7	14.7	7.4
% Social role ≥ 1	52.7	45.6	41.1
% Occupational role ≥ 1	40.0	23.5	14.2

Note: Patients with incomplete data and T1 PSE-TOT less than 3 were excluded.

patients with psychiatric symptoms at baseline. Dysfunction dropped sharply in the occupational, family, and self-care roles, and substantially in the social role, with most of the drop occurring in the first follow-up period. The functioning of patients with a recent onset seems to improve more than of those with more remote onsets of symptomatology.

Table 4.7 shows data about the extent of partial recovery from disability for moderate and severe disability levels at baseline. Four outcome categories were distinguished: (1) no disability, (2) mild disability, (3) moderate disability, and (4) severe disability. Compared to the psychopathology, the follow-up data on disability show similar recovery and improvement rates.

Synchrony of Change in Psychopathology and Disability

Finally, we examined whether symptom improvement is associated with improved function—that is, the extent of synchrony of change

Table 4.7. Social Disability Substantially Improves (Unweighted Data).

	Follow-up Disability at T2 (GSDS = TOT)				
Baseline Disability (T1)	*0 (%)*[a]	*1 (%)*	*2 (%)*	*3+ (%)*	*Total (100%)*
GSDS-TOT 2 (moderate)	44	35	12	9	43
GSDS-TOT 3+ (severe)	23	33	23	21	39
	Follow-up Disability at T3 (GSDS = TOT)				
Baseline Disability (T1)	*0 (%)*[a]	*1 (%)*	*2 (%)*	*3+ (%)*	*Total (100%)*
GSDS-TOT 2 (moderate)	66	17	11	6	35
GSDS-TOT 3+ (severe)	24	42	12	21	33

[a] GSDS–TOT equals 0—that is, no disability.

in psychopathology and social disability. We classified study subjects as having improved symptomatically if the mean of the two follow-up PSE-TOTs was reduced at least 50 percent relative to their baseline PSE-TOT. Next, they were cross-classified by baseline severity (anxiety and/or depression versus minor disorder and nonspecific distress) and improvement status (improved, unimproved) in four severity-improvement groups.

Figure 4.1 presents graphs depicting the course of disability for each of the four severity-improvement groups: (1) major disorder at baseline (depression and/or anxiety) and not improved, (2) major disorder at baseline and improved, (3) minor disorder or nonspecific distress at baseline and not improved, and (4) minor disorder or nonspecific distress at baseline and improved. Persons with improved symptomatology (reduction in (T2 + T3)/2 symptom level more than half baseline score) had meaningfully lower levels of disability at follow-up, whereas persons with nonimproved symptomatology had levels of disability that were only slightly lower than their baseline levels. At follow-up, disability among persons with improved symptoms dropped to the level found among nor-

Figure 4.1. Course of Disability for Four Severity-Improvement Groups.

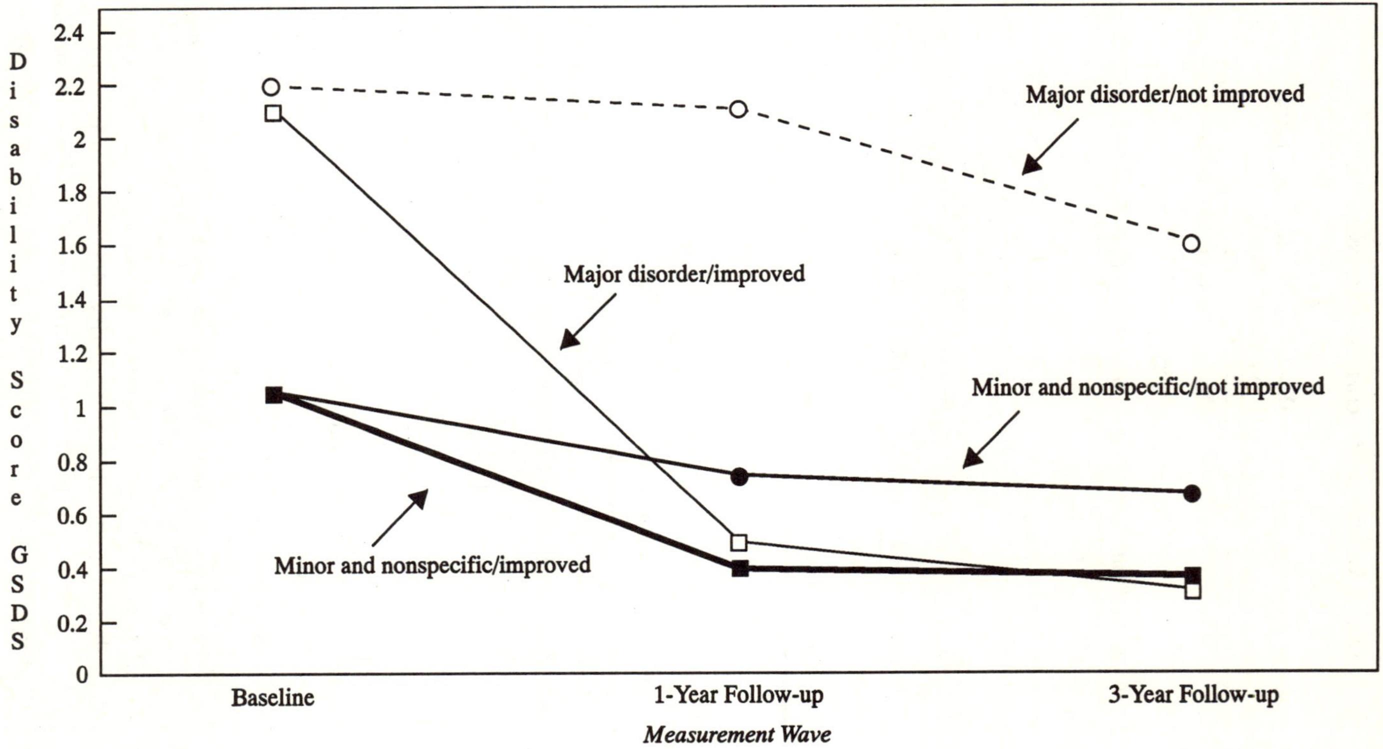

mals (PSE-TOT less than 3; see Table 4.2) for people with major as well as minor disorders at baseline.

Repeated-measures general linear models analysis was performed using SAS software to assess the statistical significance of the longitudinal differences in disability levels by symptom severity-improvement status. In this repeated-measures general linear model for the three occasions on which disability was measured, baseline severity of psychological illness and improvement status were entered as factors. The analysis of within-subject across-time effects directly tests the hypothesis that the trajectory of disability differs between persons with improved versus nonimproved symptoms. The relevant test statistic indicated a highly significant interaction effect between time and improvement status ($F = 50.1$, $p < 0.001$), confirming the hypothesis of different trajectories for improved versus nonimproved symptoms. Further, the test of between-subject effects again confirmed that severity of psychopathology was associated with level of disability across the three waves ($F = 93.0$, $p < .001$). The analysis also showed a significant main effect for time and a significant interaction effect between time and baseline severity. The main effect for time suggests that disability decreased with time across the four severity-improvement status groups. The time-by-severity interaction suggests that persons with severe baseline symptomatology had larger reductions in disability than persons with less severe initial symptomatology, as can be seen most clearly in Figure 4.1.

The analyses described above were carried out for everyone with baseline levels of three or more PSE symptoms irrespective of recency of onset and diagnosis. Therefore, we repeated the analysis to establish whether the pattern of results was similar for recency of onset: recent onset versus onset more than one year prior to the index visit. We also did this for diagnostic category: (minor) depression only, (minor) anxiety only, and comorbidity of anxiety and depression (Ormel, van den Brink, Oldehinkel, & Brilman, 1993). These stratified analyses confirmed the general hypothesis that the synchrony of change in symptom severity and disability is independent of diagnostic category and recency of onset. However, the graphs showed that the synchrony of change was somewhat weaker for anxiety than for depression and comorbidity of depression and anxiety.

Discussion

The follow-up symptom data revealed two apparently contradictory trends. Comparison of mean symptom scores and proportion of disorder across time showed substantial improvement at follow-up. However, many with disorder at baseline did not become asymptomatic. From the ninety-seven patients with PSE-TOT scores of 10+ at T1, 64 percent had PSE-TOT scores of 5 or more at the one-year follow-up. These findings suggest that most patients do improve but do not become symptom free. In other words, major disorders often become minor disorders and minor disorders become nonspecific distress, but no more than half of patients recover fully. Patients who improve most tend to be the cases with relatively recent onsets and depressions.

Differences between study samples in terms of severity, history, and diagnosis complicate the comparability among the few longitudinal studies in primary care that used standardized assessment procedures and representative samples. Follow-up studies among community samples and medical patients typically used categorical approaches and consequently reported outcome in terms of proportion of initial cases that continued to be a case at follow-up. For instance, in the ECA study, of the subjects who had major depressive disorder diagnosed at baseline interview, 20 percent were diagnosed again as having a major depression when reinterviewed one year later (Sargeant et al., 1990). We rediagnosed 18 percent of the patients with depression and/or anxiety at index consult with anxiety and/or depression one year later, remarkably similar. But this does hide the fact that only 23 percent fully recovered. In other words, categorical outcome data may suggest too favorable an outcome.

The notion of a dynamic-equilibrium model (Duncan-Jones, Fergusson, Ormel, & Horwood, 1990; Ormel & Schaufeli, 1991) may be helpful in understanding the long-term course of symptoms and disability among primary care attenders—in particular, why many patients do recover only partially. The basic assumptions of this model are that (1) each person has a distress level that is characteristic for that person, (2) internal and external events act to deflect distress levels from this characteristic level, and (3) adaptive mechanisms tend to neutralize the effects of these events and to restore the characteristic distress level. These assumptions imply that distress levels are highly stable in the absence of events. When people visit their physician for reasons of distress, their symptoms often reflect a recent and significant exacerbation of their characteristic distress and/or disability level. For some, this normal level means none or one or two symptoms only; for others, it means a minor disorder or nonspecific distress. Our data suggest that most presenting cases belong to this second category; they do not return to a symptom-free state but to their characteristic symptom level . . . until the next flare-up occurs. Our data suggest that usually this characteristic symptom level is associated with none or very minor disability. Evidence is now accumulating that most episodes of psychiatric disorder are experienced by a small group of vulnerable persons with relatively high normal symptom levels. The evidence comes from community as well as primary care studies (Cooper et al., 1969; Duncan-Jones et al., 1990). These high normal symptom levels might reflect inadequate treatment (for example, Katon, Von Korff, Lin, Bush, & Ormel, 1992), but they are more likely to reflect persistent life stresses or difficulties (for instance, Depue & Monroe, 1985; Ormel & Wohlfarth, 1991), ineffective coping strategies, and personality pathology such as high neuroticism and obsessive-compulsive tendencies (for example, Duncan-Jones et al., 1990; Hirschfeld & Klerman, 1979; Watson & Pennebaker, 1989).

A major hypothesis examined in this research was that primary care patients whose psychiatric symptoms substantially improve will show corresponding changes in disability level, while patients with unimproved or only slightly improved symptoms will on average show no improvement in disability level. This hypothesis was confirmed for patients with major depression and/or anxiety as well as for patients with mild baseline symptom levels. We also demonstrated that the synchrony in change between symptom severity and disability is largely independent of the recency of onset. The absolute drop in disability was more substantial among the patients with major disorders, especially depression or comorbidity of depression. The disability level of improved patients had returned at follow-up to approximately the same level as found among the controls. This result strengthens and extends similar findings from longitudinal work among depressed high utilizers of primary care (Von Korff et al., 1992). Given the substantial differences between the studies in sample, design, time frame, and measures, the similarity of the findings is striking.

We should stress that our study sample is not fully representative of patients with psychological illness seen in primary care settings. Our sampling scheme was nonproportionally stratified and incident cases (according to the GP!) were sampled with a much higher probability. Many of these physician-rated incident cases appeared to have onsets of more than a year prior to the index visit, but because they had never presented their psychiatric illness or were not recognized by the GP, they were rated as incident cases by the GP. Since the synchrony of change in this group of prevalent cases was as strong as among the incident cases, it is very unlikely that the nonstudied prevalent cases will have substantially different synchrony-of-change patterns. To be sure, we repeated the analysis for two major sampling groups (new GHQ+/GP+ cases; new GHQ+/GP- cases). For each group, we observed synchrony of change in symptoms and disability, suggesting that the nonproportional sampling had not resulted in gross bias. Finally, it should be noted that the findings on synchrony of change in psychopathology and disability do not allow determination of causal ordering.

The nonproportionally stratified sampling scheme may also have biased the findings on outcome. Recent-onset cases had generally slightly more favorable outcomes than cases with more remote onsets. Therefore, a truly consecutive sample or patient series, with even more prevalent cases than in our patient sample, may exhibit a less favorable outcome than we observed.

An important question is what can be done in primary care for those patients who suffer from psychiatric disorders or nonspecific distress that tends to become chronic and to be associated with disability, particularly in the case of depression. Although some work on this has already been done (for example, Katon et al., 1992; Paykel, Freeling, & Hollymen, 1988) and more is in progress, a variety of clinical trials are badly needed in which a spectrum of pharmacological interventions, psychosocial interventions, and self-help programs and materials are evaluated in terms of their ability to improve functional status.

Conclusion

In sum, our interview-based, three-wave data covering a period of more than three years show that most patients with depression, anxiety, and anxiety/depression comorbidity at index visit no longer met the case criteria at follow-up. However, many patients do not return to symptom levels found among normals. Partial recovery is found more frequently among cases with recent onsets than among cases with more remote onsets. To some extent, this is due to confounding with diagnostic category. Depressive illness has both a better outcome and a more recent onset than anxiety. Improvement in social function clearly tracked improvement in psychopathology, and this was largely independent of recency of onset and diagnosis. The robust cross-sectional and longitudinal relationship between depressive symptoms and disability indicates that experimental and quasi-experimental studies that evaluate the causal role of depression vis-à-vis disability should be undertaken as soon as possible.

References

Angst, J. (1990). Depression and anxiety: A review of studies in the community and primary care. In N. Sartorius, D. Goldberg, G. de Girolamo, J. Costa e Silva, J. Lecrubier, & H.-U. Wittchen (Eds.), *Psychological disorders in general medical settings* (pp. 146–158). Bern: Huber.

Barrett, J. E., Barrett, J. A., Oxman, T. E., & Gerber, P. D. (1988). The prevalence of psychiatric disorders in a primary care practice. *Archives of General Psychiatry, 45,* 1100–1119.

Berkman, L. F., Berkman, C. S., Kasl, S., Freeman, D. H., Leo, L., Ostfeld, A. M., Cornoni-Huntley, J., & Brody, J. A. (1986). Depressive symptoms in relation to physical health and functioning in the elderly. *American Journal of Epidemiology, 124,* 372–388.

Blacker, C. V. R., & Clare, A. W. (1987). Depressive disorder in primary care. *British Journal of Psychiatry, 150,* 737–751.

Broadhead, W. E., Blazer, D. G., George, L. K., & Tse, C. (1990). Depression, disability days, and days lost from work in a prospective epidemiologic survey. *Journal of the American Medical Association, 264,* 2524–2528.

Bronisch, T., Wittchen, H.-U., Krieg, C., Rupp, H.-U., & Von Zerssen, D. (1985). Depressive neurosis: A long-term prospective follow-up study of former inpatients. *Acta Psychiatrica Scandinavica, 71,* 237–248.

Casey, P. R., Tyrer, P. J., & Platt, S. (1985). The relationship between social functioning and psychiatric symptomatology in primary care. *Social Psychiatry, 20,* 5–9.

Ceroni, G. B., Nevi, C., & Pezolli, A. (1984). Chronicity in major depression. *Journal of Affective Disorders, 7,* 123–132.

Cooper, B., Fry, J., & Kalton, G. W. (1969). A longitudinal study of psychiatric morbidity in a general practice population. *British Journal of Preventive and Social Medicine, 23,* 210–217.

Craig, T. J., & Van Natta, P. A. (1983). Disability and depressive symptoms in two communities. *American Journal of Psychiatry, 140,* 598–601.

Depue, R. A., & Monroe, S. M. (1985). Life stress and human disorder: Conceptualization and measurement of the disordered group. In I. G. Sarason & B. R. Sarason (Eds.), *Social support: Theory, research, and application* (pp. 303–324). Dordrecht: Nijhoff.

Dohrenwend, B. S., Dohrenwend, B. P., Link, B., & Levav, I. (1983). Social functioning of psychiatric patients in contrast with community cases in the general population. *Archives of General Psychiatry, 40,* 1174–1182.

Duncan-Jones, P., Fergusson, D. M., Ormel, J., & Horwood, L. J. (1990). A model of stability and change in minor psychiatric symptoms: Results from three longitudinal studies. *Psychological Medicine, 18* (monograph suppl.), 1–28.

Finlay-Jones, R., Brown, G. W., Duncan-Jones, P., Harris, T., Murphy, E., & Prudo, R. (1980). Depression and anxiety in the community: Replication of the diagnosis of a case. *Psychological Medicine, 10,* 445–454.

Giel, R., Koeter, M. W. J., & Ormel, J. (1990). Detection and referral of primary care patients with mental health problems: The second and third filters in the pathway to psychiatric care. In D. Goldberg & Tantam (Eds.), *The public health impact of mental disorder*. Toronto: Hogrefe & Huber.

Goldberg, D., & Bridges, K. (1987). Screening for psychiatric illness in general practice: The general practitioner versus the screening questionnaire. *Journal of the Royal College of General Practitioners, 37,* 15–18.

Hankin, J. R., & Locke, B. Z. (1982). The persistence of depressive symptomatology among prepaid group practice enrollees: An exploratory study. *American Journal of Public Health, 29,* 2–10.

Hecht, H., Von Zerssen, D., & Wittchen, H.-U. (1990). Anxiety and depression in a community sample: The influence of comorbidity on social functioning. *Journal of Affective Disorders, 18,* 137–144.

Hirschfeld, R. M. A., & Klerman, G. L. (1979). Personality attributes and affective disorders. *American Journal of Psychiatry, 136,* 67–70.

Katon, W., Von Korff, M., Lin, E., Bush, T., & Ormel, J. (1992). Adequacy and duration of antidepressant treatment in primary care. *Medical Care, 30*(1), 67–76.

Keller, M. B., Klerman, G. L., Lavori, P. W., Coryell, W., Endicott, J., & Taylor, J. (1984). Long-term outcome in major depression. *Journal of the American Medical Association, 252,* 788–792.

Kessler, L. G., Cleary, P. D., & Burke, J. D. (1985). Psychiatric disorders in primary care: Results of a follow-up study. *Archives of General Psychiatry, 42,* 583–587.

Koeter, M. W. J., & Ormel, J. (1991). *Handleiding van de Nederlandse Versie van de General Health Questionnaire.* Lisse: Swets & Zeitlinger.

Link, B. (1982). Mental patient status, work, and income: An examination of the effect of a psychiatric label. *American Sociological Review, 47,* 202–215.

Mann, A. H., Jenkins, R., & Belsey, E. (1981). The twelve-month outcome of patients with neurotic illness in general practice. *Psychological Medicine, 11,* 535–550.

Marks, J. N., Goldberg, D., & Hillier, V. F. (1979). Determinants of the ability of general practitioners to detect psychiatric illness. *Psychological Medicine, 9,* 337–353.

Mechanic, D. (1978). *Medical sociology* (2nd ed.). New York: Free Press.

Murphy, J. M., Olivier, D. C., Sobol, M., Monson, R. R., & Leighton, A. H. (1986). Diagnosis and outcome: Depression and anxiety in a general population. *Psychological Medicine, 16,* 117–126.

Ormel, J., Brink, W. van den, Koeter, M. W. J., Giel, R., Meer, K. V., Willige, G. van de, & Wilmink, F. W. (1990). Recognition, management, and outcome of psychological disorders in primary care: A naturalistic follow-up study. *Psychological Medicine, 20,* 909–923.

Ormel, J., Brink, W. V., Oldehinkel, A. J., & Brilman, E. I. (1993). *Outcome of psychiatric disorders in primary care: A 3-wave 3-year prospective study of psychopathology and social disability.* Manuscript submitted for publication.

Ormel, J., & Schaufeli, W. (1991). Stability and change of psychological distress and their relationship with self-esteem and locus of control. *Journal of Personality and Social Psychology, 60,* 288–299.

Ormel, J., & Wohlfarth, T. (1991). How neuroticism, long-term difficulties, and life situation change influence psychological distress: A longitudinal model. *Journal of Personality and Social Psychology, 60,* 744–755.

Parker, G., Holmes, S., & Manicavasagar, V. (1986). Depression in general practice attenders: Caseness, natural history, and predictors of outcome. *Journal of Affective Disorders, 10,* 27–35.

Paykel, E. S., Freeling, P., & Hollyman, J. A. (1988). Are tricyclic antidepressants useful for mild depression? A placebo controlled trial. *Pharmacopsychiatry, 21,* 15–18.

Regier, D. A., Burke, J. D., Manderscheid, R. W., & Burns, B. J. (1985). The chronically mentally ill in primary care. *Psychological Medicine, 15,* 265–273.

Sargeant, J. K., Bruce, M. L., Florio, L. P., & Weissman, M. M. (1990). Factors associated with 1-year outcome of major depression in the community. *Archives of General Psychiatry, 47,* 519–526.

Schulberg, H. C., McClelland, M., & Gooding, W. (1987). Six-month outcomes for medical patients with major depressive disorders. *Journal of General Internal Medicine, 2,* 312–317.

Shapiro, S., Skinner, E. A., Kessler, L. G., Von Korff, M., German, P. S., Tischler, G. L., Leaf, P. J., Benham, L., Cottler, L., & Regier, D. A. (1984). Utilization of health and mental health services: Three Epidemiologic Catchment Area sites. *Archives of General Psychiatry, 41,* 971–978.

Shepherd, M., Cooper, B., Brown, A. C., & Kalton, G. W. (1966). *Psychiatric illness in general practice.* London: Oxford University Press.

Stoudemire, A., Frank, R., Hedemark, N., Kamlet, M., & Blazer, D. (1986). The economic burden of depression. *General Hospital Psychiatry, 8,* 387–394.

van den Brink, W., Leenstra, A., Ormel, J., & Willige, G. van de (1991). Mental health intervention programs in primary care: Their scientific basis. *Journal of Affective Disorders, 21,* 273–284.

Von Korff, M., Ormel, J., Katon, W., & Lin, E. H. B. (1992). Disability and depression among high utilizers of health care: A longitudinal analysis. *Archives of General Psychiatry, 49,* 91–100.

Von Korff, M., Shapiro, S., Burke, J. D., Teitelbaum, M., Skinner, E. A., German, P., Turner, R. W., Klein, L., & Burns, B. (1987). Anxiety and depression in a primary care clinic: Comparison of DIS, GHQ, and practitioner assessments. *Archives of General Psychiatry, 44,* 152.

Watson, D., & Pennebaker, J. W. (1989). Health complaints, stress, and distress: Exploring the central role of negative negativity. *Psychological Review, 96,* 234–254.

Weissman, M. M. (1975). The assessment of social adjustment. *Archives of General Psychiatry, 32,* 357–365.

Wells, K. B., Stewart, A., Hays, R. D., Burnam, M. A., Rogers, W., Daniels, M., Berry, S., Greenfield, S., & Ware, J. (1989). The functioning and well-being of depressed patients: Results from the Medical Outcomes Study. *Journal of the American Medical Association, 262*(7), 914–919.

Wiersma, D., DeJong, A., & Ormel, J. (1988). The Groningen Social Disability Schedule: Development, relationship with ICIDH, and psychometric properties. *International Journal of Rehabilitation Research, 11,* 213–224.

Wilmink, F. W. (1989). *Patient, physician, psychiatrist: Assessment of mental health problems in primary care.* Unpublished doctoral dissertation, University of Groningen.

Wing, J. K., Cooper, J., & Sartorius, N. (1974). *The measurement and classification of psychiatric symptoms.* Cambridge, England: Cambridge University Press.

Wittchen, H.-U., & Von Zerssen, D. (1987). *Verlaufe behandelter und unbehandelter Depressionen und Angststörungen. Eine klinisch-psychiatrisch und epidemiologisch Verlaufsuntersuchung.* Berlin: Springer-Verlag.

Wohlfarth, T. D., van den Brink, W. V., Ormel, J., Koeter, M. W., & Oldehinkel, A. J. (1993). The relationship between social dysfunctioning and psychopathology among primary care attenders. *British Journal of Psychiatry, 163,* 37–44.

World Health Organization. (1980). International classification of impairments, disability, and handicaps. Geneva: Author.

Part Two

Co-occurring Mental and Medical Disorders

Jeanne Miranda
Patricia A. Arean
Richard L. Rickman

5

Relationship of Mental and Medical Disorders in Primary Care

As documented in previous chapters of this book, high rates of mental disorders are found in primary care patients. This chapter will focus on causal relationships between mental and medical disorders. Currently, mental and medical disorders are assumed to be caused by complex interactions among many factors, including personality type, social milieu, biological predisposition, and stressful life events. Although searching for specific causal links between mental and medical disorders is somewhat reductionistic, evaluating possible causal pathways between the two is useful. This linkage has particular relevance for planning treatment interventions, as well as giving meaning to epidemiologic data in the field.

This chapter will consider the following possible links between mental and physical disorders: (1) direct causal relationships between specific mental and medical disorders (in this case, either type of disorder causing the other, such as hypothyroidism directly causing depression, or a reciprocal relationship existing between the two), and (2) indirect relationships (such as the stress of arthritis leading to depression). In rare cases, mental and medical disorders may be related because of underlying common factors such as arteriosclerosis causing both dementia and coronary heart disease. This chapter will focus on both direct and indirect links between mental and medical disorders.

Prevalence of Psychiatric Disorders in Medical Patients

Prior to addressing links between mental and medical disorders, we should touch on the prevalence of comorbidity. Depression and, to a lesser degree, anxiety have been studied in three settings: (1) in primary care medical settings where patients frequently have chronic medical disorders, (2) in acute care settings where patients have suffered severe disorders, and (3) in neurological settings where patients have central nervous system involvement, which frequently affects mental status.

Diagnosing psychiatric illness in the medically ill has been controversial, particularly because of symptom overlap. For example, if a patient with cancer complains of loss of appetite, should this symptom be ascribed to the malignancy or depression? Similarly, if a cardiac patient complains of palpitations, sweating, and nausea, are these symptomatic of anxiety or cardiac illness? Symptoms of depression that can easily be caused by medical illness include anorexia, appetite/weight disturbance, psychomotor agitation/retardation, insomnia/hypersomnia, decreased libido, and fatigue. Similarly, symptoms of anxiety that can arise from medical illness include dyspnea, dizziness, palpitations, and nausea. As a result, studies measuring only symptoms of depression or anxiety and using cutoff scores established in healthy populations probably overdiagnose psychiatric distress. On the other hand, diagnostic criteria for a disorder are more likely to be accurate. For example, to meet diagnostic criteria for major depression requires severe, persistent low mood, as well as other symptoms, only some of which are likely to stem entirely from a physical ailment. Therefore, diagnostic criteria are preferable for determining psychiatric disorder in primary care patients.

Chronic Medical Illness

Depression is the most common mental disorder found in medical patient populations. Anxiety disorders, although less studied, are also prevalent in medical patients.

Approximately 4.8 to 9.2 percent of ambulatory medical patients have major depression, and 7.1 have anxiety disorders (Von Korff et al., 1987). These mental disorders are particularly common among primary care patients with chronic medical conditions. For example, 18.2 percent of diabetic patients have current depression (Marcus, Wing, Guare, Blair, & Jawad, 1992; Mayou, Peveler, Davies, Mann, & Fairburn, 1991), and 22 percent have anxiety disorders (Popkin, Callies, Lentz, Colon, & Sutherland, 1988). Similarly, cardiac disease has been linked with anxiety disorders; nearly 9.2 percent of cardiac patients have symptoms of panic (Barsky, 1992; Goldberg et al., 1990). Even higher rates of mental disorders are found among hospitalized medical patients, with 22 to 33 percent reporting depression (see the review by Katon & Sullivan, 1990). In sum, mental disorders—particularly depression and anxiety—are very common among primary care and hospitalized medical patients.

Acute Medical Illnesses

Depression is also a frequent concomitant of acute, severe medical disorders. For example, 20 to 30 percent of oncology patients report depression, with pancreatic cancer patients having the highest rates (Massie & Holland, 1987). Similarly, 18 percent of patients report major depressive disorder following myocardial infarction (Schleifer et al., 1989). Thus, acute medical illnesses have been linked to mental disorders.

Neurological Illnesses

Depression is frequent in patients with central nervous system disorders; 30 to 50 percent of cerebral vascular accident patients experience depression following the accident (Starkstein & Robinson, 1989). Similarly, patients with other central nervous system disorders have high rates of depression—nearly 21 percent for Parkinson's disease (Starkstein & Robinson, 1989) and 14 percent for multiple sclerosis (Joffe, Lippert, Gray, Sawa, & Horvath, 1987).

In summary, depression and anxiety are common in medical patients. In particular, patients with chronic medical conditions and acute, severe disorders report high rates of depression and anxiety. Finally, patients with specific disorders, such as pancreatic cancer or stroke, have unusually high rates of comorbidity.

Direct Causal Links

Physiological disorders may directly cause psychological illness or vice versa. Similarly, medications for one type of disorder may directly cause the other. These potential links may account for a significant amount of co-occurrence. For example, Kinzie, Lewinsohn, Maricle, and Teri (1986) examined comorbidity in a community sample of persons aged fifty and over who met Research Diagnostic Criteria for depression. The depressive symptoms were determined to have a direct medical cause in 38 percent of the sample and a direct psychological cause as a result of loss or injury in 8 percent. Similarly, 22 percent were considered to be depressed as a direct result of depressogenic medications. Evidence for these direct causal links between mental and medical disorders will be discussed in this section.

Direct Impact of Medical Illness on Mental Health

Physiological changes associated with medical disorders may cause depression and anxiety. Evidence for this link has been evaluated by examining temporal links between disorders as well as by evaluating comparative data among disorders. Recently, more sophisticated studies of underlying mechanisms have been reported.

Chronic Medical Illness. In general, the rates of psychiatric disorder are high among primary care patients with chronic medical disorders. Two chronic disorders have been studied in particular: diabetes mellitus and coronary disease. Depression is common in diabetics and is unrelated either to severity of illness (Wilkinson et al., 1988) or complications, such as neuropathy, retinopathy, and nephropathy (Lustman, Griffith, & Clouse, 1988). Although the rates of depression are high among diabetics, no causal mechanisms have been identified.

An anxiety disorder—panic attacks—has been linked with coronary heart disease. Interestingly, recent research suggests that among patients presenting in cardiac clinics, those with panic symptoms are less likely to actually evidence heart disease; some 38 to 45 percent are found to have a normal cardiac examination (Bass & Wade, 1984; Beitman, Lamberti, & Mukerji, 1987). Thus, panic may be related to heart disease by misdiagnosis of panic as noted above, by symptom overlap (palpitations, sweating, shortness of breath), or by oversensitivity of coronary patients to physiological changes (Barsky, 1992). Overall, no direct causal mechanisms have been found linking psychiatric distress to these cardiac illnesses. The two are likely to be related through complex interactions related to the stress of medical illness, symptom overlap, physiological changes, and sensitivity to these physiological changes.

Medications for both chronic and acute illnesses may cause depression. The most common drugs associated with depression are the antihypertensives, including reserpine, methyldopa, thiazides, spironolactone, and clonidine; oral contraceptives; H_2-blockers such as cimetidine and ranitidine; and beta-blockers, particularly propranolol (Cassem, 1988). In general, onset of depression coincides with beginning the drug and ceases shortly after withdrawing the medication.

Acute Medical Disorders. Psychiatric morbidity has been related to two acute, severe medical disorders, cancer and myocardial infarction. Pancreatic cancer has the strongest causal association to psychiatric symptomatology among oncology disorders (Holland et al., 1986; Joffe, Rubinow, Denicoff, Maher, & Sindelar, 1986). Depression and psychological changes are often the first symptoms to signal the presence of this cancer, even in the absence of other disease-related symptoms. The causal mechanism is most likely associated with decreased serotonin available in the central nervous system. This is because pancreatic tumors metabolize tryptophan, which decreases serotonin, and cells from this tumor bind to serotonin receptors. Clearly, physiological changes that accompany pancreatic cancer cause depression.

Treatments for cancer may also have depressogenic effects. Vincristine, L-asparaginase, and other neurotoxins have been found to produce depressive symptoms (Massie & Holland, 1987). The effects of the treatments, such as malnutrition, anorexia, and pain, may also cause psychological distress.

The relationship of depression to myocardial infarction is less clear; however, depression appears to be related to acute myocardial infarction in at least two ways. In a careful review of the literature, Fielding (1991) cites numerous studies that document the presence of depression in a substantial number of patients with acute myocardial infarction, even in the absence of angina. This would suggest that depression either is a causal factor in development of the infarction or that a third factor causes both. In addition, a substantial number of patients become depressed following myocardial infarction, possibly related to both hospitalization and adjustment to the coronary illness. In sum, no direct causal links have been established, but depression is present in a substantial number of patients both before and after myocardial infarction.

Neurological Disorders. Cerebral vascular accidents are often followed by depression. The depression is related to location of the lesion (that is, left parietal/occipital, left inferior frontal, right superior frontal, and right temporal) rather than degree of disability (Robinson, Kubos, Starr, Rao, & Price, 1984). In particular, lesions affecting the left basal ganglia and left frontal ganglia predict depression (Robinson et al., 1984; Starkstein, Robinson, & Price, 1987; Starkstein et al., 1991). In fact, patients with left anterior lesions are likely to have major depression only in the presence of typical occipital asymmetry; reverse asymmetry—that is, reversed hemisphere dominance—does not predict depression. Finally, patients with poststroke anxiety are likely to have cortical lesions, whereas patients with poststroke depression are likely to have subcortical lesions.

Poststroke depression is hypothesized to be due to destruction of biogenic amine pathways that run anteriorly through the deep layers of the cortex, resulting in depletion of noradrenalin (Glick, Ross, & Hough, 1982; Mayberg et al., 1988). This pathway has been verified in animal studies where specific sites can be lesioned (Castellano, Diaz-Palarea, Rodriguez, & Barroso, 1987). This literature convincingly addresses a direct causal link between specific cortical injuries following stroke and psychiatric distress.

Parkinson's disease—a disorder of the basal ganglia—is also associated with depression. In fact, many patients experience depression prior to the onset of motor symptoms with this disorder, and treatment with levodopa alleviates the depression (Starkstein & Robinson, 1989). Proposed mechanisms causing the depression are depletion of dopamine in the mesocorticolimbic system (Folstein, Robinson, Folstein, & McHugh, 1985) and serotonin depletion (Mayeux et al., 1986). Hemispheric dominance, again, has been found to play a role in the development and severity of depression. Those with left hemispheric disturbances tend to be more depressed than those with opposite-sided symptoms (Starkstein & Robinson, 1989).

Multiple sclerosis is another central nervous system disorder with findings suggesting direct biological links with depression. Schiffer and Babigian (1984) were able to demonstrate that patients with multiple sclerosis were more likely to be depressed than patients with amyotrophic lateral sclerosis, a disorder with very similar presenting features and symptoms. The depression is hypothesized to be due to demyelination of the biogenic amine pathways that directly affect the limbic system.

To summarize, substantial evidence links psychiatric morbidity to particular medical disorders through specific biological mechanisms. In particular, central nervous system lesions and pancreatic cancer result in biologically induced depression or anxiety. Other disorders, particularly more chronic medical conditions, show high rates of psychiatric disorder without clear direct causal mechanisms.

Direct Impact of Mental Disorders on Medical Disorders

Psychiatric patients have high rates of medical disorders (Hall, Gardner, Stickney, LeCann, & Popkin, 1980); however, the medical disorder is generally seen as causing or exacerbating the mental illness rather than vice versa. Psychiatric disorders do complicate medical illness; medical patients who are psychiatrically distressed die earlier than their nondistressed counterparts (Lustman, Griffith, & Clouse, 1988). One plausible explanation is that psychiatric disorders interfere with the ability of these patients to identify and treat their medical disorders. For example, studies have found that between 33 and 60 percent of psychiatric patients have undiagnosed physical diseases (Hall et al., 1980). Although psychiatric patients frequently have concomitant medical disorders, no clear data are available to implicate psychiatric illness directly in causing medical disorders.

Although psychiatric disorders have not been shown to cause medical illness, psychological characteristics have been implicated as potential causal factors, when combined with conditions such as genetic predisposition and environmental factors. For example, negative emotions such as anger, hostility, anxiety, and depression are consistently related to heart disease (Booth-Kewley & Friedman, 1987). These psychological factors are believed to exert their influence on coronary disease through cardiovascular reactivity. Similarly, suppressed anger, although not sufficient for the development of hypertension, is likely an important causal factor when combined with genetic and environmental input (for example, Niaura & Goldstein, 1992; Taylor & Aspinwall, 1990).

In sum, mental disorders have not been shown to directly cause medical illness. However, in combination with other factors, negative emotions are implicated in cardiovascular diseases.

Indirect Causal Links

Mental and medical disorders can be linked through indirect causes. The most widely studied indirect causal link between mental and medical disorders is stress. Stress is the psychological state that exists when a person perceives that demands exceed current resources (Lazarus & Folkman, 1984). Medical illnesses can clearly be seen as stressful life events that influence subsequent medical and mental health. In contrast, psychological factors can cause an individual to perceive a life event as stressful (Lazarus & Folkman, 1984).

Indirect Impact of Medical Illness on Mental Health

Psychiatric practitioners have generally considered medical illnesses to be stressful events that automatically lead to depression and anxiety (Bowlby, 1980). In fact, the exclusionary criteria of the *Diagnostic and Statistical Manual-III-R* exclude the diagnosis of major depression as a psychiatric illness if the symptoms follow onset of a medical illness. However, not all patients become depressed or anxious following medical illness. Two factors—coping skills and social support—appear to mediate the relationship between the stress of physical illness and psychological distress.

Coping strategies mediate the relationship between the stress of physical illness and mental disorder. Those patients who use an active style of coping fare better psychologically than do those who use a more passive coping style. For example, Revenson and Felton (1989) found that patients with rheumatoid arthritis who coped well with their illness used active problem-solving coping styles. On the other hand, similar patients who became depressed coped with the problems of their illness through passive emotion-focused problem solving, such as wish-fulfilling fantasy or self-blame. Similarly, patients with chronic chest pain and psychiatric disturbance were less likely to use problem-focused coping than their non–psychiatrically distressed counterparts (Vitaliano, Katon, Maiuro, & Russo, 1989).

Social networks also influence whether patients become psychiatrically distressed as a response to medical illness. Having emotional and practical support from others in coping with medical illness clearly has a direct impact on the ability to adapt to illness (Auerbach, 1989). Thus, both active coping style and social support can moderate the impact of medical illness on mental health.

Indirect Impact of Mental Disorder on Medical Illness

Psychiatric disorder is clearly related to morbidity and mortality. Mortality rates among psychiatric patients are one and a half to two times higher than among community residents, even after controlling for coexisting factors such as age and alcoholism (Babigian & Odoroff, 1969). For example, pneumonia constitutes a leading cause of death among the elderly (Yoshikawa, 1983); however, within the first year after psychiatric admission, fifty times more deaths from pneumonia occur among elderly psychiatric patients than among their nonpsychiatrically impaired counterparts.

Psychiatric impairment may lead to medical illness through poor health-related behaviors. Research has shown that psychiatric impairment increases the likelihood of engaging in poor health behaviors (Moore, Stunkard, & Srole, 1962; Kandel & Davies, 1986;

Ross & Hayes, 1988). Poor health behaviors, including obesity, cigarette smoking, excessive alcohol consumption, and failure to exercise regularly, have been shown to increase morbidity and mortality (Hamburg, Elliott, & Parron, 1982; Breslow & Enstrom, 1980). Thus, psychiatric impairment may lead to poor health behaviors that complicate or bring on increased morbidity and mortality.

Psychiatric distress has been implicated in the cause of gastrointestinal disorders, such as peptic ulcer disease and inflammatory bowel disease. Experimental evidence links stressors to increased acid and pepsin secretion; cross-sectional studies tend to substantiate this finding (Tennant, 1988). However, in the absence of well-controlled longitudinal studies, definitive statements about the role of stress in causing gastrointestinal disorders are not possible.

The clearest connections between psychiatric distress and medical illness involve the release of hormones, particularly catecholamines and corticosteroids, by the endocrine system. An intense episode of distress with extremely high levels of hormones can cause the heart to beat erratically and may lead to sudden death (Sarafino, 1990). More frequently, however, chronically high levels of distress lead to two factors: (1) increased growth of plaques on artery walls (McKinney, Rovang, Buell, & Eliot, 1984; Schneiderman & Gruhn, 1983), ultimately increasing risk of heart attack and stroke, and (2) adverse immunological changes (Kiecolt-Glaser & Glaser, 1988).

Conclusion

The links between mental and medical disorders are both biologically and psychologically based and can be either direct or indirect. These complex causal linkages are important considerations in designing research in primary care settings. A few final comments will focus on the implications of comorbidity for epidemiologic and treatment research in primary care.

Epidemiologic research in primary care settings has been carried out to establish the prevalence of psychiatric disorders in medical patients. Since particularly high prevalence rates of specific psychological disorders are found in specific medical patient populations, causal mechanisms should be evaluated. For specific disorders, such as pancreatic cancer, mechanisms have been clarified. However, for the more common chronic disorders, such as diabetes, causal mechanisms have not been established. Further work in this area is needed.

Treatment outcome research should also consider comorbidity of mental and medical disorders. Two nonrandomized treatment-of-depression trials in medical patients have shown that physicians' standard treatments, including adequate trials of tricyclic antidepressants, are not effective at six-month and one-year evaluations (Magruder-Habib et al., 1989; Schulberg, McClelland, & Gooding, 1987). Perhaps these treatments fail to account for the complex interactions between medical and mental illness. Clearly, future treatment-outcome research should carefully evaluate the impact of medical illness on treatment of depression.

Finally, the linkage between mental illness and poor health behaviors should lead to specific research in improving health behaviors among patients with psychiatric distress. This might include evaluating smoking cessation among psychiatric inpatients, treating depression concomitantly with weight loss programs, and so on. Specific, targeted programs to increase health behaviors for patients with psychiatric distress should be developed and evaluated.

References

Auerbach, S. M. (1989). Stress management and coping research in the health care setting: An overview and methodological commentary. *Journal of Consulting and Clinical Psychology, 57*(3), 388–395.

Babigian, H. M., & Odoroff, C. L. (1969). The mortality experience of a population with psychiatric illness. *American Journal of Psychiatry, 126*(4), 470–480.

Barsky, J. (1992). Palpitations, cardiac awareness, and panic disorder. *American Journal of Medicine, 92* (Suppl. 1A), 31S–34S.

Bass, C., & Wade, C. (1984). Chest pain with normal coronary arteries: A comparative study of psychiatric and social morbidity. *Psychological Medicine, 14,* 51–61.

Beitman, B. D., Lamberti, J. W., & Mukerji, V. (1987). Panic disorder in patients with angiographically normal coronary arteries. *Psychosomatics, 28,* 480–484.

Booth-Kewley, S., & Friedman, H. S. (1987). Psychological predictors of heart disease: A quantitative review. *Psychological Bulletin, 101,* 343–362.

Bowlby, J. (1980). *Loss, sadness, and depression* (Vol. 3). New York: Basic Books.

Breslow, L., & Enstrom, J. E. (1980). Persistence of health habits and their relationship to mortality. *Preventive Medicine, 9*(4), 469–483.

Cassem, E. H. (1988). Depression secondary to medical illness. In A. J. Frances & R. E. Hales (Eds.), *Review of psychiatry* (pp. 256–273). Washington, DC: American Psychiatric Press.

Castellano, M. A., Diaz-Palarea, M. D., Rodriguez, M., & Barroso, J. (1987). Lateralization in male rats and dopaminergic system: Evidence of right-side population bias. *Physiology and Behavior, 40*(5), 607–612.

Fielding, R. (1991). Depression and acute myocardial infarction: A review and reinterpretation. *Social Science Medicine, 32*(9), 1017–1027.

Folstein, M. F., Robinson, R., Folstein, S., & McHugh, R. R. (1985). Depression and neurological disorders: New treatment opportunities for elderly depressed patients. *Affective Disorders, 1*(Suppl. 1), 811–814.

Glick, S. D., Ross, D. A., & Hough, L. B. (1982). Lateral asymmetry of neutrotransmitters in human brain. *Brain Research, 234*(1), 53–63.

Goldberg, R., Morris, P., Christion, F., Badger, J., Chabot, S., & Edlund, M. (1990). Panic disorder in cardiac outpatients. *Psychosomatics, 31*(2), 168–173.

Hall, R. C., Gardner, E. R., Stickney, S. K., LeCann, A. F., & Popkin, M. K. (1980). Physical illness manifesting as psychiatric disease: 2. Analysis of a state hospital inpatient population. *Archives of General Psychiatry, 37*(9), 989–995.

Hamburg, D. A., Elliott, G. R., & Parron, D. L. (1982). *Health and behavior: Frontiers of research in the biobehavioral sciences.* Washington, DC: National Academy Press.

Holland, J. C., Korzun, A. H., Tross, S., Silberfarb, P., Perry, M.,

Comis, R., & Oster, M. (1986). Comparative psychological disturbance in patients with pancreatic and gastric cancer. *American Journal of Psychiatry, 143*(8), 982–986.

Joffe, R. T., Lippert, G. P., Gray, T. A., Sawa, G., & Horvath, Z. (1987). Mood disorder and multiple sclerosis. *Archives of Neurology, 44*(4), 376–378.

Joffe, R. T., Rubinow, D. R., Denicoff, K. D., Maher, M., & Sindelar, W. F. (1986). Depression and carcinoma of the pancreas. *General Hospital Psychiatry, 8*(4), 241–245.

Kandel, D. B., & Davies, M. (1986). Adult sequelae of adolescent depressive symptoms. *Archives of General Psychiatry, 43,* 255–262.

Katon, W., & Sullivan, M. D. (1990). Depression and chronic medical illness. *Journal of Clinical Psychiatry, 51*(6), 3–11.

Kiecolt-Glaser, J. K., & Glaser, R. (1988). Psychological influences on immunity: Making sense of the relationship between stressful life events and health. *Advances in Experimental Medicine and Biology, 245,* 237–247.

Kinzie, J. D., Lewinsohn, P., Maricle, R., & Teri, L. (1986). The relationship of depression to medical illness in an older community population. *Comprehensive Psychiatry, 27*(3), 241–246.

Lazarus, R. S., & Folkman, S. (1984). *Stress, appraisal, and coping.* New York: Springer.

Lustman, P. J., Griffith, L. S., & Clouse, R. E. (1988). Depression in adults with diabetes: Results of 5-yr. follow-up study. *Diabetes Care, 11*(8), 605–612.

McKinney, M. E., Rovang, K., Buell, J. C., & Eliot, R. S. (1984). Sex-related differences in first-stage impedance cardiographic variables. *Biofeedback and Self Regulation, 9*(3), 365–370.

Magruder-Habib, K., Zung, W. W. K., Feussner, J. R., Alling, W. C., Saunders, W. B., & Stevens, H. A. (1989). Management of general medical patients with symptoms of depression. *General Hospital Psychiatry, 11,* 201–206.

Marcus, M. D., Wing, R. R., Guare, J., Blair, E. H., & Jawad, A. (1992). Lifetime prevalence of major depression and its effect on treatment outcome in obese type II diabetic patients. *Diabetes Care, 15*(2), 253–255.

Massie, M. J., & Holland J. C. (1987). The cancer patient with pain:

Psychiatric complications and their management. *Medical Clinics of North America, 71*(2), 243-258.

Mayberg, H. S., Robinson, R. G., Wong, D. F., Parikh, R., Bolduc, P., Starkstein, S. E., Price, T., Dannals, R. F., Links, J. M., & Wilson, A. A. (1988). PET imaging of cortical S2 serotonin receptors after stroke: Lateralized changes and relationship to depression. *American Journal of Psychiatry, 145*(8), 937-943.

Mayeux, R., Stern, Y., Williams, J. B. W., Cote, L., Frantz, A., & Dyrenfurth, I. (1986). Clinical and biochemical features of depression in Parkinson's disease. *American Journal of Psychiatry, 143,* 756-759.

Mayou, R., Peveler, R., Davies, B., Mann, J., & Fairburn, C. (1991). Psychiatric morbidity in young adults with insulin-dependent diabetes mellitus. *Psychological Medicine, 21*(3), 639-645.

Moore, M. A., Stunkard, A., & Srole, L. (1962). Obesity, social class, and mental illness. *Journal of the American Medical Association, 181,* 962-966.

Niaura, R., & Goldstein, M. G. (1992). Psychological factors affecting physical condition: Cardiovascular disease literature review: 2. Coronary artery disease and sudden death and hypertension. *Psychosomatics, 33,* 146-155.

Popkin, M. K., Callies, A. L., Lentz, R. D., Colon, E. A., & Sutherland, D. E. (1988). Prevalence of major depression, simple phobia, and other psychiatric disorders in patients with long-standing type I diabetes mellitus. *Archives of General Psychiatry, 45,* 64-68.

Revenson, T. A., & Felton, B. J. (1989). Disability and coping predictors of psychological adjustment to rheumatoid arthritis. *Journal of Consulting and Clinical Psychology, 57*(3), 344-348.

Robinson, R. G., Kubos, K. L., Starr, L. B., Rao, K., & Price, T. R. (1984). Mood disorders in stroke patients: Importance of location and lesion. *Brain, 107,* 81-93.

Ross, C. E., & Hayes, D. (1988). Exercise and psychologic well-being in the community. *American Journal of Epidemiology, 127*(4), 762-771.

Sarafino, E. P. (1990). *Health psychology: Biopsychosocial interactions.* New York: Wiley.

Schiffer, R. B., & Babigian, H. M. (1984). Behavioral disorders in multiple sclerosis, temporal lobe epilepsy, and amyotrophic lateral sclerosis: An epidemiologic study. *Archives of Neurology, 41*(10), 1067–1069.

Schleifer, S. J., Macari-Hinson, M. M., Coyle, D. A., Slater, W. R., Kahn, M., Gorlin, R., & Zucker, H. D. (1989). The nature and course of depression following myocardial infarction. *Archives of Internal Medicine, 149*(8), 1785–1789.

Schneiderman, H., & Gruhn, J. (1983). Metachronous axillary and splenic lymphangiomatosis: Demonstration of immunoreactive factor VIII-related antigen. *American Journal of Clinical Pathology, 79*(5), 625–627.

Schulberg, H., McClelland, M., & Gooding, W. (1987). Six month outcome for medical patients with major depressive disorders. *Journal of General Internal Medicine, 2,* 312–317.

Starkstein, S. E., Bryer, J. B., Berthier, M. L., Cohen, B., Price, T. R., & Robinson, R. G. (1991). Depression after stroke: The importance of cerebral hemisphere asymmetries. *Journal of Neuropsychiatry Clinical Neuroscience, 3*(3), 276–285.

Starkstein, S. E., & Robinson, R. G. (1989). Affective disorders and cerebral vascular disease. *British Journal of Psychiatry, 154,* 170–182.

Starkstein, S. E., Robinson, R. G., & Price, T. R. (1987). Comparison of cortical and subcortical lesions in the production of post-stroke mood disorders. *Brain, 110*(4), 1045–1059.

Taylor, S. E., & Aspinwall, L. G. (1990). Psychosocial aspects of chronic illness. In G. M. Herek, P. T. Costa, & G. R. Vandenbos (Eds.), *Psychological aspects of serious illness: Chronic conditions, fatal diseases, and clinical care.* Washington, D.C.: American Psychological Association.

Tennant, C. (1988). Psychosocial causes of duodenal ulcer. *Australian and New Zealand Journal of Psychiatry, 22,* 195–201.

Vitaliano, P. P., Katon, W., Maiuro, R. D., & Russo, J. (1989). Coping in chest pain patients with and without psychiatric disorders. *Journal of Consulting and Clinical Psychology, 57*(3), 333–343.

Von Korff, M., Shapiro, S., Burke, J. D., Teitelbaum, M., Skinner, E. A., German, P. Turner, R. W., Klein, L., & Burns, B. (1987). Anxiety and depression in a primary care clinic: Comparison of

Diagnostic Interview Schedule, General Health Questionnaire, and practitioner assessments. *Archives of General Psychiatry, 44,* 152–156.

Wilkinson, G., Borsey, D. Q., Leslie, P., Newton, R. W., Lind, C., & Ballinger, C. B. (1988). Psychiatric morbidity and social problems in patients with insulin-dependent diabetes mellitus. *British Journal of Psychiatry, 153,* 38–43.

Yoshikawa, T. T. (1983). Geriatric infectious diseases: An emerging problem. *Journal of the American Geriatrics Society, 31*(1), 34–39.

Nicholas Long
Barbara Starfield
Kelly Kelleher

6

Co-occurrence of Medical and Mental Disorders in Pediatric Primary Care

Relatively little is known about the extent and nature of the co-occurrence of physical and mental health disorders in children seen in primary care settings. However, sufficient empirical evidence exists to reach three conclusions: (1) considerable overlap exists in the occurrence of mental health and physical health problems, particularly for children with frequent acute medical illnesses (Starfield, Weiner, Mumford, & Steinwachs, 1991); (2) at least for older children and adolescents, children who eventually receive a mental health diagnosis have higher use of medical services, which may decrease after psychiatric care (Kelleher & Starfield, 1990); and (3) there is a clear association between the number of acute medical illnesses and the number of chronic medical and psychosocial problems in children seen in primary care facilities (Starfield, Katz, et al., 1984).

There is one area of research in which the interrelationships among physical and mental health disorders have been explored: chronic childhood illnesses and maladjustment. We will present an overview of that literature and then provide our suggestions for a future research agenda in this area.

Chronic Illness and Co-occurring Mental Health Problems

It is evident that the care of children and adolescents with chronic medical conditions is a major component of primary care practice. Gortmaker and Sappenfield (1984) report that at least 13 percent of pediatric primary care visits are by children with a chronic medical disorder. It is estimated that overall, 10 to 12 percent of children in the United States have a chronic medical disorder (Hobbs, Perrin, & Ireys, 1985). The overall prevalence of chronic medical disorders in the pediatric population appear to be relatively stable (Collins, 1988) but may be increasing as a result of better survival due to ever-improving technology (for example, Meadows & Silber, 1985).

What is not evident is the nature of the relationship between chronic medical disorders and psychiatric status. Most investigators and reviewers examining the relationship between childhood chronic illness and co-occurring psychiatric morbidity have concluded that children with chronic medical conditions are at increased risk for behavioral and emotional problems (for instance, Bedell, Giordani, Amour, Tavormina, & Boll, 1977; Breslau, 1985; Garrison & McQuiston, 1989; Shapiro, 1983). However, several investigators have questioned the assumption that psychiatric disorders are significantly more common in individuals with chronic illnesses (Cassileth et al., 1984; Drotar et al., 1981; Tavormina, Kastner, Slater, & Watt, 1976).

Differing opinions on the relationship between chronic childhood illness and psychiatric problems reflect inconsistent findings across various clinical studies. Some of this inconsistency is due to methodological differences. Studies vary in how chronic illness is defined, in the degree to which they rely on recognition of psychosocial problems by primary care providers, and in the assessment of psychiatric status (Starfield et al., 1980).

Definitional Issues in Chronic Illness

Beyond the issue of differences in the definition of chronic illness, researchers in this area are struggling with whether the type of chronic illness is related to psychosocial outcomes. Pless and Pinkerton (1975) have advocated a noncategorical approach to chronic conditions on the assumption that there is no predictable association between the type of chronic illness and the prevalence of psychosocial problems. There is evidence that the degree of child behavioral and emotional problems does not differ significantly across certain different chronic conditions (Stein & Jessop, 1982; Wallander, Varni Babani, Banis, & Wilcox, 1988), even though chronically ill children have a generally increased risk of such problems. These findings suggest that there are more similarities than differences across chronic medical disorder groups regarding psychosocial problems of children. However, the investigators associated with the Ontario Child Health Study (Cadman, Boyle, Szatmari, & Offord, 1987) believe that differences across chronic medical disorder groups may exist when specific psychiatric diagnoses—as opposed to psychosocial problems more broadly conceived—are examined.

Recognition of Mental Health Disorders

Inadequate recognition of mental health problems among children, whether or not they have chronic medical illnesses, by primary care providers is not trivial, either for research or in everyday primary care practice. Data from the National Ambulatory Medical Care Survey, which documents the frequency of diagnosed disorders occurring in a representative sample of visits to office-based physicians in the United States, indicate that only 1 percent of all visits by children have a primary diagnosis of a mental health problem; if second- and third-listed diagnoses are included, roughly 3 percent of all visits by children are related to mental health problems (Starfield et al., 1980). The preponderance of mental health diagnoses are made by mental health providers, even though mental health specialists account for a small proportion of ambulatory visits (Hankin, Kessler, Goldberg, Steinwachs, & Starfield, 1983). One large national study of practices indicated that 60 percent of all diagnoses of mental disorders among individuals under age twenty are made in non-primary care settings. Another 20 percent are made by pediatricians, and the remaining 20 percent are made by general and family physicians (Starfield et al., 1984). By comparison, community-based studies of children find that at least 15 percent of children and youth have problems classifiable as mental disorders (Costello, 1989).

The lack of recognition of mental health disorders among nonpsychiatrist physicians has several possible explanations:

- Psychiatric diagnostic nomenclature is inadequate to allow the consistent collection of information about the occurrence of child mental health disorders in primary care settings. The International Classification of Diseases, which was developed to code causes of death, does not yet permit the coding of diagnoses as they occur in primary care practice situations, even though it has been expanded over time to permit the coding of problems identified during hospitalizations and ambulatory care. The standard psychiatric nomenclatures of the *Diagnostic and Statistical Manuals* (DSM) are often not useful in primary care, though attempts are currently being made to construct a manual that will be more relevant to primary care (Frances, Pincus, Widiger, Davis, & First, 1990; Regier, Kessler, Burns, & Goldberg, 1979).
- The training of most primary care practitioners, whose medical education has focused most heavily on organic disease with known pathophysiological processes, generally lacks focus on mental health conditions. This relative lack of training is likely to result in poor recognition of mental health symptoms and a lack of confidence in the efficacy of treatment when they are recognized.
- Poor communication may also play a role. Patients are more comfortable presenting physical symptoms than psychological symptoms, since physical problems are less apt to convey a sense of personal inadequacy. A physician who has not established a good relationship with a patient is even less likely to elicit a complaint with such connotations.
- Because there is a co-occurrence between mental health and physical problems, primary care physicians may choose to focus on the physical condition as the primary problem. Such an explanation is consistent with the finding that the majority of mental health diagnoses in office-based practice are listed as

secondary to physical health diagnoses where multiple diagnoses happen to be recorded.

- The limited or nonexistent reimbursement from third-party payers reinforces other tendencies among providers to disregard mental health problems.

Assessment of Psychiatric Status

The assessment of psychiatric status by investigators is perhaps the most critical issue to address in studies that seek to examine the relationship between chronic illness and psychiatric problems. In the studies performed to date, two major measurement problems exist. The first is the lack of precision in the assessment of psychiatric disorders. Various terms are used to identify mental health concerns: *psychosocial problems, psychosocial adjustment, psychological problems, psychological adjustment, psychiatric problems, psychiatric disorders,* and *mental disorders.* Investigators measure these concepts in many ways and use the terms interchangeably. And even though most investigators focus on the term *adjustment problems,* the term lacks specificity and does not necessarily denote psychiatric diagnoses.

The lack of assessment precision reflects the clinical realities of studying children with chronic medical illnesses. Most clinical settings do not have enough children in any specific chronic medical disorder group to draw valid conclusions regarding diagnosable psychiatric disorders. Multisite studies have rarely been conducted and are clearly needed to address the problem. As a result, some investigators study behavioral and emotional problems (for example, peer relationship problems, self-esteem problems, school problems) instead of disorders, believing that psychiatric symptoms may be a result of and/or may be exacerbating the chronic medical illness and are therefore important to examine, despite the fact that they are insufficient by themselves to reach diagnostic thresholds. Primary care providers regard evaluation of the impairment resulting from subdiagnostic clusters of psychiatric symptoms experienced by children and adolescents with chronic medical conditions as important. A second related and equally serious measurement problem is the source of information on the psychiatric status of the children being studied. Most studies have relied on parent-completed questionnaires of children's behavioral and emotional status, even though little interrater reliability exists in reporting child psychiatric symptoms. Ideally, studies in this area should assess children's psychiatric symptomatology from multiple sources: the children, their parents, their siblings, and, where appropriate, their teachers.

Chronic Medical Disorders and Mental Health Problems

Even with the methodological shortcomings of existing studies, the weight of evidence supports the existence of a significant relationship between chronic childhood medical disorders and psychosocial problems. A recent meta-analytic study and a few large epidemiological studies report an increased risk of emotional and behavioral disorder among children with chronic medical conditions. The meta-analytic study investigated the relationship of "psychological adjustment" to pediatric physical disorders (Lavigne and Faier-Routman, 1992). These investigators reviewed approximately five hundred studies obtained through a comprehensive literature review. A total of ninety studies met the inclusion criteria for the meta-analysis. These criteria included (1) a sample of children or adolescents with a chronic illness, (2) use of a quantifiable outcome measure, and (3) outcome data presented in a manner to allow calculation of effect size through comparison with a control group or normative data and to allow correlates of adjustment to be converted to Pearson correlations. The results of the meta-analysis supported the view that children with chronic medical disorders are at significant risk of behavioral and emotional problems. However, this study did not distinguish psychological problems from diagnosable psychiatric disorders.

Large epidemiological studies have underscored the relationship between chronic childhood medical disorders and psychiatric problems. The Ontario Child Health Study was an epidemiological survey of 3,294 children four to sixteen years of age in the general community (Cadman et al., 1987). Data were collected on the relationship of psychiatric disorders and social adjustment problems among children with chronic illness, medical conditions, and long-term disability in contrast to children free of chronic health problems. After making adjustments for age and gender differences, children with both chronic illness and associated physical disability were at a risk of diagnosable psychiatric disorders three times greater than healthy children. Children with a chronic medical condition but no disability were found to be at a twofold risk of psychiatric disorder. Other large epidemiological studies—including the Isle of Wight studies, the Rochester Child Health studies, and the National Health Survey-Child Health Supplement—also indicate that children with long-term illnesses are at approximately twice the risk of behavioral and emotional problems as children who do not have significant health problems (Gortmaker, Walker, Weitzman, & Sobol, 1990; Rutter, Tizard, & Whitmore, 1970).

Despite the increased risk of mental health problems among children with chronic illness, many such children have no evidence of concurrent mental illness. In fact, most have no significant behavioral or emotional dysfunction. It is becoming increasingly clear that a direct relationship between chronic childhood medical disorders and psychiatric problems does not exist (Garrison & McQuiston, 1989). Rather, it is likely that chronic illness functions as a nonspecific life stressor to which a wide range of responses is possible. The specific response to the stress is undoubtedly a function of various factors.

Correlates of Psychiatric Comorbidity in Chronic Illness

The factors that affect a child's response to stress include the characteristics of the disease, external factors in the child's environment (such as parental psychiatric status and family functioning), and personality factors related to resiliency.

Disease Factors

Early investigators of disease characteristics believed that psychiatric status was primarily a function of the chronic medical disorder's severity and resulting level of impairment. Approximately 75 percent to 80 percent of children with chronic medical disorders are believed to be only mildly to moderately affected by the medical disorder (Haggerty, 1984). Therefore, relatively few children with a chronic medical disorder should experience behavioral and/or emotional problems if these problems are a result of the severity of their chronic physical disorders. However, it is now becoming apparent that severity of the disorder and functional status alone do not account for the considerable variation in the presence of behavioral and emotional problems in these populations (Hurtig, Koepke, & Park, 1989; Daniels, Moos, Billings, & Miller, 1987; Steinhausen, Schindler, & Stephan, 1983). For example, in a recent study of children with sickle cell disease, illness severity (as assessed by frequency of hospitalization and emergency room visits, frequency and intensity of pain crises, and duration of illness) was not significantly related to child psychological status as assessed by IQ, self-esteem, social and personal adjustment, behavioral problems, school performance, and peer relations (Hurtig, Koepke, & Park, 1989). In another study, children with spina bifida were found to have significantly more behavior and social competence problems than expected for children in general, but their psychosocial status was not significantly related to level of disability or physical problems (Wallander, Feldman, & Varni, 1989). Another recent study examined the relationship between disability parameters, chronic strain, and adaptation of physically handicapped children and their mothers (Wallander, Varni Babani, Banis, et al., 1989). They found that both the children and the mothers displayed adaptation problems but that adaptation was not significantly related to the children's disability status or the related chronic strain. However, a few studies differ in their conclusions. For example, Billings, Moos, Miller, and Gottlieb (1987) found that disease severity for a group of children with juvenile rheumatoid arthritis was significantly related to psychosocial functioning. The results of the Ontario Child Health Study also suggest that disability status is related to the risk for psychiatric disorders (Cadman et al., 1987). Other reviewers have reported that children with chronic medical disorders that involve physical incapacitation may be at higher risk for psychiatric problems (Drotar & Bush, 1985; Pless, 1984).

Recent evidence suggests that the critical variable related to children's psychiatric status may not be objective measures of disease severity but rather family members' perception of disease severity (DeMaso et al., 1991). DeMaso and colleagues examined the relationship between maternal perceptions of medical disorder severity, objective measures of disease severity, and children's emotional adjustment in a group of children with congenital heart disease. They found that objective measures of disease severity accounted for 3 percent of the variance in children's emotional adjustment, whereas maternal perceptions of disease severity accounted for 33 percent of the variance. Perrin, MacLean, and Perrin (1989) found that children whose parents rated their asthma as either mild or severe had lower adjustment scores than those children whose parents rated the asthma as moderate.

Other disorder-related variables that have been found to be significantly correlated with behavioral and emotional problems include the presence of disease-related visible impairments and invasive interventions. A study examining survivors of end-stage renal disease found that maladjustment (distorted body image, social immaturity, low self-esteem) was directly related to the presence of impairments that are visible to others (Beck, Nethercut, Crittenden, & Hewins, 1986). An important question that deserves further study is the relative impact of actual physical incapacitation and disease visibility on behavioral and emotional problems.

Certain interventions for specific chronic medical disorders have also been found to be associated with psychological problems. Cousens, Waters, Said, and Stevens (1988) conducted a meta-analysis involving seventeen studies and concluded that children undergoing central nervous system irradiation show substantial cognitive deficits. These deficits were especially pronounced for children who received treatment at younger ages. The implication of these cognitive deficits for later psychiatric morbidity is unclear. Long-term survivors of childhood cancer show a fourfold increase in school problems and somatic complaints of unknown origin (Mulhern, Wasserman, Friedman, & Fairclough, 1989). These investigators found that children who were treated with irradiation, who were older at diagnosis, or were from single-parent homes were at greatest risk for psychological problems. In reviewing the literature in this area, Eiser (1990) found that cognitive deficits have been found to be greater for children diagnosed at younger ages when immediate follow-up data are collected. However, long-term follow-up data tend to suggest greater deficits for children who were older at diagnosis (Eiser, 1990). It is also important to note that children with "brain-related" illnesses have been reported to have poorer psychosocial outcomes than children with non-brain-related disorders (Rutter et al., 1970; Breslau, 1985).

In summary, specific characteristics of chronic medical disorders do appear to be related to children's behavioral and emotional problems. However, these factors are not likely to account for a majority of the variance in regard to the behavioral and emotional status of children with chronic medical disorders. What is most obvious from the research reviewed is the need for uniform definitions of terms that clearly define the manifestations of disease, such as physical disability or functional status.

Parental Factors

Parental factors have also been hypothesized to be significantly related to behavioral and emotional manifestations in children with chronic medical disorders. This hypothesis is not surprising, given the important role of parents in helping their child adjust to a chronic medical disorder. For example, Johnson (1985) discussed the major tasks involved in parenting a chronically ill child. These included (1) illness management and helping the child assume this responsibility, (2) helping the child cope with the illness and also encouraging normal development, and (3) normalizing family functioning while also managing the life-style disruptions secondary to the illness. Therefore, parental maladjustment would appear to have the potential for being a major mediating variable regarding psychiatric sequelae in chronically ill children.

While both paternal and maternal psychiatric adjustment are probably important mediating variables (Blotcky, Raczynski, Gurwich, & Smith, 1985), maternal variables would appear to be especially significant, since in our society mothers tend to bear most of the day-to-day responsibility of caring for the chronically ill and disabled child (for example, Carey, 1982; Wilkin, 1979). Consequently, most of the studies examining the role of parental factors have focused on maternal variables; relatively few have focused on the role of paternal variables.

A recent study of children with rheumatic disease and their unaffected siblings found that children with both depressed mothers and high family stress were at much higher risk for the development of multiple psychological problems (Daniels, Moos, Billings, & Miller, 1987). Jessop, Riessman, and Stein (1988) examined the relationship between the health status of children with a variety of chronic medical disorders and maternal psychiatric symptoms. They found no significant relation between burden of the child's physical condition, as rated by the health providers, and maternal psychiatric symptoms. However, they did find a significant relationship between the mental health status of the mother and the child's functional status.

High levels of maternal depression have been found in many families that have a child with a chronic medical condition (Breslau, Staruch, & Mortimer, 1982). Some preliminary evidence also suggests that maternal depression is significantly related to chronically ill children's behavioral and emotional dysfunction (Walker, Ortiz-Valdes, & Newbrough, 1989). A large literature indicates, with few exceptions, that maternal depression is associated with child maladjustment in a variety of non-chronically ill populations (Billings & Moos, 1986; Radke-Yarrow, Cummings, Kuczynski, & Chapman, 1985; Richters & Pellegrini, 1989; Weintraub, Neale, & Liebert, 1975; Weintraub, Prinz, & Neale, 1978; Weissman et al., 1987). An early review of research in this area concluded that children of depressed parents were at considerable risk for a wide range of psychological difficulties (Beardslee, Bemporad, Keller, & Klerman, 1983). School-age children of depressed parents are generally found to have higher levels of both externalizing and internalizing problems (see Downey & Coyne, 1990), as judged by teachers (Lee & Gotlib, 1989a, 1989b; Richters & Pelligrini, 1989), parents (Breslau, Davis, & Prabucki, 1988; Lee & Gotlib, 1989a, 1989b; Richters & Pelligrini, 1989), or children themselves (Breslau, Davis, & Prabucki, 1988; Hirsch, Moos, & Reischl, 1985). Children of depressed parents have also been found to have deficits in social competence (Hammen et al., 1987) and academic competence not due to intellectual limitations (Billings & Moos, 1983; Hammen et al., 1987; Weissman et al., 1987). The increased interest in the parenting practices of depressed parents reflects a growing interest in the interpersonal context of depression (Downey & Coyne, 1990). Parental depression has been found to be related to both poor marital adjustment and to a less positive child-rearing approach (Christensen, Phillips, Glasgow, & Johnson, 1983). Several studies suggest that depressed mothers are inconsistent in discipline strategies with their children (Stoneman, Brody, & Burke, 1989; Susman, Trickett, Iannotti, Hollenbeck, & Zahn-Waxler, 1985; Zelkowitz, 1982). Maternal depression has also been associated with various child-rearing styles including increased punitiveness (Longfellow, Zelkowitz, & Saunders, 1982; Zelkowitz, 1982), less tolerance (Zelkowitz, 1982), and less nurturance, warmth, and affection (Longfellow, Zelkowitz, & Saunders, 1982). Susman and colleagues (1985) also found that depressed mothers tended to foster guilt and anxiety as a means of controlling the behavior of their children.

The important issue for future research is to determine whether maternal depression has a quantitatively or qualitatively different impact on children with chronic illness than on children without such illness. It may be that the impact is the same but that parental dysfunction is more prevalent in mothers of children with chronic illness or that children already vulnerable, due to their chronic illness, may be especially susceptible.

Family and Social Factors

Clinicians working with chronically ill children have long reported their observation of marital distress in families with chronically ill children. However, early studies of divorce rates in families with and without a chronically ill child typically found no differences (see Sabbeth & Leventhal, 1984). Although evidence of increased marital distress does exist, few well-controlled studies have examined the relationship between marital distress and psychiatric status in the chronically ill child. Kovacs and her colleagues (1985) found a relationship between marital discord and child psychiatric disorder in a group of children with insulin-dependent diabetes mellitus. A more recent study examined the adaptation of children with congenital or acquired limb deficiencies as a function of family variables (Varni, Rubenfeld, Talbot, & Setoguchi, 1989) and found that family conflict and family cohesion were significantly related to child adaptation, whereas degree of limb loss, age, gender, and socioeconomic status were not.

Little evidence suggests that the impact of marital conflict on children's mental health is limited to those with chronic illness. Grych and Fincham (1990) have recently reviewed the literature examining the relation between marital conflict and child maladjustment in the non-chronically ill population. Their review indicates that marital conflict has been associated with child psychiatric symptomatology, including conduct disorder (Johnson & O'Leary, 1987; Jouriles, Murphy, & O'Leary, 1989; Wierson, Forehand, & McCombs, 1988), aggression (Jacobson, 1978; Johnston, Gonzalez, & Campbell, 1987), antisocial behavior (Emery & O'Leary, 1984; Peterson & Zill, 1986), depression (Johnson & O'Leary, 1987; Peterson & Zill, 1986), and anxiety/withdrawal (Wierson, Forehand, & McCombs, 1988). In addition to externalizing and internalizing behavior problems, marital conflict has been associated with children's social competence (Emery & O'Leary, 1984), cognitive competence, and grade-point average (Wierson, Forehand, & McCombs, 1988). Of the nineteen studies reviewed by Grych and Fincham (1990), fifteen supported a significant relation between marital conflict and child psychological status.

Other family variables that have been found to be related to the psychiatric status of chronically ill children include socioeconomic status, household composition, marital status, and family coping style (Stein & Jessop, 1984; Cadman, Boyle, & Offord, 1986; Cadman, Boyle, Szatmari, & Offord, 1987; Haggerty, Roghmann, & Pless, 1975; Shapiro, 1983). For example, McGauhey and colleagues (1991) showed that adverse social conditions place children, especially children born at low birthweight, at much higher risk of all types of problems, including physical and mental illness as well as disability.

Since most of these factors also are associated with mental health problems in children without chronic illness, the documented increase in risk among children with chronic illness may be due to a greater prevalence of these stressors in their families rather than to an increased impact of the social factors. It is likely that children born into and reared in socioeconomically disadvantaged families are at double jeopardy (Escalona, 1982). Again, the issue that needs to be addressed is whether the relationship between family variables and child psychiatric status is different for the chronic illness population.

Child Factors

Many early investigations in this area attempted to identify certain disease-specific personality types. This line of research has not been very successful. For example, the evidence is lacking for an "asthma personality" (Creer, 1987) or a "diabetic personality" (Johnson, 1984; Kovacs et al., 1985; Rodin, 1983).

A child's level of cognitive functioning may be related to psychiatric status associated with chronic illness. Poor academic performance and cognitive deficits are associated with various disorders. For example, children with sickle cell anemia have been found to score significantly lower on reading and spelling achievement tests than matched "healthy" children (Fowler et al., 1988). These investigators also found that children with sickle cell disease performed less well on tests measuring visual-motor skills and attentional skills. It is interesting to note that these results were not significantly related to most measures of disease severity. In another study, boys with hemophilia were often found to be achieving below expectations in math and reading. This underachievement did not appear to be related to disease severity, school absenteeism, or level of intelligence (Woolf et al., 1989). As noted previously, irradiation treatment in children with cancer has also been associated with cognitive deficits (Cousens et al., 1988). It is possible that cognitive/academic dysfunction plays a mediating role in the development of psychiatric disorders in chronically ill children.

A child's age may also be an important mediating variable regarding psychiatric morbidity. For example, older children with juvenile rheumatoid arthritis display greater social maladjustment than younger children with the same medical problem (Billings et al., 1987). Similar age effects have been found in other diagnostic groups, including those with sickle cell anemia (Hurtig & White, 1986). Some studies have also found boys to display more maladjustment than girls (Hurtig, Koepke, & Park, 1989; Hurtig & White, 1986; Morgan & Jackson, 1986).

A Research Agenda

Despite the attention devoted to exploring the relationships between mental health and chronic physical illness, many questions remain. Little is known, for example, about the directionality of the association. One possibility is that mental health problems, particularly those that are of the type manifested by nonspecific affective symptoms or behavior problems, are generalized manifestations of unresolved stress. If so, and if such stress results from physical disorder, mental health problems could be a consequence of physical disorder acting as a trigger superimposed on susceptibility to psychiatric disorders. Alternatively, in some cases mental health problems could be a cause of physical disorder, by exposing individuals to situations where they are made more vulnerable to such disorders. A third possibility is that both mental and physical disorders are a concomitant response to the same threat to health (for example, environmental or social stressors), which acts to increase susceptibility to both kinds of problems, as suggested by Ross and Duff (1982). To address these possibilities, two factors are critical to future research designs: theoretical or conceptual models and longitudinal designs.

Recently there has been greater focus on the need to develop theoretical models to guide research in this area. Vandvik and Eckblad (1991) have advanced a conceptual model that postulates the biopsychosocial interrelationships among predisposing, provoking, modifying, and outcome variables (Figure 6.1). This model incorporates variables that buffer and others that potentiate the impact of biological and psychosocial stress variables. Such a theoretical model combined with a longitudinal research design would greatly improve our understanding of the relationship between chronic childhood illness and psychiatric disorder.

An equally important area to explore is the adaptation of parents with chronically ill children, particularly since the literature is so clear on the effect of parental psychiatric state on the child. Wallander, Varni Babani, Banis, et al., (1989) have proposed a conceptual model to account for the variance in adaptation of parents of chronically ill and disabled children (Figure 6.2). This model includes various risk factors (disease/disability parameters, func-

Figure 6.1. Conceptual Model for Research on Mothers of Physically Handicapped Children.

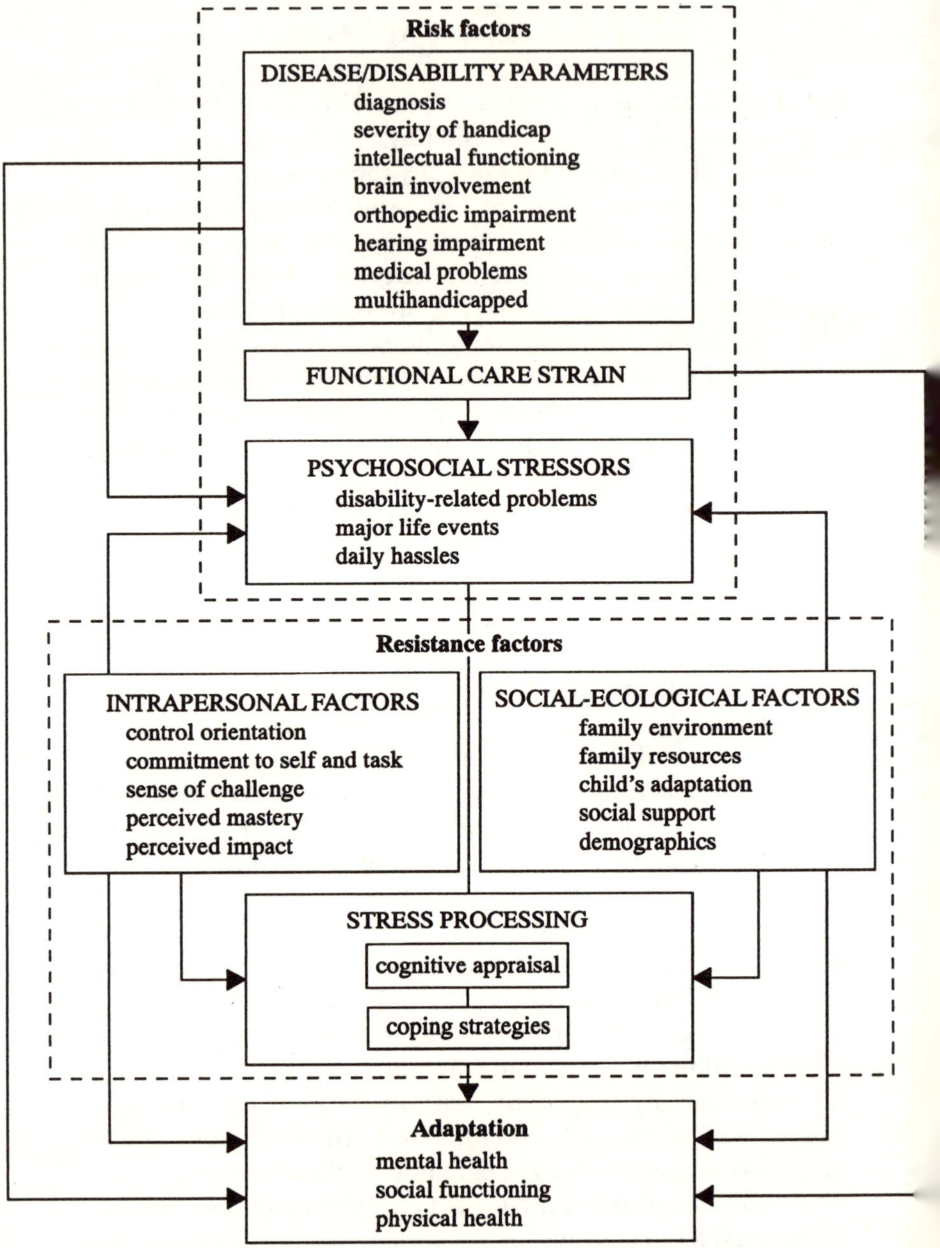

Source: Wallander, Varni Babani, DeHaan, Wilcox, & Banis, 1989, p. 373. Used by permission.

Figure 6.2. A Biopsychosocial Model of Multifactorial Diseases.

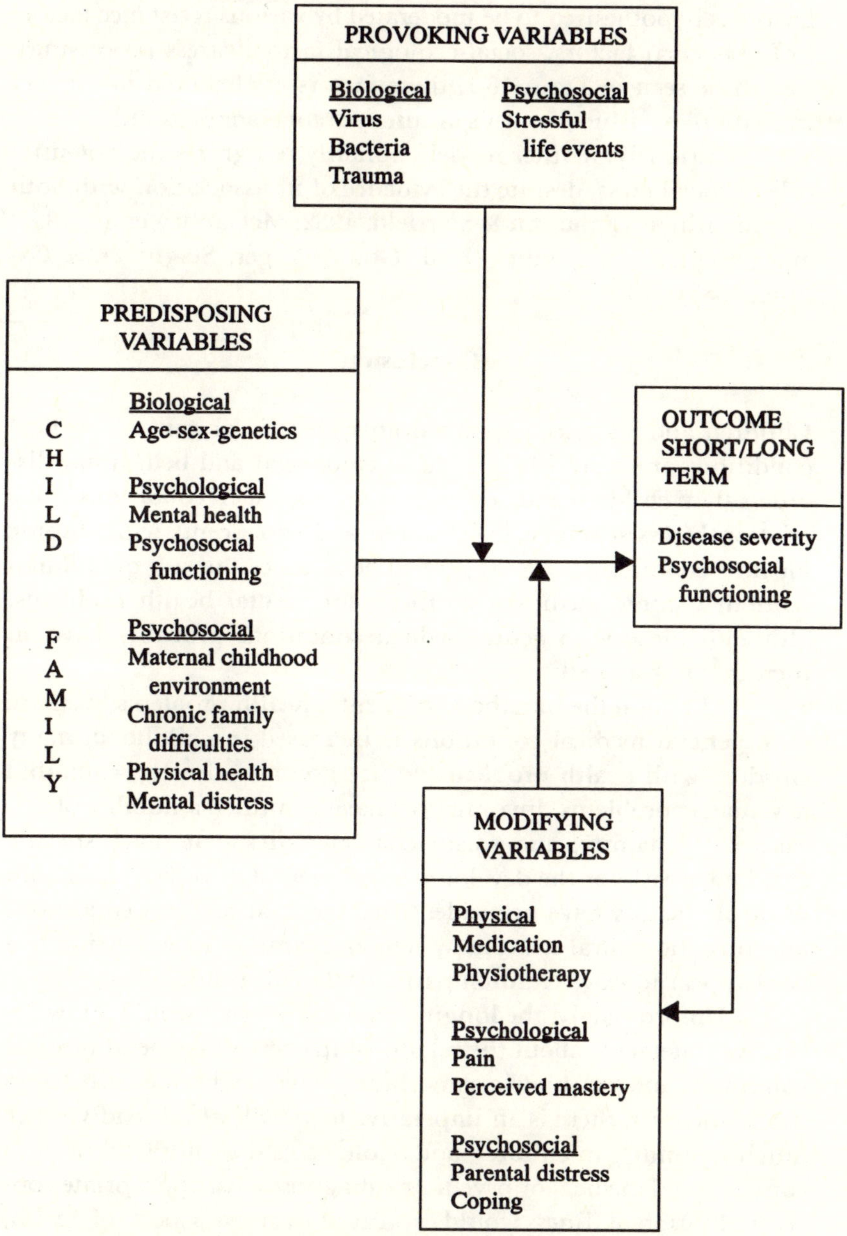

Source: Vandvik & Eckblad, 1991, p. 55. Used by permission.

tional care strain, psychosocial stressors). The impact of these risk factors is hypothesized to be moderated by various resistance factors (intrapersonal factors, social-ecological factors, stress processing). As can be seen in Figure 6.1, these factors are believed to interact in a complex fashion in determining parental adaptation.

Curiously, neither model explicitly recognizes the potential role of social class, despite the evidence of its association with both chronic illness (Egbuonu & Starfield, 1982; McGauhey et al., 1991) and psychiatric morbidity (Bird, Gould, Yager, Staghezza, & Canino, 1989).

Conclusion

Children and adolescents with nonpsychiatric or general medical conditions are more likely to have emotional and behavioral disorders than children and adolescents without such conditions. This relationship is strongest for children and adolescents with chronic medical conditions, who appear to be at twice the risk of children without chronic medical conditions for mental health problems, although those with acute medical conditions probably have an increased risk as well.

Although the likelihood of mental health problems for those with general medical conditions is increased in childhood, many children with health problems do not go on to develop comorbid psychiatric problems. Investigators have identified a number of disease, child, family, and social characteristics that place specific children at risk for the development of mental disorders. Although multiple factors have been identified, general medical conditions affecting the central nervous system and families experiencing discord appear to leave children particularly vulnerable.

Unfortunately, the longitudinal studies that would allow definitive statements about the relationships between general medical conditions and psychiatric comorbidity have not been conducted to date. Moreover, there is an imperative to view health broadly, since much morbidity in children and adolescents does not lend itself to conventional medical or psychiatric diagnoses. An appropriate conceptualization of illness would capture at least five aspects of health, in addition to medical diagnoses: physical activity and physical fitness, physical and mental symptomatology, general perceptions of health and self-esteem, extent of achievement of developmental and social expectations, and manifestations of activities and situations that pose a threat to subsequent health. Many of these domains are especially important to primary care providers, who must address outcomes of importance to patients and their families.

References

Beardslee, W., Bemporad, J., Keller, M. B., & Klerman, G. L. (1983). Children of parents with a major affective disorder: A review. *American Journal of Psychiatry, 140,* 825–832.

Beck, A. L., Nethercut, G. E., Crittenden, M. R., & Hewins, J. (1986). Visibility of handicap, self-concept, and social maturity among young adult survivors of end-stage renal disease. *Journal of Developmental and Behavioral Pediatrics, 7,* 93–96.

Bedell, J. R., Giordani, B., Amour, J. L., Tavormina, J., & Boll, T. (1977). Life stress and the psychological and medical adjustment for chronically ill children. *Journal of Psychosomatic Research, 21,* 237–242.

Billings, A. G., & Moos, R. H. (1983). Comparison of children of depressed and nondepressed parents: A social environmental perspective. *Journal of Abnormal Child Psychology, 11,* 483–486.

Billings, A. G., & Moos, R. H. (1986). Children of parents with unipolar depression: A controlled 1-year follow-up. *Journal of Abnormal Child Psychology, 14,* 149–166.

Billings, A. G., Moos, R. H., Miller, J. J., & Gottlieb, J. E. (1987). Psychosocial adaptation in juvenile rheumatic disease: A controlled evaluation. *Health Psychology, 6,* 343–359.

Bird, H. R., Gould, M. S., Yager, T., Staghezza, B., & Canino, G. (1989). Risk factors for maladjustment in Puerto Rican children. *Journal of American Academy of Child Adolescent Psychiatry, 28,* 847–850.

Blotcky, A. D., Raczynski, J. M., Gurwich, R., & Smith, K. (1985). Family influences on hopelessness among children in the cancer experience. *Journal of Pediatric Psychology, 10,* 479–494.

Breslau, N. (1985). Psychiatric disorder in children with physical disabilities. *Journal of the American Academy of Child Psychiatry, 24,* 87–94.

Breslau, N., Davis, G., & Prabucki, K. (1988). Depressed mothers as informants in family history research—Are they accurate? *Psychiatry Research, 24,* 345–359.

Breslau, N., Staruch, K. S., & Mortimer, E. A. (1982). Psychological distress in mothers of disabled children. *American Journal of Diseases in Children, 136,* 682–686.

Cadman, D., Boyle, M. H., & Offord, D. R. (1986). Chronic illnesses, medical conditions and limitations in Ontario children. *Canadian Medical Association Journal, 9,* 117–121.

Cadman, D., Boyle, M. H., Szatmari, P., & Offord, D. R. (1987). Chronic illness, disability, and mental and social well-being: Findings of the Ontario Child Health Study. *Pediatrics, 79,* 805–813.

Carey, G. E. (1982). Community care—Care by whom? Mentally handicapped children living at home. *Public Health, 96,* 269–278.

Cassileth, B. R., Lusk, E. J., Strouse, T. B., Miller, D. S., Brown, L. L., Cross, P. A., & Tenaglia, A. N. (1984). Psychosocial status in chronic illness: A comparative analysis of six diagnostic groups. *New England Journal of Medicine, 311,* 506–511.

Christensen, A., Phillips, S., Glasgow, R. E., & Johnson, S. M. (1983). Parental characteristics and interactional dysfunction in families with child behavior problems: A preliminary investigation. *Journal of Abnormal Child Psychology, 11,* 153–166.

Collins, J. G. (1988, May 24). Prevalence of selected chronic conditions, United States, 1986–88 (DHHS Publication No. (PHS) 93-1510). Hyattsville, MD: U.S. Department of Health and Human Services.

Costello, E. J. (1989). Developments in child psychiatric epidemiology. *Journal of the American Academy of Child Adolescent Psychiatry, 147,* 349–352.

Cousens, P., Waters, B., Said, J., & Stevens, M. (1988). Cognitive effects of cranial irradiation in leukemia: A survey and meta-analysis. *Journal of Child Psychology and Psychiatry, 29,* 839–852.

Creer, T. L. (1987). Psychological and neuropsychological aspects of childhood asthma. In D. G. Tinkelman, C. J. Falliers, & C. K. Napitz (Eds.), *Childhood asthma: Pathophysiology and treatment.* New York: Marcel Dekker.

Daniels, D., Moos, R., Billings, A., & Miller, J. (1987). Psychosocial risk and resistance factors among children with chronic illnesses, healthy siblings, and healthy controls. *Journal of Abnormal Child Psychology, 15,* 295–308.

DeMaso, D. R., Campis, L. K., Wypij, D., Bertram, S., Lipshitz, M., & Freed, M. (1991). The impact of maternal perceptions and medical severity on the adjustment of children with congenital heart disease. *Journal of Pediatric Psychology, 16,* 137–149.

Downey, G., & Coyne, J. C. (1990). Children of depressed parents: An integrative review. *Psychological Bulletin, 108,* 50–76.

Drotar, D., & Bush, M. (1985). Mental health issues and services. In N. Hobbs & J. M. Perrin (Eds.), *Issues in the care of children with chronic illness: A sourcebook on problems, services, and policies.* San Francisco: Jossey-Bass.

Drotar, D., Doershuk, C. F., Stein, R. C., Boat, T. F., Boyer, W., & Matthews, L. (1981). Psychosocial functioning of children with cystic fibrosis. *Pediatrics, 67,* 338–343.

Egbuonu, L., & Starfield, B. (1982). Child health and social status. *Pediatrics, 69,* 550–555.

Eiser, C. (1990). Psychological effects of chronic disease. *Journal of Child Psychology and Psychiatry, 31,* 85–98.

Emery, R. E., & O'Leary, K. D. (1984). Marital discord and child behavior problems in a nonclinic sample. *Journal of Abnormal Child Psychology, 12,* 411–420.

Fowler, M. G., Whitt, J. K., Lallinger, R. R., Nash, K. B., Atkinson, S. S., Wells, R. J., & McMillan, C. (1988). Neuropsychologic and academic functioning of children with sickle cell anemia. *Journal of Developmental and Behavioral Pediatrics, 9,* 213–220.

Frances, A., Pincus, H. A., Widiger, T. A., Davis, W. W., & First, M. B. (1990). DSM-IV: Work in progress. *American Journal of Psychiatry, 147,* 1439–1448.

Garrison, W., & McQuiston, S. (1989). *Chronic illness during childhood and adolescence: Psychological aspects.* Newbury Park, CA: Sage.

Gortmaker, S. L., & Sappenfield, W. (1984). Chronic childhood disorders: Prevalence and impact. *Pediatric Clinics of North America, 31,* 3–18.

Gortmaker, S. L., Walker, D. K., Weitzman, M., & Sobol, A. M. (1990). Chronic conditions, socioeconomic risks, and behavioral problems in children and adolescents. *Pediatrics, 85,* 267–276.

Grych, J. H., & Fincham, F. D. (1990). Marital conflict and children's adjustment: A cognitive-contextual framework. *Psychological Bulletin, 108*(2): 267–290.

Haggerty, R. (1984). Foreward to symposium on chronic disease in children. *Pediatric Clinics of North America, 31,* 1–2.

Haggerty, R., Roghmann, K. J., & Pless, I. B. (1975). *Child health and the community*. New York: Wiley.

Hammen, C., Gordon, G., Burge, D., Adrian, C., Jaenicke, C., & Hiroto, G. (1987). Maternal affective disorders, illness, and stress: Risk for children's psychopathology. *American Journal of Psychiatry, 144,* 736–741.

Hankin, J. R., Kessler, L. G., Goldberg, I. D., Steinwachs, D. M., & Starfield, B. H. (1983). A longitudinal study of offset in the use of nonpsychiatric services following specialized mental health care. *Medical Care, 21*(11), 1099–1110.

Hirsch, B. J., Moos, R. F., & Reischl, T. M. (1985). Psychosocial adjustment of adolescent children of a depressed, arthritic, or normal parent. *Journal of Abnormal Psychology, 94,* 154–164.

Hobbs, N., Perrin, J. M., & Ireys, H. T. (1985). *Chronically ill children and their families: Problems, prospects, and proposals from the Vanderbilt study*. San Francisco: Jossey-Bass.

Hurtig, A., Koepke, D., & Park, K. (1989). Relation between severity of chronic illness and adjustment in children and adolescents with sickle cell disease. *Journal of Pediatric Psychology, 14,* 117–132.

Hurtig, A. L., & White, L. S. (1986). Psychosocial adjustment in children and adolescents with sickle cell disease. *Journal of Pediatric Psychology, 11,* 411–428.

Jacobson, D. S. (1978). The impact of marital separation/divorce on children: 2. Interparent hostility and child adjustment. *Journal of Divorce, 2,* 3–19.

Jessop, D. J., Riessman, C. K., & Stein, R. E. (1988). Chronic childhood illness and maternal mental health. *Journal of Developmental and Behavioral Pediatrics, 9*(3), 147–156.

Johnson, P. L., & O'Leary, K. D. (1987). Parental behavior patterns and conduct disorders in girls. *Journal of Abnormal Child Psychology, 15,* 573–581.

Johnson, S. B. (1984). Knowledge, attitudes, and behavior: Correlates of health in childhood diabetes. *Clinical Psychology Review, 4,* 503–524.

Johnson, S. B. (1985). The family and the child with chronic illness. In D. C. Turk & R. D. Kerns (Eds.), *Health, illness, and families: A life span perspective.* New York: Wiley.

Johnston, J. R., Gonzalez, R., & Campbell, L. E. (1987). Ongoing postdivorce conflict and child disturbance. *Journal of Abnormal Child Psychology, 15,* 497–509.

Jouriles, E. N., Murphy, C. M., & O'Leary, K. D. (1989). Interspousal aggression, marital discord, and child problems. *Journal of Consulting and Clinical Psychology, 57,* 453–455.

Kelleher, K., & Starfield, B. (1990). Health care use by children receiving mental health services. *Pediatrics, 85,* 114–118.

Kovacs, M., Feinberg, T. L., Paulauskas, S., Finkelstein, R., Pollock, M., & Crouse-Novak, M. (1985). Initial coping responses and psychosocial characteristics of children with insulin-dependent diabetes mellitus. *Journal of Pediatrics, 106,* 827–834.

Lavigne, J. V., & Faier-Routman, J. (1992). Psychological adjustment to pediatric physical disorders: A meta-analytic review. *Journal of Pediatric Psychology, 17*(2), 133–157.

Lee, C. M., & Gotlib, I. H. (1989a). Clinical status and emotional adjustment of children of depressed mothers. *American Journal of Psychiatry, 146,* 478–483.

Lee, C. M., & Gotlib, I. H. (1989b). Maternal depression and child adjustment: A longitudinal analysis. *Journal of Abnormal Psychology, 98,* 78–85.

Longfellow, C., Zelkowitz, P., & Saunders, E. (1982). The quality of mother-child relationships. In D. Belle (Ed.), *Lives in stress: Women and depression* (pp. 163–176). Newbury Park, CA: Sage.

McGauhey, P. J., Starfield, B., Alexander, C., & Ensminger, M. (1991). The social environment and vulnerability of low birthweight children: A social-epidemiological perspective. *Pediatrics, 88,* 943–953.

Meadows, A., & Silber, J. (1985). Delayed consequences of therapy for childhood cancer. *Cancer, 35,* 271–286.

Morgan, S. A., & Jackson, J. (1986). Psychological and social concomitants of sickle cell anemia. *Journal of Pediatric Psychology, 11,* 429–440.

Mulhern, R. K., Wasserman, A. L., Friedman, A. G., & Fairclough, D. (1989). Social competence and behavioral adjustment of children who are long-term survivors of cancer. *Pediatrics, 83,* 18–25.

Perrin, J. M., MacLean, W. E., & Perrin, E. C. (1989). Parental perceptions of health status and psychologic adjustment of children with asthma. *Pediatrics, 83,* 26–30.

Peterson, J. L., & Zill, N. (1986). Marital disruption, parent-child relationships, and behavior problems in children. *Journal of Marriage and the Family, 48,* 295–307.

Pless, I. (1984). Clinical assessment: Physical and psychological functioning. *Pediatric Clinics of North America, 31,* 33–46.

Pless, I., & Pinkerton, P. (1975). *Chronic childhood disorders: Promoting patterns of adjustment.* London: Kimpton.

Radke-Yarrow, M., Cummings, E. M., Kuczynski, L., & Chapman, M. (1985). Patterns of attachment in two- and three-year-olds in normal families and families with parental depression. *Child Development, 56,* 884–893.

Regier, D. A., Kessler, L. G., Burns, B. J., & Goldberg, I. D. (1979). The need for a psychosocial classification system in primary-care settings. *International Journal of Mental Health, 8,* 16–29.

Richters, J., & Pellegrini, D. (1989). Depressed mothers' judgments about their children: An examination of the depression-distortion hypothesis. *Child Development, 60,* 1068–1075.

Rodin, G. M. (1983). Psychosocial aspects of diabetes mellitus. *Canadian Journal of Psychiatry, 28,* 219–223.

Ross, C. E., & Duff, R. S. (1982). Medical care, living conditions, and children's well being. *Social Forces, 61,* 457–474.

Rutter, M., Tizard, J., & Whitmore, K. (Eds.). (1970). *Education, health, and behavior.* London: Longman.

Sabbeth, B. F., & Leventhal, J. M. (1984). Marital adjustment to chronic childhood illness: A critique of the literature. *Pediatrics, 73*(6), 762–768.

Shapiro, J. (1983). Family reactions and coping strategies in response to the physically ill or handicapped child: A review. *Social Science Medicine, 17,* 913–931.

Starfield, B., Gross, E., Wood, M., Pantell, R., Allen, C., Gordon, I. B., Moffatt, P., Drachman, R., & Katz, H. (1980). Psychosocial and psychosomatic diagnoses in primary care of children. *Pediatrics, 66,* 159–167.

Starfield, B., Hoekelman, R., McCormick, M., Benson, P., Mendenhall, R., Moynihan, C., & Radecki, S. (1984). Who provides health care to children in the United States? *Pediatrics, 74,* 991–997.

Starfield, B., Katz, H., Gabriel, A., Livingston, G., Benson, P., Hankin, J., Horn, S., & Steinwachs, D. (1984). Morbidity in childhood: A longitudinal view. *New England Journal of Medicine, 310,* 824–829.

Starfield, B., Weiner, J., Mumford, L., & Steinwachs, D. (1991). Ambulatory care groups: A categorization of diagnoses for research and management. *Health Services Research, 26,* 53–74.

Stein, R., & Jessop, D. (1982). A noncategorical approach to chronic childhood illness. *Public Health Reports, 97,* 354–362.

Stein, R., & Jessop, D. (1984). Relationship between health status and psychological adjustment among children with chronic conditions. *Pediatrics, 73,* 169–174.

Steinhausen, H., Schindler, H., & Stephan, H. (1983). Correlates of psychopathology in sick children. *Journal of the American Academy of Child Psychiatry, 22,* 559–564.

Stoneman, Z., Brody, G. H., & Burke, M. (1989). Marital quality, depression, and inconsistent parenting: Relationship with observed mother-child conflict. *American Journal of Orthopsychiatry, 59*(1), 105–117.

Susman, E. J., Trickett, P. K., Iannotti, R. J., Hollenbeck, B. E., & Zahn-Waxler, C. (1985). Child-rearing patterns in depressed, abusive, and normal mothers. *American Journal of Orthopsychiatry, 55,* 237–251.

Tavormina, J. B., Kastner, L. S., Slater, P. M., & Watt, S. L. (1976). Chronically ill children: A psychologically and emotionally deviant population? *Journal of Abnormal Child Psychology, 4,* 99–110.

Vandvik, I. H., & Eckblad, G. (1991). Mothers of children with recent onset of rheumatic disease: Associations between maternal distress, psychosocial variables, and the disease of the children. *Journal of Developmental and Behavioral Pediatrics, 12,* 84–91.

Varni, J. W., Rubenfeld, M. A., Talbot, D., & Setoguchi, Y. (1989). Family functioning, temperament, and psychologic adaptation in children with congenital or acquired limb deficiencies. *Pediatrics, 84,* 323–330.

Walker, L., Ortiz-Valdes, J., & Newbrough, J. (1989). The role of maternal employment and depression in the psychological adjustment of chronically ill, mentally retarded, and well children. *Journal of Pediatric Psychology, 14,* 357–370.

Wallander, J. L., Varni, J. W., Babani, L., Banis, H. T., & Wilcox, K. T. (1988). Children with chronic physical disorders: Maternal reports of their psychological adjustment. *Journal of Pediatric Psychology, 13,* 197–212.

Wallander, J. L., Feldman, W. S., & Varni, J. W. (1989). Physical status and psychosocial adjustment in children with spina bifida. *Journal of Pediatric Psychology, 14,* 89–102.

Wallander, J. L., Varni, J. W., Babani, L., Banis, H. T., DeHaan, C. B., & Wilcox, K. T. (1989). Disability parameters, chronic strain, and adaptation of physically handicapped children and their mothers. *Journal of Pediatric Psychology, 14,* 23–42.

Wallander, J. L., Varni Babani, L., DeHaan, C. B., Wilcox, K. T., & Banis, H. T. (1989). The social environment and the adaptation of mothers of physically handicapped children. *Journal of Pediatric Psychology, 14,* 371–387.

Weintraub, S., Neale, J. M., & Liebert, D. E. (1975). Teacher ratings of children vulnerable to psychopathology. *American Journal of Orthopsychiatry, 45,* 838–845.

Weintraub, S., Prinz, R. J., & Neale, J. M. (1978). Peer evaluation of the competence of children vulnerable to psychopathology. *Journal of Abnormal Child Psychology, 6,* 461–473.

Weissman, M. M., Gammon, G. D., John, K., Merikangas, K., Warner, V., Prusoff, B. A., & Sholomskas, D. (1987). Children of depressed parents: Increased psychopathology and early onset of major depression. *Archives of General Psychiatry, 44,* 847–853.

Wierson, M., Forehand, R., & McCombs, A. (1988). The relationship of early adolescent functioning to parent-reported and adolescent-perceived interparental conflict. *Journal of Abnormal Child Psychology, 16,* 707–718.

Wilkin, D. (1979). *Caring for the mentally handicapped child.* London: Croom Helm.

Woolf, A., Rappaport, L., Reardon, P., Ciborowski, J., D'Angelo, E., & Bessette, J. (1989). School functioning and disease severity in boys with hemophilia. *Journal of Developmental and Behavioral Pediatrics, 10,* 81–85.

Zelkowitz, P. (1982). Parenting philosophies and practices. In D. Belle (Ed.), *Lives in stress: Women and depression* (pp. 154–162). Newbury Park, CA: Sage.

Part Three

Presentation and Recognition of Mental Disorders

7

W. Eugene Broadhead

Presentation of Psychiatric Symptomatology in Primary Care

The presentation of psychiatric symptoms in primary care raises at least four issues. First, in primary care, psychiatric symptoms often present intermixed with an array of somatic and psychological symptoms that are not part of the established criteria for the patient's actual mental disorder diagnosis and that may mask or obscure it. Second, the presentations of some mental disorder diagnoses, well described in psychiatric settings, may be different in primary care. Third, a significant number of patients have mental disorder symptoms accompanied by social or occupational dysfunction but do not meet either the duration criteria or the severity criteria for any officially recognized psychiatric disorder. Fourth, primary care physicians in both rural and urban areas often take care of patients from diverse cultural backgrounds who have ways of expressing emotional distress that may differ significantly from behavioral patterns in the dominant culture, from which many of

Note: Preparation of this chapter was supported in part by National Institute of Mental Health grant R01 MH45750.

the diagnostic criteria have been derived. Each of these aspects in turn has implications for future primary care mental health research, including new nosologies (or classification systems), new instrumentation, new research methods, and perhaps new approaches to research funding.

Mixing and Masking Mental Disorder Symptoms

Panic disorder, depression, and mixed anxiety-depression are three of the mental disorders that can present in primary care settings with prominent symptoms that hinder rather than aid the diagnosis of the underlying mental disorder. While medical and psychiatric comorbidity also play a part in the often confusing presentations of mental disorders in primary care (Schulberg, McClelland, & Burns, 1987), this discussion will only focus on symptoms believed to originate from the primary mental disorders themselves.

Panic Disorder

Panic disorder is notorious for its frequent presentation with somatic symptoms that often involve multiple organ systems and that are dramatic enough to bring the patient to a hospital emergency room or to the primary care physician's office for relief and reassurance (Grant, Katon, & Beitman, 1983). The public health significance of panic disorder is demonstrated by its lifetime prevalence of from 1.6 to 2.0 percent (Wittchen, 1986; Canino et al., 1987), its significant functional morbidity (Markowitz, Weissman, Ouellette, Lish, & Klerman, 1989), and the 20 percent suicide attempt rate of its sufferers (Weissman, Klerman, Markowitz, & Ouellette, 1989). The prevalence of panic disorder in primary care may be as high as 6 to 10 percent (Ballenger, 1987). Its frequent somatic symptoms—particularly chest pain, tachycardia, shortness of breath, and diaphoresis (Grant et al., 1983; Katon, 1990)—present so acutely and dramatically that the physician must evaluate the patient for multiple and possibly life-threatening medical conditions. Acute myocardial infarction, congestive heart failure, thyroid disorders, pulmonary embolism, and asthma are notable examples (Raj & Sheehan, 1987). This confusing presentation of psychiatric symptoms intermixed with serious somatic symptoms feeds into the primarily biomedical model of Western medicine, in which somatic symptoms drive diagnostic evaluations. As a result of this approach, panic disorder frequently goes unrecognized. The potential magnitude of this problem is revealed in one study of 100 panic disorder patients in which 70 percent had seen at least ten physicians for their panic symptoms before receiving a correct diagnosis (Sheehan, Ballenger, & Jacobsen, 1980).

To competently study the diagnosis and management of panic disorder in primary care, investigators should be familiar with the pathophysiology and symptomatology of panic disorder and the processes by which it is diagnosed or not diagnosed in the primary care setting.

Depression

Depression is another prevalent mental disorder in primary care settings that can be masked by somatic symptoms. Lesse (1983) described masked depression as a state closely resembling depression in which the patient does not express the overt symptoms of "sadness, melancholy, dejection, despair, despondency, or gloominess" usually associated with depression. These patients instead complain of many of the nonmood symptoms of depression and also manifest a large number of hypochondriacal, psychosomatic, or somatic symptoms, most of which do not respond to somatic treatments (Lesse, 1968, 1980, 1983). Lesse (1983) asserted that masked depression was responsive to tricyclic antidepressant therapy and was the most common type of depression seen by nonpsychiatric physicians. Barrett, Barrett, Oxman, and Gerber (1988), using stricter research criteria requiring impairment of social or occupational functioning attributable to the patients' symptoms, supported Lesse's assertion that masked depression was the most common type of depression in nonpsychiatry practice. In a rural internal medicine practice, they found that 6.4 percent of the patients had masked depression, as compared to the next most common depressive diagnoses, mixed anxiety-depression (4.1 percent), episodic minor depression (3.6 percent), and both treated and untreated major depression (2.2 percent).

A series of studies in family practice settings in Iowa found that depressed patients demonstrated a significant increase in the frequency of office visits, pain complaints, functional complaints, and anxiety symptoms in the period approximately seven months prior to the diagnosis of a depressive episode (Wilson, Widmer, Cadoret, & Judiesch, 1983; Cadoret, Widmer, & Troughton, 1980; Widmer & Cadoret, 1979).

Bridges and Goldberg (1985) showed that, of British general practice patients with undiagnosed mental disorders, 53 percent were somatizers. In a later study (Goldberg & Bridges, 1988), these investigators found that patients with DMS-III diagnoses presented to their general practitioners for care with somatic complaints 80 percent of the time.

Katon and Russo (1989) studied 197 medical patients. They determined that, of those patients with major depression, 50 percent of men and 42 percent of women met abridged criteria for somatization disorder (Escobar, Burnam, Karno, Forsythe, & Golding, 1987). Katon and Russo concluded that major depression, rather than somatoform disorders, is associated with the somatization seen in primary care patients. However, their heterogeneous sample of referred patients from a variety of specialized pain and chronic medical condition clinics and inpatient wards may have resulted in an overestimate of the magnitude of this problem, because most of these patients had disorders strongly linked to depression and somatization.

Finally, in a review of the literature on somatic presentations of psychiatric illness in primary care settings, Goldberg and Bridges (1988) stated that somatization is the most common reason that psychiatric illness goes unrecognized in general medical settings.

The importance of unexplained somatic symptoms in primary care must be addressed if patients with masked or early depression are to be identified, adequately studied, and treated. Research designs in primary care settings should not use traditional psychiatric diagnoses but rather should take into account the role somatic symptoms play in the presentation of depression (American Psychiatric Association, 1987). Precautions should be taken to obtain true primary care samples and to avoid samples of convenience that may not be representative of primary care.

This brief review of somatic symptoms and depression must

end with one caveat that is particularly important in the primary care setting. Many patients presenting with the somatic complaints of a bona fide medical illness are also depressed (Goldberg & Bridges, 1988; Bridges & Goldberg, 1985). And not all the somatic complaints of patients with depression in primary care are secondary to their depressions. There is great potential for a depressive disorder to mask an underlying medical diagnosis—a fact that investigators and clinicians working in this area should never lose sight of.

Mixed Anxiety-Depression

Reviews of the literature discuss the various merits of classification of anxiety and depression as secondary or primary, or as mixed syndromes in psychiatric populations (Stavrakaki & Vargo, 1986; Katshnig, Nutzinger, David, & Nouzak, 1986; Winokur, 1988; Liebowitz et al., 1990). However, little data exist on mixed anxiety-depression in primary care settings, where its presentation is likely to be quite different than in a referral psychiatric or mental health clinic.

Any observer of primary care physicians' chart notations will uncover the difficulty inherent in making a precise diagnosis of anxiety or depression in the primary care setting: a large number of patients with psychiatric symptoms will have notations of some variation of "anxiety-depression" or "depression-anxiety." Two family practice and general practice studies of the General Health Questionnaire in primary care found that, of those patients with recognized mental disorders, 31 percent and 68 percent were classified by clinicians and investigators as having mixed anxiety-depression (Goldberg, 1979). One study in an internal medicine setting showed 25 percent of all patients to have significant coexistent anxiety and depression symptoms (Walker, Novack, Brynes, & Kaiser, 1982). Barrett et al. (1988) used Research Diagnostic Criteria (Spitzer, Endicott, & Robins, 1978) for mixed anxiety-depression and found a prevalence of 4.1 percent in a rural internal medicine group practice. In a study of twenty-five general practices in the Netherlands, Ormel et al. (1990) determined that 4.9 percent of the patients had depression and anxiety symptoms.

The phenomenon of mixed "anxiety-depression" is a genuine concern for primary care physicians that the DSM-III-R does not address. Research into the recognition and management of mental disorders in primary care should not take place without a knowledge of diagnostic groups used by primary clinicians such as anxiety-depression. Efforts to improve recognition may need to include attempts to distinguish anxiety from depression in the clinical interview and to develop coherent ways of handling mixed states that do not depend on one or more of the symptom complexes meeting criteria for major disorders.

Comparisons Between Primary Care and Psychiatry

Few studies directly compare primary care patients to psychiatry outpatients with the same disorders using defined and reproducible diagnostic criteria. Sireling, Freeling, Paykel, and Rao (1985) compared eighty-three newly referred outpatient psychiatry patients with depression to fifty-three general practice patients with major depression who were treated with tricyclic antidepressants. The psychiatry patients were more likely than the general practice major depressives to have primary depressions (that is, with no previous history of another diagnosis), endogenous depressions, and retarded depressions. They were also more likely to have simple depression (no other diagnosis in the previous year) and situational depression (depression related to external events).

Coulehan, Schulberg, Block, and Zettler-Segal (1988) compared twenty-one major depressives (according to DSM-III-R criteria) drawn from primary medical care centers and sixty-six major depressives from community mental health centers and found that the primary care group was more likely to be black, unmarried, and of lower income than the community mental health group. There were no differences by age, gender, education, depression screening scores, social adjustment, or use of mental health facilities or medical physicians in the prior six months. With the exception of a greater frequency of loss of libido in the community mental health group, a comparison of DSM-III-R symptoms of major depression revealed no differences in the frequency of affective, neurovegetative, and cognitive symptoms. Finally, there was no difference in current somatic symptoms between the two groups.

In a comparison of seven major depressives (by DSM-III criteria) in a family practice site to thirty-eight major depressives in a psychiatry outpatient clinic, Williamson and Yates (1989) found that only the frequency of psychomotor retardation, indecisiveness, and a feeling of worthlessness were more prevalent in the psychiatry outpatient group. A history of depression, other psychiatric history, or a family history of depression was higher in the psychiatry patients (50 to 55 percent) than in the depressed family practice patients (29 percent), though this was not significant statistically. Family practice patients had a significantly higher mean number of chronic diseases (2.6 medical disorders) than the psychiatry patients (0.8). The depressed family practice patients initially presented with vaguer complaints such as "physical exam, general yuck, hurt finger," while the psychiatric patients' initial presentations were more psychologically focused or identifiable as potentially psychiatric—"depressed, anxious, confused, can't cope." A standardized general review of medical symptoms showed no difference in the number of symptoms between the depressed family practice and depressed psychiatry patients. Though the mean scores for the severity of depression were similar and not significantly different, the clinical impressions of the investigators were that, with the exception of one family practice patient severely ill with rheumatoid arthritis, the family practice patients were *less* severely depressed.

The potential differences in severity, demographic profile, and presentation between primary care and psychiatric depressions demonstrated by these three studies may affect research on these disorders in primary care. Even if diagnostic standards are kept the same as in these examples, screening criteria, sampling criteria, and parameters to follow for clinical outcomes may be altered by a knowledge of the disorders' characteristics in primary care settings. Further research comparing the natural history of mental disorders in primary care and psychiatry settings is needed.

Syndromal Symptoms

The DSM-III-R and its predecessors tend to reflect the symptom presentations of a patient population that is more severely ill and has a more classical presentation than patients seen in primary care. Primary care presentations of less-well-defined and milder symptom complexes have been given a variety of labels, including "minor," "subthreshold," "subsyndromal," "subclinical," "subdefinitional," and "symptoms without disorder." None adequately describes this group of syndromes, yet the terms appear to have developed because the predominant classification system in the United States—the DSM-III-R—does not recognize them as discrete disorders.

Minor Depression

Physicians working in primary care settings often prescribe tricyclic drugs for patients whom they diagnose as depressed but who do not meet DSM-III-R criteria (Broadhead, Clapp-Channing, Finch, & Copeland, 1989; Tollefson, Hughes, Derro, Teubner-Rhodes, & Tuason, 1983; Sireling, Paykel, Freeling, & Rao, 1985). Perhaps these cases of depression only appear to not meet diagnostic criteria and are actually cases of major depression that have been misdiagnosed for lack of a rigorous diagnostic interview by the physician. We have few data on this hypothesis beyond conjecture. On the other hand, the hypothesis that a minor or subsyndromal level of depression exists is becoming well documented.

Snaith (1987) made a careful argument for the concept of mild depression, a disorder that he felt general practitioners were more likely to treat. He argued for criteria that would distinguish mild or minor depression from other mild depressive syndromes that might fall under the DSM-III-R residual category of Depressive Disorder Not Otherwise Specified, to which minor depression is currently relegated. New criteria would aid in the diagnosis of mild depressions and might facilitate research to provide guidance on when these patients would need treatment and what forms of treatment would work best. Several such criteria have been proposed, including Research Diagnostic Criteria (Spitzer et al., 1978). These criteria generally include depressed mood or anhedonia and one or more additional depressive symptoms of two weeks or more duration in a patient who does not meet criteria for major depression, dysthymia, or adjustment disorder with depressed mood.

Using criteria similar to those Snaith has proposed, other

investigators have documented the prevalence of a syndrome of minor depression in both epidemiologic surveys (Broadhead, Blazer, George, & Tse, 1990; Myers & Weissman, 1980; Blazer, Hughes, & George, 1987; Blazer & Williams, 1980; Blazer et al., 1989) and primary care settings. The prevalence of Research Diagnostic Criteria minor depression in primary care settings has ranged from 3.4 to 5.4 percent versus a prevalence of 2.2 to 5.8 percent for major depression (Hoeper, Nycz, Cleary, Regier, & Goldberg, 1979; Blacker, Clare, & Thomas, 1987; Barrett et al., 1988). In one study using the Present State Examination, "borderline depression" or "minor depression" was present at a prevalence of 1.9 versus 2.3 percent for major depression (Ormel et al., 1990).

Does "subsyndromal" or "minor depression" result in a significant impairment of functioning in the patients' everyday lives? Wells, Stewart, and Hays (1989) found that patients with depressive symptoms (but not major depression) had, on the average, worse physical, social, and role functioning, more sickbed days, and poorer well-being than other medical patients without chronic conditions. They were worse off than the patients in seven chronic disease groups on all these parameters. Only patients with advanced coronary heart disease scored more poorly. Broadhead et al. (1990) uncovered a similar higher rate of disability days in persons with minor depression over persons without depressive symptoms.

Minor depression is a syndrome that may have multiple etiologies, but its high prevalence in primary care and its significant morbidity make it a potentially large clinical problem. Treatment has not been established. Hence great opportunity exists for research on this syndrome to determine its causes and correlates and to evaluate potential primary care treatments. But a major stumbling block to research in this area is the lack of a currently acceptable and standardized nosology that would permit findings to be compared across studies.

Mixed Anxiety-Depression and Masked-Depression

Mixed anxiety-depression and masked depression were discussed earlier. While masked depression is almost by definition "subsyndromal," depending on the definition, mixed anxiety-depression may fall into the subsyndromal category if both its depression and anxiety components do not meet DSM-III-R criteria. Again, the point for the primary care mental health researcher or clinician is that these are incompletely described but discernible entities. They are not adequately addressed by the existing official nosologies, and standardized assessment instruments are not yet available for them. New nosologies and instruments are necessary for the study of these two common syndromes in primary care.

Brief Recurrent Depression

Angst, Merikangas, Scheidegger, and Wicki (1990) have described a syndrome of depression with symptom and impairment criteria identical to those of major depression, but requiring one or two distinct episodes per month for over one year. The community prevalence of 7 percent, the degree of social and work impairment similar to major depression, and the suicide attempt rate of 11.4 versus 7.7 percent for major depression indicate that brief recurrent depression—though "subdefinitional" with respect to DSM-III-R—is not a minor disorder but one that may have significant impact on primary care. Only further research with this syndrome will determine its validity in the clinical setting of primary care. A study of brief recurrent depression in a primary care setting to establish prevalence, levels of impairment, and medical comorbidity would be a reasonable next step.

Panic Disorder Versus Panic Symptoms

The prevalence, presentations, and morbidity of panic disorder have been discussed earlier in this chapter (Markowitz et al., 1989); panic attacks without the disorder present similar problems. The community prevalence of panic attacks that do not meet criteria for panic disorder is from 2.3 to 4.5 percent versus 1.5 to 1.6 percent for panic disorder (Klerman, Weissman, Ouellette, Johnson, & Greenwald, 1991). In one family practice setting, the prevalence of panic attacks was 8.7 versus 16 percent for panic disorder (Katon, Vitaliano, Russo, Jones, & Anderson, 1987). Persons with panic attacks have fewer mean panic symptoms than those with panic disorder—

4.7 versus 7.3—which may hamper recognition. But they are just as likely to have agoraphobia and major depression. Persons with panic attacks are almost as likely as those with panic disorder to report a feeling of poor health; to make emergency room visits, office visits to nonpsychiatric physicians, or psychiatric visits; to use minor tranquilizers, sleeping pills, or antidepressants; and to be admitted to general hospitals or psychiatric hospitals for emotional problems. People with panic attacks are also more likely than controls to be financially dependent and unemployed and not looking for work due to their emotional problems (Klerman et al., 1991). While individuals with panic disorder have a 20 percent lifetime prevalence for suicide attempts, this rate is 12 percent in patients with panic attacks (Weissman et al., 1989). Katon et al. (1987) found that panic disorder patients had coexisting major depressions 75 percent of the time, compared to 46 percent of those with panic attacks. Panic disorder patients had an average of 4.8 phobias and panic attack patients had 3.3; both were significantly different from controls (1.2 phobias). In addition, the persons with panic attacks scored similarly to those with panic disorder on a battery of psychological and functional status questionnaires.

The current criteria for panic disorder have been derived from the symptoms of patients in a specialty setting. Yet patients with less severe symptoms have noticeable impairment in their psychological, physical, financial, and social lives. If we are to study mental disorders in primary care settings, we must adapt and/or develop methods for this patient population.

Somatization Syndromes in Primary Care

Several studies support the existence of a syndrome of somatization below the current threshold of thirteen symptoms of the DSM-III-R. Escobar et al. (1987) found that respondents who met abridged criteria for somatization (four symptoms for males and six symptoms for females) when compared to controls were heavier users of health services, preferred medical over psychiatric sources of care, and were more likely to report recent sick leave or restricted activity. DeGruy, Columbia, and Dickinson (1987), using "borderline somatization disorder" criteria of ten or more symptoms, found a prevalence in a family practice setting of 4 percent. These patients were more likely than controls to live in households with children but no spouse, to be in the lower social classes, and to have 50 percent more office visits and total charges, thicker and heavier charts, and almost 70 percent more medical diagnoses than controls. Katon et al. (1987) found similar evidence for a "spectrum of severity" below the threshold for somatization disorder, but with significant impairment, comorbidity with depression, and health care utilization.

Despite these findings of morbidity in patients with "subthreshold" somatization disorder, the usefulness of abridged criteria is questionable given the high prevalence of major depression in primary care patients who meet these criteria (Katon & Russo, 1989), the observation that somatic symptoms serve as a "harbinger" of depression (Wilson et al., 1983), and the major role of somatic symptoms in masking depression (Bridges & Goldberg, 1985). Next steps in this area might include longitudinal follow-up of patients with various levels of somatization symptoms who are not depressed and treatment trials of those who are depressed to see to what extent these syndromes are or are not interrelated.

Cultural Issues

The presentation of mental disorders varies across cultures (Kleinman, 1980; Marsella, Sartorius, Jablensky, & Fenton, 1985; Binitie, 1975; Ebigno, 1982; Marsella, 1987). Primary care physicians often serve immigrant and minority populations in rural areas and the inner city and tend to learn cross-cultural approaches to psychiatry from their patients or from older colleagues, if they are lucky. Sensitivity to cross-cultural differences will make future primary care mental health research relevant to a significant and growing proportion of our society that does not always express mental disorders in the same fashion as does the dominant culture. The dominant culture, we should remember, developed both the currently accepted diagnostic criteria (DSM-III-R) and the scientific literature on which the U.S. Public Health Service Agency for Health Care Policy and Research will base its guidelines for therapy.

Susto

Susto is a folk illness of Latino peoples resembling a mental disorder (Trotter, 1985). It is common throughout Latin America, in the Southwestern states of Arizona, New Mexico, and Texas (Trotter, 1985), and in Cuban refugee camps in the United States (Foreman, 1985). *Susto* means fright; within its cultural context, the illness is believed to result from frightening or traumatic experiences that dislodge the soul from the body. The afflicted individual, or *asustado,* suffers a myriad of symptoms that overlap the Western syndromes of anxiety, depression, and somatization but are diagnostic of none. The *asustado* may report anorexia, weight loss, debility (Collado-Ardon, Rubel, O'Nell, & Murray, 1983), nighttime insomnia, daytime drowsiness, irritability, exaggerated startle reflex, diarrhea, depression (Trotter, 1985), restlessness, and sudden, spontaneous outbursts of hysteria and fainting (Foreman, 1985). In a seven-year study (Rubel & O'Nell, 1979; Collado-Ardon et al., 1983; Rubel, O'Nell, & Collado-Ardon, 1991), fifty ambulatory *asustados* in three Mexican communities were compared to ambulatory adult patient controls matched by age, gender, and community affiliation. The *asustados* suffered higher levels of social stress but similar levels of psychological symptoms. Nevertheless, they were more likely to receive an emotional disorder diagnosis from the study physicians than the controls. The *asustados* had more medical illnesses and more severe and life-threatening illnesses than controls. Eight of forty-seven (17 percent) *asustados* died after seven years, while none of the controls died.

The prevalence of *susto* is as high as 10 percent in susceptible populations. Efforts by Western medicine to treat it are unsuccessful, yet the culture from which it is derived can offer an etiology, a diagnosis, preventive measures, and therapy (Foreman, 1985). While milder cases may be treated at home by a family member, more severe cases may require the services of a *curandero* or folk healer (Trotter, 1985). Treatments may involve heat, massage, bed rest, drug therapies including hallucinogens, sweeping the body with a branch of herbs, prayers combined with the patient calling out for the soul to return, and finally a recitation of the details of the event suspected of causing the soul to leave the body (Klein, 1978; Foreman, 1985; Trotter, 1985).

Primary care investigators interested in the mental health of Latinos must be aware of the existence of *susto* and the culture that affects the patients' conceptualizations of the illness and their approaches to treating it. Standardized ways of diagnosing this syndrome are necessary before it can be reliably studied. The natural history of *susto* and its treatment in the United States need further evaluation.

Somatization in African Americans

Rates of depression are reported as lower in blacks than whites (Somervell, Leaf, Weissman, Blazer, & Bruce, 1989). However, they are based on diagnoses dependent largely on psychological symptoms (DSM-III-R) and not on the somatic symptoms that predominate in the presentation of depression in African Americans as well as others who have non-Western cultural roots (Kleinman, 1980; Marsella, Sartorius, Jablensky, & Fenton, 1985; Binitie, 1975; Ebigno, 1982; Marsella, 1987; Miller, Knapp, & Daniels, 1968; Simon, Fleiss, Gurland, & Stiller, 1973). Broadhead and Reinhard (1991) found that depressed African Americans in a rural North Carolina family practice had similar rates of somatic symptoms to whites but had significantly fewer of the psychological symptoms necessary to make a diagnosis of depression. Furthermore, as discussed above, the presence of somatic symptoms decreases the likelihood of depression being diagnosed (Bridges & Goldberg, 1985). These factors make it likely that many blacks with depression are in fact undiagnosed and may be seeking care for somatic symptoms that cannot be alleviated without recognition and treatment of their depression.

Are current criteria (DSM-III-R) appropriate for diagnosing depression in rural African Americans? Helzer et al. (1985) have shown that most people who missed the diagnosis of major depression in a validity study of the Diagnostic Interview Schedule (Robins, Helzer, Croughan, & Ratcliff, 1981) missed it by only one symptom. This suggests that the demarcation between those with and without major depression is not distinct, as the DSM-III-R would suggest. Patients with the same disorder who somatize and do not psychologize may simply miss being diagnosed as depressed under the current nosology. Primary care investigators must evaluate the appropriateness of their methods and measurements to the cultures of their research subjects. Only then will research on African Americans or other groups with similar expressions of emotional distress be useful and relevant to their health care.

"Nerves"

"Nerves" is a frequent complaint of patients visiting medical practices in the Southeastern United States. As Nations, Camino, and Walker (1988) point out, this is not simple nervousness but an ethnomedical complaint associated with significant anxiety, depression, and disability. They describe "nerves" as follows: "The acute attack is described as a wave of tension which breaks over the patient in a fit of body shaking and quivering, stomach pains and nausea, headaches, heart tremors, shortness of breath, chest pains, dizziness, trembling in the extremities, blurred vision, and hot flashes; it then calms into a state of lethargy, sadness, tension, insomnia, and feelings of weariness, of weight pressing on the chest, arms, and head, and obsessive worrying" (p. 1248). When compared to controls, patients with "nerves" had higher Holmes-Rahe stress scores (187 versus 119), higher Beck Depression Inventory scores (7.6 versus 2.5), and higher scores on the General Health Questionnaire (13.0 versus 5.8).

Nations et al. (1988) believe that these patients would fall under the DSM-III-R category of Depressive Disorder Not Otherwise Specified if a diagnosis were made. Unfortunately, conventional clinicians evaluate symptoms for potential medical ailments; finding none, they leave these patients with the message that nothing is wrong. The patients then frequently seek out the help and guidance of a variety of lay healers, ranging from lay ministers to readers and advisers. These individuals offer an unorthodox form of social support and fairly sophisticated supportive counseling, which provides some relief from the patient's symptoms but no cure.

Investigators of mental disorders in primary care must be

aware of ethnomedical disorders, of which "nerves" is only one. While some of these may be classifiable as variants of DSM-III-R disorders, their existence as illnesses within the culture may affect their presentation, the patients' compliance with therapy, and the patients' participation in alternative therapies—all of which are ripe for further investigation.

Conclusion

The presentations of mental disorders in primary care are clearly different than in psychiatry. This must affect the primary care mental health researcher's approach to this population. Most mental health researchers in primary care settings are not primary care clinicians. The investigator without clinical experience in primary care should consider the primary care experience of others in order to improve the likelihood of valid or generalizable research findings. This may take place, for example, through the input of practicing primary care clinicians on the research team.

Some of the specific issues before primary care mental health investigators are the following: (1) the problem of traditional diagnostic criteria for mental disorders being confounded by symptoms of physical conditions, (2) the potential for different presentations of a single psychiatric disorder in primary care setting vis-à-vis outpatient or inpatient psychiatry, (3) the existence of syndromes that do not meet diagnostic criteria for any specific disorders in the current nosology but that are accompanied by significant morbidity, and (4) the existence of folk illnesses or ethnomedical complaints that are likely to appear in primary care physicians' offices.

A knowledge of the unique issues surrounding the presentation of mental disorders in primary care necessitates that primary care researchers design realistic and appropriate sampling methods to capture most of those suffering from a disorder that has a different presentation and may even involve different referral patterns and help-seeking behavior (for example, panic disorder or masked depression) than in psychiatry. Study instrumentation—whether it be through structured lay interviews like the Diagnostic Interview Schedule (Robins et al., 1981) or clinical interviews—must be adapted to reflect the "subsyndromal" syndromes and their apparent morbidity before their validity as clinical entities in primary care can be fully evaluated. Finally, we should acknowledge that we live in a multicultural society and are obligated to listen to what our patients tell us. Neither as clinicians nor as researchers should we shove a symptom into one pigeonhole when the patient intends it for another.

A primary care nosology could facilitate this research. The Primary Care version of the DSM-IV was developed by the American Psychiatric Association to serve this purpose. Field trials to evaluate and standardize this nosology are needed. Such syndromes as masked depression and folk illnesses should not be shrugged off as irrelevant because they are not recognized by the currently accepted nosology. Rather, these syndromes should be teased apart so that we may develop a better understanding of their presentations and natural history. This may require something akin to a paradigm shift (Kuhn, 1970), in which members of the study sections that approve funding for mental health research begin to accept the desirability of changing the current research nosologies and of investigating phenomena using research methods that may be unique to the primary care milieu.

This teasing apart or dissection of primary care presentations may not only require comparisons of associated features (for example, occurrence and frequency of symptoms), functional status, health care utilization, and mortality rates to evaluate the degree of their clinical relevance. Depending on their severity, it might also be desirable to pursue a biological approach to sort out possible etiologies, mechanisms of action affecting their presentation, and the interrelationships of these disorders. This research might include family history and genetic linkage studies (Hill, Wilson, Elston, & Winokur, 1988), a variety of provocative endocrine tests (Kathol, Sherman, Winokur, Lewis, & Schlesser, 1983), electroencephalography (Lewis & Winokur, 1983), hematological markers (Kronfol, Turner, Nasrallah, & Winokur, 1984), platelet [3H]-imipramine binding, and nuclear magnetic resonance imaging (Husain et al., 1991). Finally, primary care mental health investigators should consider employing ethnographic or qualitative techniques to help us identify the pertinent research questions and perhaps help us develop approaches that more accurately reflect the circumstances of our patients' lives. Just as the primary care mental health researcher from a non-primary care discipline must adapt to the primary care environment to understand the presentations of mental disorders in primary care, all researchers in primary care mental health may need to reach into other disciplines (biological psychiatry, cultural anthropology, and others) to learn what these presentations mean.

References

American Psychiatric Association. (1987). *Diagnostic and statistical manual of mental disorders* (3rd ed., rev.). Washington, DC: Author.

Angst, J., Merikangas, K., Scheidegger, P., & Wicki, W. (1990). Recurrent brief depression: A new subtype of affective disorder. *Journal of Affective Disorders, 19,* 87–98.

Ballenger, J. C. (1987). Unrecognized prevalence of panic disorder in primary care, internal medicine, and cardiology. *American Journal of Cardiology, 60,* 39J–47J.

Barrett, J. E., Barrett, J. A., Oxman, T. E., & Gerber, P. D. (1988). The prevalence of psychiatric disorders in a primary care practice. *Archives of General Psychiatry, 45,* 1100–1106.

Binitie, A. (1975). A factor-analytical study of depression across cultures (Africa and Europe). *British Journal of Psychiatry, 127,* 559–563.

Blacker, C. V., Clare, A. W., & Thomas, J. (1987). *Depression in primary care.* Paper presented at Mental Disorders in General Health Care Settings Research Conference, Seattle, WA.

Blazer, D., Hughes, D. C., & George, L. K. (1987). The epidemiology of depression in an elderly community population. *Gerontologist, 27,* 281–287.

Blazer, D., & Williams, C. D. (1980). Epidemiology of dysphoria and depression in an elderly population. *American Journal of Psychiatry, 137,* 439–444.

Blazer, D., Woodbury, S., Hughes, D. C., George, L. K., Manton, K. G., Bachar, J. R., & Fowler, N. (1989). A statistical analysis of the classification of depression in a mixed community and clinical sample. *Journal of Affective Disorders, 16,* 11–20.

Bridges, K. W., & Goldberg, D. P. (1985). Somatic presentation of DSM-III psychiatric disorders in primary care. *Journal of Psychosomatic Research, 29,* 563–569.

Broadhead, W. E., Blazer, D. G., George, L. K., & Tse, C. K. (1990). Depression, disability days, and days lost from work in a prospective epidemiologic survey. *Journal of the American Medical Association, 264*(19), 2524–2528.

Broadhead, W. E., Clapp-Channing, N. E., Finch, J. N., & Copeland, J. A. (1989). Effects of medical illness and somatic symptoms on treatment of depression in a family medicine residency practice. *General Hospital Psychiatry, 11,* 194–200.

Broadhead, W. E., & Reinhard, C. G. (1991, September). *Somatic symptoms of depression in black and white patients in a rural North Carolina family practice.* Paper presented at the Classification and Treatment of Mental Disorders in General Medical Settings Research Conference, Bethesda, MD.

Cadoret, R. J., Widmer, R. B., & Troughton, E. P. (1980). Somatic complaints—harbinger of depression in primary care. *Journal of Affective Disorders, 2,* 61–70.

Canino, G. J., Bird, H. R., Shrout, P. E., Rubio-Stipec, M., Bravo, M., Martinez, R., & Sesman, M. (1987). The prevalence of specific psychiatric disorders in Puerto Rico. *Archives of General Psychiatry, 44,* 727–735.

Collado-Ardon, R., Rubel, A. J., O'Nell, C. W., & Murray, R. H. (1983). A folk illness (Susto) as an indicator of real illness. *Lancet, 2,* 1362.

Coulehan, J. L., Schulberg, H. C., Block, M. R., & Zettler-Segal, M. (1988). Symptom patterns of depression in ambulatory medical and psychiatric patients. *Journal of Nervous and Mental Disease, 176*(5), 284–288.

deGruy, F., Columbia, L., & Dickinson, P. (1987). Somatization disorder in a family practice. *Journal of Family Practice, 25,* 45–51.

Ebigno, P. (1982). Development of a culture-specific screening scale of somatic complaints indicating psychiatric disturbance. *Culture in Medicine and Psychiatry, 6,* 29–43.

Escobar, J. I., Burnam, M. A., Karno, M., Forsythe, A., & Golding,

J. M. (1987). Somatization in the community. *Archives of General Psychiatry, 44,* 713–718.

Escobar, J. I., Golding, J. M., Hough, R. L., Karno, M., Burnam, M. A., & Wells, K. B. (1987). Somatization in the community: Relationship to disability and use of services. *American Journal of Public Health, 77,* 837–840.

Foreman, J. T. (1985). Susto and the health needs of the Cuban refugee population. *Topics in Clinical Nursing, 7,* 40–47.

Goldberg, D. (1979). Detection and assessment of emotional disorders in primary-care setting. *International Journal of Mental Health, 8,* 30–48.

Goldberg, D. P., & Bridges, K. (1988). Somatic presentations of psychiatric illness in primary care settings. *Journal of Psychosomatic Research, 32*(2), 137–144.

Grant, B., Katon, W., & Beitman, B. (1983). Panic disorder. *Journal of Family Practice, 5,* 907–914.

Helzer, J. E., Robins, L. N., McEvoy, L. T., Spitznagel, E. L., Stoltzman, R. K., Farmer, A., & Brockington, I. F. (1985). A comparison of clinical and Diagnostic Interview Schedule diagnoses: Physician reexamination of lay-interviewed cases in the general population. *Archives of General Psychiatry, 42,* 657–666.

Hill, E. M., Wilson, A. F., Elston, R. C., & Winokur, G. (1988). Evidence for possible linkage between genetic markers and affective disorders. *Society of Biological Psychiatry, 24,* 903–917.

Hoeper, E. W., Nycz, G. R., Cleary, P. D., Regier, D. A., & Goldberg, I. D. (1979). Estimated prevalence of RDC mental disorders in primary medical care. *International Journal of Mental Health, 8,* 6–15.

Husain, M. M., Knight, D. L., Doraiswamy, P. M., Figiel, G. S., McDonald, W. M., Boyko, O. B., Krishnan, K. R., & Nemeroff, C. B. (1991). Platelet [3H]-imipramine binding and leukoencephalopathy in geriatric depression. *Biological Psychiatry, 29*(7), 665–670.

Kathol, R. G., Sherman, B. M., Winokur, G., Lewis, D., & Schlesser, M. (1983). Dexamethasone suppression, protirelin stimulation, and insulin infusion in subtypes of recovered depressive patients. *Psychiatry Research, 9,* 99–106.

Katon, W. (1990). Chest pain, cardiac disease, and panic disorder. *Journal of Clinical Psychiatry, 51*(Suppl. 5), 27–30.

Katon, W., & Russo, J. (1989). Somatic symptoms and depression. *Journal of Family Practice, 29,* 65–69.

Katon, W., Vitaliano, P. P., Russo, J., Jones, M., & Anderson, K. (1987). Panic disorder: Spectrum of severity and somatization. *Journal of Nervous and Mental Disease, 175,* 12–19.

Katshnig, H., Nutzinger, D., David, H. P., & Nouzak, A. (1986). Anxiety and the clinical course of depression. *Clinical Neuropharmacology, 9,* 146–148.

Klein, J. (1978). Susto: The anthropological study of diseases of adaptation. *Social Science and Medicine, 12,* 23–28.

Kleinman, A. (1980). *Patients and healers in the context of culture.* Berkeley: University of California Press.

Klerman, G. L., Weissman, M. M., Ouellette, R., Johnson, J., & Greenwald, S. (1991). Panic attacks in the community: Social morbidity and health care utilization. *Journal of the American Medical Association, 265,* 742–746.

Kronfol, Z., Turner, R., Nasrallah, H., & Winokur, G. (1984). Leukocyte regulation in depression and schizophrenia. *Psychiatry Research, 13,* 13–18.

Kuhn, T. S. (1970). *The structure of scientific revolutions* (2nd ed.). Chicago: University of Chicago Press.

Lesse, S. (1968). Masked depression: A diagnostic and therapeutic problem. *Diseases of the Nervous System, 29,* 169–173.

Lesse, S. (1980). Masked depression: The ubiquitous but unappreciated syndrome. *Psychiatric Journal of the University of Ottawa, 5,* 269–273.

Lesse, S. (1983). The masked depression syndrome: Results of a seventeen-year clinical study. *American Journal of Psychotherapy, 37,* 456–475.

Lewis, D. A., & Winokur, G. (1983). The familial classification of primary unipolar depression: Biological variation of distinct subtypes. *Comprehensive Psychiatry, 24,* 495–501.

Liebowitz, M. R., Hollander, E., Schneier, F., Campeas, R., Fallon, B., Welkowitz, L., Cloitre, M., & Davies, S. (1990). Anxiety and depression: Discrete diagnostic entities? *Journal of Clinical Psychopharmacology, 10,* 61S–66S.

Markowitz, J. S., Weissman, M. M., Ouellette, R., Lish, J. D., & Klerman, G. L. (1989). Quality of life in panic disorder. *Archives of General Psychiatry, 46,* 984-992.

Marsella, A. J. (1987). *The measurement of depression: The measurement of depressive experience and disorder across cultures.* New York: Guilford Press.

Marsella, A. J., Sartorius, N., Jablensky, A., & Fenton, F. R. (1985). Cross-cultural studies of depressive disorders: An overview. In A. Kleinman & B. Good (Eds.), *Culture and depression: Studies in the anthropology and cross-cultural psychiatry of affect and disorder.* Berkeley: University of California Press.

Miller, C., Knapp, S. C., & Daniels, C. W. (1968). MMPI study of Negro mental hygiene clinic patients. *Journal of Abnormal Psychology, 73,* 168–173.

Myers, J. K., & Weissman, M. M. (1980). Use of a self-report symptom scale to detect depression in a community sample. *American Journal of Psychiatry, 137,* 1081–1084.

Nations, M. K., Camino, L. A., & Walker, F. B. (1988). "Nerves": Folk idiom for anxiety and depression. *Social Science and Medicine, 26,* 1245–1259.

Ormel, J., van den Brink, W., Koeter, M. W., Giel, R., van der Meer, K., van de Willige, G., & Wilmink, F. W. (1990). Recognition, management, and outcome of psychological disorders in primary care: A naturalistic follow-up study. *Psychological Medicine, 20,* 909-923.

Raj, A., & Sheehan, D. V. (1987). Medical evaluation of panic attacks. *Journal of Clinical Psychiatry, 48,* 309–313.

Robins, L. N., Helzer, J. E., Croughan, J., & Ratcliff, K. S. (1981). National Institute of Mental Health Diagnostic Interview Schedule: Its history, characteristics, and validity. *Archives of General Psychiatry, 38,* 381–389.

Rubel, A. J., & O'Nell, C. W. (1979). Difficulties of presenting complaints to physicians: Susto illness as an example. *Bulletin of the Pan American Health Organization, 13,* 134–138.

Rubel, A. J., O'Nell, C. W., & Collado-Ardon, R. (1991). *Susto: A folk illness.* Berkeley: University of California Press.

Schulberg, H. C., McClelland, M., & Burns, B. J. (1987). Depression and physical illness: The prevalence, causation, and diagnosis of comorbidity. *Clinical Psychology Review, 7,* 145–167.

Sheehan, D. V., Ballenger, J., & Jacobsen, G. (1980). Treatment of endogenous anxiety with phobic, hysterical, and hypochondriacal symptoms. *Archives of General Psychiatry, 37,* 51–59.

Simon, R. J., Fleiss, J. L., Gurland, B. J., & Stiller, P. R. (1973). Depression and schizophrenia in hospitalized black and white mental patients. *Archives of General Psychiatry, 28,* 509–512.

Sireling, L. I., Freeling, P., Paykel, E. S., & Rao, B. M. (1985). Depression in general practice: Clinical features and comparison with out-patients. *British Journal of Psychiatry, 147,* 119–126.

Sireling, L. I., Paykel, E. S., Freeling, P., & Rao, B. M. (1985). Depression in general practice: Case thresholds and diagnoses. *British Journal of Psychiatry, 147,* 113–119.

Snaith, R. P. (1987). The concepts of mild depression. *British Journal of Psychiatry, 150,* 387–393.

Somervell, P. D., Leaf, P. J., Weissman, M. M., Blazer, D. G., & Bruce, M. L. (1989). The prevalence of major depression in black and white adults in five United States communities. *American Journal of Epidemiology, 130,* 725–735.

Spitzer, R. L., Endicott, J., & Robins, E. (1978). Research diagnostic criteria: Rationale and reliability. *Archives of General Psychiatry, 35,* 773–782.

Stavrakaki, C., & Vargo, B. (1986). The relationship of anxiety and depression: A review of the literature. *British Journal of Psychiatry, 149,* 7–16.

Tollefson, G., Hughes, E., Derro, R. A., Teubner-Rhodes, D., & Tuason, V. (1983). Depressive syndromes in a primary care setting: Evaluation, classification, and outcome. *Comprehensive Psychiatry, 24,* 144–153.

Trotter, R. T. II. (1985). Folk medicine in the Southwest. *Postgraduate Medicine, 78,* 167–179.

Walker, F. B., Novack, D. H., Brynes, G., & Kaiser, D. L. (1982). Recognition of anxiety and depression by residents in a general medicine clinic. *Journal of Medical Education, 57,* 195–197.

Weissman, M. M., Klerman, G. L., Markowitz, J. S., & Ouellette, R. (1989). Suicidal ideation and suicide attempts in panic disorder and attacks. *New England Journal of Medicine, 321,* 1209–1214.

Wells, K. B., Stewart, A., & Hays, R. D. (1989). The functioning and well-being of depressed patients: Results of the Medical Outcomes Study. *Journal of the American Medical Association, 262,* 914–919.

Widmer, R. B., & Cadoret, R. J. (1979). Depression in family practice: Changes in pattern of patient visits and complaints during subsequent developing depression. *Journal of Family Practice, 9,* 1017–1021.

Williamson, P. S., & Yates, W. R. (1989). The initial presentation of depression in family practice and psychiatric outpatients. *General Hospital Psychiatry, 11*(3), 188–193.

Wilson, D. R., Widmer, R. B., Cadoret, R. J., & Judiesch, K. (1983). Somatic symptoms: A major feature of depression in family practice. *Journal of Affective Disorders, 5,* 199–207.

Winokur, G. (1988). Anxiety disorders: Relationships to other psychiatric illness. *Psychiatric Clinics of North America, 11,* 287–293.

Wittchen, H.-U. (1986). Epidemiology of panic attacks and panic disorders. In I. Hand & H.-U. Wittchen (Eds.), *Panic and phobias* (pp. 18–28). New York: Springer-Verlag.

Rolando Castillo
Howard Waitzkin
Javier I. Escobar

8

Somatic Symptoms and Mental Health Disorders in Immigrant and Refugee Populations

Culture and the language and idioms specific to that culture can be powerful forces shaping individuals' perceptions of their world and themselves. Language, in particular, can stand as a barrier to interactions among peoples of different ethnic and cultural backgrounds, not only because of the obvious issue of interpretability, but also because language circumscribes the cognitive choices an individual has to define and interpret life experiences (Angel & Thoits, 1987). In the context of health and mental health care, divergent cultural backgrounds between those seeking and those providing care can be a critical barrier to appropriate and timely treatment.

The issue of culture is particularly salient today, because changing sociodemographic conditions in the United States have

Note: This work was supported in part by grants from the National Institute of Mental Health (R01 MH47536) and the Health Resource and Services Administration (5 D28 PE 19154). We are indebted to members of the Primary Care Research Seminar at the University of California, Irvine, for constructive suggestions, and to Yvette Ramirez and Michelle Stone for help with manuscript preparation.

created new conditions for providing health and mental health services, especially in primary care. During the last decade, immigration to the United States from Mexico, other Latin American countries, and Southeast Asia has increased substantially. The Mexican community has increased by 56 percent since 1980; Latinos from El Salvador, Guatemala, and other Latin American countries have increased by 64 percent (Table 8.1). Even larger increases have occurred in the Asian population (U.S. Bureau of the Census, 1983, 1992). The majority of these immigrants have settled in California (Table 8.2).

Many immigrants from Central America and Southeast Asia come to this country as refugees from regions experiencing multiple economic and political changes due to war.* For example, El Salvador's civil war has displaced 10 percent of the population,

Table 8.1. Minority Groups in the United States, by Nationality.

	1980	*1990*	*Percent Change*
	Hispanics		
Mexican	8,678,632	13,495,938	56
Puerto Rican	2,004,961	2,727,754	37
Cuban	806,223	1,043,932	30
Other	3,113,867	5,086,435	64
	Asians		
Chinese	812,178	1,645,472	103
Filipino	781,894	1,406,770	77
Japanese	716,331	847,562	19
Asian Indian	387,223	815,447	111
Korean	357,393	798,849	124
Vietnamese	245,025	614,547	151

Source: Data from U.S. Bureau of the Census, 1983, 1992.

*For the purposes of this chapter, *refugees* are individuals who have emigrated from their home country because of severely stressful circumstances, including but not limited to war, torture, forced relocation, or similar changes that comprised extreme threats to safety or survival. *Immigrants* are individuals who have emigrated from their home country because of perceived economic advantages, professional advancement, desire to join other family members, or other reasons that did not involve extreme threats to safety or survival.

Table 8.2. Geographic Distribution of Refugees in the United States by Selected Settings in the Mid 1980s.

Setting	*Percentage of Total Southeast Asian Refugees*	*Percentage of Total Central American Refugees*
California	40.1	46.9
Florida	1.6	8.4
Illinois	3.3	3.8
Louisiana	1.9	9.4
Arizona	0.3	1.4
New York	3.5	9.4
Texas	7.2	11.3
Washington, DC	0.2	9.4
43 other states	41.9	
Total	100.0	100.0

Source: Data from Berryman & Berryman, 1988; Haines, 1989.

and between 750,000 and one million Salvadorans have fled their homeland (Aron, 1992). Nearly all Central American refugees experience difficulties acculturating to American society (Cervantes, Salgado de Snyder, & Padilla, 1989), and many have previously experienced warfare, political persecution, economic hardship, incarceration, or injury (Vargas, 1984). Southeast Asian refugees come not only with substantial premigration trauma, but also with limited prior exposure to Western culture, which may exacerbate their premigration trauma.

It is in this context that we examine mental health issues for immigrants and refugees in primary health care. But we set the stage by exploring the ways in which culture can affect the expression of mental disorders and the recognition and treatment of those disorders.

Cross-Cultural Issues in Treating Mental Disorders

Clark (1983) and Barker (1992) have articulated how culture affects medical care interactions and can impose barriers to appropriate and effective care when those seeking care and those providing it come from different backgrounds. They make five specific points.

The first two focus on recognition and treatment issues and the final three on how illnesses are defined and expressed.

First, language barriers and cultural differences in communication patterns can create obstacles in patient-practitioner interactions. For example, simply interpreting spoken language poses a challenge in primary care encounters. Lay interpreters who accompany monolingual patients often are family members or friends who lack training in procedures of accurate interpretation. In addition to having limited knowledge of medical terminology, lay interpreters may experience cultural inhibition or embarrassment in explaining patients' symptoms or in conveying practitioners' requests for information. Because of these difficulties, the participation of trained, professional interpreters is highly desirable but is frequently not feasible to obtain in primary care settings (Haffner, 1992; Hardt, 1991; Putsch, 1985).

Nonverbal communication barriers, based in cultural difference, also may impede patient-physician interaction. For instance, handshaking and smiling are viewed as highly desirable behaviors to be initiated by practitioners in Latino culture. On the other hand, similar behaviors may be experienced as inappropriate or offensive by Southeast Asian immigrants (Hoang & Erickson, 1982). In encounters with patients from a different culture, the impact of varying patterns of demeanor and decorum may prove difficult to predict for clinicians without prior knowledge of these patterns.

Second, cultural differences in medical roles and responsibilities can create a broad barrier in primary care encounters. For instance, a "lay referral system" for alternative forms of healing usually comprises an important part of a culture's approach to illness. Thus, medical practitioners treating Southeast Asian or Latino immigrants may remain unaware of or insensitive to their patients' use of herbal remedies, traditional healers, special foods, or other forms of alternative healing (Hoang & Erickson, 1982; Mull & Mull, 1983; Nguyen, 1985). A lay referral system, imported from the country of origin, may continue to provide alternative therapies in the United States, alongside the techniques of scientifically oriented medicine. Although practitioners often do not become aware of these parallel healing practices, even when they do become aware, integration of alternative medical roles and responsibilities into the primary care setting may prove challenging.

Third, explanatory models of disease can differ greatly across cultures. Medical anthropologists have described cross-cultural differences in explanatory models for physical symptoms and signs (Kleinman, 1988; Rubel, O'Nell, & Collado-Ardon, 1984). Attempts by professionals practicing modern medicine to explain patients' medical problems may lead to explanations that have little meaning in the context of a patient's culture. In particular, the divergence between scientific and "ethnomedical" explanatory models often creates tension as practitioners fail to take into account patients' understanding of illness as rooted in spiritual forces, supernatural processes, or other culturally shaped events. Cultures also differ markedly in the acceptability of psychological disturbance as an explanation for the experience of distress. As discussed further below, such cultural differences help account for the patterning of somatic symptoms as a response to extreme stress among refugees.

Fourth, contextual factors that are culturally patterned may create further barriers to professional-client interaction. These contextual factors include dietary customs, socialization of children, sexual activities, exercise, work habits, rituals, and other cultural traditions that impact on health and illness. Contextual factors such as culturally prescribed responses to the experience of physical threats to survival during war or civil unrest may determine the patterning of symptoms that refugees present to primary care practitioners. For a refugee experiencing the extreme stress of war, inability to protect or to grieve for loved ones who die can create a difficult gap between reality and cultural expectations. When practitioners are unaware of such contextual patterns, major misunderstandings of patients' physical symptoms may persist.

Fifth, cultural differences exist in the emotional impact and stigma of illness. While some cultures attach stigma to certain diseases like cancer or tuberculosis, in many instances emotional disturbance becomes particularly stigmatized. For example, partly because of stigma, Southeast Asian and Latino cultures tend to interpret psychological or psychophysiological symptoms as manifestations of somatic disorder. Likewise, in some Latino subcultures emotional disturbances are viewed as both precursors to and consequences of physical disease (Clark, 1983). Such cultural interpretations of a close relationship between psychic and somatic experiences may prove difficult to comprehend for practitioners grounded in Anglo-American cultural patterns.

These final three points—differences in explanatory models, contextual factors, and emotional impact—are critical to an understanding of the presentation of symptoms in primary care practices by immigrant and refugee groups. Underlying these ideas is the very real tendency of immigrant groups and those not familiar with psychiatric vocabulary to manifest distress in a somatic form (Katon, Kleinman, & Rosen, 1982). A substantial proportion, estimated at more than 25 percent, of patients' visits to primary care physicians involve somatic complaints referable to underlying psychological distress (Katon, Ries, & Kleinman, 1984a).

Somatic Presentation of Distress: Somatization

Clusters of somatic complaints or reactions to somatic symptoms that interfere with an individual's functioning have been termed *somatoform disorders.* Four types of somatoform disorders appear in the *Diagnostic and Statistical Manual of Mental Disorders* (DSM-III-R): conversion, hypochondriasis, psychogenic pain, and somatization. These somatoform disorders presume no other primary psychiatric disorder but may manifest clinical features that overlap with anxiety and depression. *Conversion* symptoms are defined as an alteration in physical functioning or complaints suggesting a physical disorder, but without a pathophysiological explanation. *Hypochondriasis* is an abnormal response to a normal sensation; it is interpreted as being pathological—that is, as an amplified response to a minor abnormal sensation. *Psychogenic pain* constitutes pain that is inconsistent with or out of proportion to physical findings.

Somatization disorder is characterized by multiple, recurrent somatic symptoms for which no medical explanation can be found (Monson & Smith, 1983). These "unfounded" physical complaints tend to be associated with psychopathology, poor treatment response, substantial disability, and frequent utilization of medical services (Escobar, 1987; Escobar, Burnam, et al., 1987). As defined by the DSM-III-R, an individual must present with at least thirteen from a list of thirty-five possible physical symptoms to reach diagnostic levels. The symptoms are in six areas: gastrointestinal, regional pain, cardiopulmonary, neurological, sexual, and reproductive. A closer look at the DSM-III-R indicates that somatization is a long-standing pattern of illness behavior, a way of life dominated by medical experiences and possibly disturbed personal relationships (American Psychiatric Association, 1987).

The diagnosis of the somatoform disorders, of which somatization is one, is not straightforward. Epidemiologic studies of the prevalence of somatoform symptoms have yielded differing findings, depending on the operational definition used. Based on data from the Epidemiologic Catchment Area (ECA) program, some investigators have estimated a prevalence of 0.13 percent for the full somatization disorder in the general population (Swartz, Landerman, George, Blazer, & Escobar, 1990). The ECA's survey instrument may underestimate prevalence; a careful clinical examination is likely to be more accurate (Smith, 1990). Using an abridged somatization construct, researchers have estimated a much higher prevalence in specific settings—4.4 percent of the general population in the Los Angeles area (Escobar, Burnam, et al., 1987) and 18 to 20 percent in Puerto Rico (Escobar, Golding, et al., 1987).

Diagnosing somatoform disorders in primary care can be especially difficult. This is, in part, because DSM-III-R categories are not mutually exclusive. However, it may also be that the nature of somatization, as presented in primary care settings, is phenomenologically different from that seen in psychiatric settings (Kaplan, Lipkin, & Gordon, 1988).

The research on prevalence in primary care settings does suggest that the prevalence of somatization is probably higher among patients who seek primary care than estimates from population-based surveys indicate. For instance, a study conducted in a family practice setting found that 5 percent of patients who sought primary care manifested the full somatization disorder and an additional 4 percent showed "borderline" somatization (more than ten but fewer than thirteen symptoms) (deGruy, Columbia, & Dickinson, 1987). According to an influential study that used looser diagnostic criteria, at least 25 percent of patients who visit primary care physicians present with somatic complaints that are due primarily to psychosocial distress (Katon, Ries, & Kleinman, 1984a). Somatization occurs less frequently in men than women (deGruy, Columbia, et al., 1987; deGruy, Crider, et al., 1987; Smith, Monson, & Livingston, 1985). Patients of lower socioeconomic status tend to somatize more than those of higher socioeconomic status (deGruy, Columbia, et al., 1987; deGruy, Crider, et al., 1987; Kleinman, 1982; Barsky, 1979).

The research on the treatment of somatization has shown that management of somatization can prove difficult and expensive (Smith, Monson, & Ray, 1986a). A study in a family practice setting found that outpatients with somatization showed about 51 percent more office visits and charges for services than matched controls and that their physicians reported lower satisfaction in caring for somatizers (deGruy, Columbia, et al., 1987). In a study at a university hospital, inpatients with somatization manifested a higher proportion of negative findings on work-up of their presenting complaints than matched controls (deGruy, Crider, et al., 1987). Earlier studies have indicated that per capita expenditures for hospital services among patients with somatization greatly exceed the average per capita amount in the United States (Smith et al., 1986a).

The diagnosis and treatment of somatization disorder is further complicated by the substantial comorbidity existing between somatization and other psychiatric disorders. A recent review of data from the ECA study suggested that more than 60 percent of subjects that the Diagnostic Interview Schedule (DIS) survey identified with abridged somatization also manifested at least one other DIS diagnosis (Escobar, Swartz, Rubio-Stipic, & Manu, 1991). Major depression or dysthymia occurred in 41 percent of women with abridged somatization and 26 percent of men, phobias in 38 percent of women and 33 percent of men, and panic disorder in 9 percent of women and 8 percent of men.

In clinical studies, comorbidity varies, but the strongest association is between somatization and depression. Table 8.3 summarizes recent findings about this association. According to Smith's (1990) review, depression is present in 80 to 90 percent of patients with full-blown somatization disorder who are seen in psychiatric inpatient or outpatient settings. Zoccolillo and Cloninger's (1986)

Table 8.3. Depression as Comorbidity with Somatization.

Reference	*Percent of Patients with Somatization Who Manifested Depression*	*Clinical Setting*
Smith, 1990	80–90	Psychiatric inpatients or outpatients
Zoccolillo & Cloninger, 1986	52	Psychiatric outpatients
Katon et al., 1984b	48	Psychiatric liaison service
Miranda et al., 1991	39	Medical outpatients

study of psychiatric outpatients with clinically diagnosed somatization disorder revealed depression as a comorbid condition in 52 percent of subjects. Although patients with somatoform symptoms in primary care settings may show somewhat less depression, it is likely that a majority of patients with somatization disorder have a present or past history of depression (Smith, 1990). In a study of medical and surgical patients with clinically diagnosed somatization seen on a psychiatry liaison service, Katon and co-workers (1984b) found that 48 percent manifested major depression. Among medical outpatients, Miranda, Perez-Stable, Muñoz, Hargreaves, and Henke (1991) observed that, in patients with somatization measured by the abridged index, 39 percent also showed evidence of depression. While not reporting percentages, Westermeyer, Bouafuely, Neider, and Callies (1989) found in their longitudinal study of Hmong refugees that somatization (measured by four separate scales) and depression (measured by the Zung scale) showed Pearson correlation coefficients between .28 and .49, all statistically significant. Preliminary evidence from a clinical study of patients with chronic fatigue indicates that, among a small proportion of patients with somatoform symptoms who also manifest depression, improvement in somatoform symptoms follows treatment with antidepressant medication (P. Manu and J. I. Escobar, unpublished data).

Other comorbid conditions have been observed in these clinical studies, generally at a somewhat lower prevalence (Table 8.4). Among psychiatric outpatients with somatization disorder, Liskow,

Table 8.4. Other Conditions of Comorbidity with Somatization.

	Percent of Patients with Somatization Who Manifest:			
Reference	*Phobic Disorder*	*Panic Disorder*	*Anxiety Disorder*	*Clinical Setting*
Liskow et al., 1986	39	45		Psychiatric outpatients
Zoccolillo & Cloniger, 1986		10		Psychiatric outpatients
Katon et al., 1984b		4		Psychiatric liaison service
Smith, 1990		26	34	Psychiatric outpatients

Othmer, Penick, De Souza, and Gabrielli (1986) found that 39 percent met criteria for phobic disorders and 45 percent for panic disorder. In Zoccolillo and Cloninger's (1986) study of psychiatric outpatients with somatization disorder, the co-occurrence of panic disorder was 10 percent; in Katon and co-workers' (1984b) research on psychiatry liaison patients with clinically diagnosed somatization, the rate of panic disorder was 4 percent. Smith's (1990) study of patients from primary care settings with somatization disorder found that 34 percent showed generalized anxiety disorder, 26 percent manifested panic disorder, and 66 percent showed some diagnosable anxiety disorder.

Somatization and Cross-Cultural Issues

Even though much research has recently appeared examining the prevalence and treatment of somatization and comorbid conditions presented in primary care settings (Smith, 1990), cross-cultural issues and issues related to the possible sociogenesis of somatization and comorbid conditions (Kaplan et al., 1988) have largely been ignored.* However, the history of research in this area shows the

**Sociogenesis* refers to symptoms that are manifestations of socioeconomic, environmental, or political stress, particularly in relation to experiences of war.

importance of culture and acculturation for expression of symptoms and use of services (for example, Zola, 1966; Pliskin, 1987; Lin, Carter, & Kleinman, 1985).

Studies of Latino populations in the United States show culture-specific rates of somatization, with prevalence varying among subgroups of the Latino population (Mexican-American, Puerto Rican, and Cuban-American) (Angel & Guarnaccia, 1989). In some studies, sociocultural factors have been found to affect levels of somatization and other emotional disorders, especially among Mexican-American women (Kirmayer, 1984; Escobar, Gomez, & Tuason, 1983). In other studies, no effect of ethnicity on somatization among males has been found. Particularly among older Mexican-American men, denial and minimization of symptoms are likely to occur, which may be related to cultural patterns such as "machismo" and stoicism (Bach-y-Rita, 1982).

Epidemiologic evidence suggests that the association between somatization and depression may vary substantially by ethnic group. For instance, using data from both the ECA and the Hispanic Health and Nutrition Examination Survey (HHANES), different investigators have found that this association tends to be stronger among Puerto Rican respondents than among other Latino ethnic groups (Angel & Guarnaccia, 1989; Escobar & Canino, 1989).

The presentation of somatoform complaints appears to differ substantially among immigrants to the United States from Latin America and Southeast Asia (Lin et al., 1985). Predictably the degree of acculturation to a new culture after immigration may prove to be an important variable that mediates the relationship between culture and somatization (Angel & Thoits, 1987). However, for immigrants from war-torn countries, acculturation is not the only variable requiring close examination.

The study of somatization also needs to consider the possible sociogenesis of symptoms, particularly among those who immigrate to this country as political refugees. There is little indication in the DSM-III-R of the possibility that physical symptoms may be at least partly sociosomatic in nature—that is, manifestations of socioeconomic, environmental, or political stress, particularly in relation to experiences of war. A recent review has categorized the mechanisms of somatization according to currently held neurobiological, psychodynamic, behavioral, and sociocultural theories (Kaplan et al., 1988); though helpful, this review does not refer to somatization in refugees or to the impact of extremely stressful experiences on the development and presentation of somatoform symptoms.

The refugee experience can include some of the most stressful events that any individual can encounter. Experiences in the country of origin (such as political persecution, torture, forced migration, human atrocities, and separation from or loss of family members) may precede stressful experiences in the country of refuge (such as attempts to find political asylum, hardships in refugee camps, new family relations, different language, lack of relevant work skills, and elimination of social support systems) (Smith, 1982). Such experiences may result in the development of substantial personal impediments—including individual psychopathology—and also manifestations of physical symptoms with no organic basis. Anxiety, depression, and delayed grief may emerge as specific emotional reactions to refugee trauma (Keller, 1975). The development of both emotional and somatic responses to traumatic experiences may be delayed until a refugee reaches the country of resettlement. A schematic model of delayed somatic response to refugee trauma, adapted from Muecke's work (1983), appear in Table 8.5.

Somatic symptoms among refugees frequently reach diagnostic levels for somatization disorder (Lin et al., 1985). The severity of the refugee's traumatic experience before and during migration plays a vital role in shaping symptom expression and sociocultural adaptation in the country of settlement. For many refugee populations, this conversion of psychological distress into somatic complaints—as would be predicted by Clark (1983) and Barker (1992)—is a more socially acceptable form for psychological symptoms (Barsky, 1979) and avoids the stigma attached to symptoms of mental illness (Kleinman, 1982).

Comorbidity Among Refugees

One comorbid condition, which may be directly related to the refugees' traumatic life experiences and until recently has been ignored

Table 8.5. Schematic Model of Delayed Somatic Response to Refugee Trauma.

Components of Refugee Trauma by State of Refugee Life History	*Emotional Response*	*Somatic Response*
Country of Origin	Delayed	Delayed
Persecution		
Forced migration		
Witness to human atrocities		
Separation from or loss of family members		
Country of Refuge	Delayed	Delayed
Limbo experience		
Finding asylum		
Refugee		
Separation from or loss of family members		
Hasty marriages and affiliation with new families in refugee camps		
Country of Resettlement	Anxiety	Psychosomatic conditions
Alien culture	Delayed grief	
Religion, language, and skills may no longer be relevant	Depression	
	PTSD	Somatic problems with no identifiable cause
Previous social support system may not exist		
Frequent isolation from compatriots		
Low English-speaking ability		
Wrong skills for North American economy: cannot find employment; welfare dependency		
Children may be more skilled than parents; parent-child role reversal and tension		
Marital conflicts		
Single-parent households		

Source: Adapted from Muecke, 1983.

by researchers is post-traumatic stress disorder (PTSD). The American Psychiatric Association's official diagnostic manual (American Psychiatric Association, 1987) indicates that victims of extraordinary experiences such as natural disasters, accidents, torture, and war-related incidents are predisposed to PTSD, but the relationship between somatization and PTSD has received little attention.

During the last ten years, warlike conditions have forced people from several parts of Central America to flee their countries suddenly, unprepared and without social supports. In a recent study, Cervantes and colleagues (1989) assessed PTSD in a community sample of Central American and Mexican immigrants. The investigators reported that 52 percent of Central American immigrants who had experienced major stress and 49 percent of Central American immigrants without major stress manifested PTSD, as compared to 25 percent of Mexican immigrants. Although they found no significant differences among the three groups of subjects in somatization, the Pearson correlation coefficient between PTSD and somatization in the overall sample was statistically significant at .35. While the high rates of PTSD observed in part may reflect the instrument used, the data indicate that a high prevalence of PTSD may occur among Central American, and to a lesser extent, Mexican immigrants.

Until recently, studies of PTSD have focused on the psychological difficulties of Vietnam veterans (Helzer, Robins, & McEvoy, 1987; Breslau & Davis, 1987). Yet the emotional effects of torture and violent behavior persist among many other groups who have survived traumatic events (Mollica et al., 1990). Although no systematic data on PTSD among adult Central American refugees in primary care settings are yet available, studies of Southeast Asian refugees indicate that exposure to violence may result in the development of PTSD, whose frequency appears to vary for different cultural groups. Some refugees with PTSD present predominantly somatoform complaints (Mollica et al., 1990; Hondius & van Willigen, 1989) rather than explicitly emotional symptoms. Refugee populations share common experiences such as violent death of loved ones, imprisonment, harassment, torture of self or family members, sexual abuse, and family or marital breakdown (Ortiz, 1985). Notably, in at least some studies, the stressful experience of sexual or related forms of abuse appears to characterize the developmental history of a substantial proportion of nonrefugee women with somatoform disorders (Morrison, 1989; Harrop-Griffiths et al., 1988).

Several epidemiologic studies provide data on prevalence of PTSD in the general population and among target groups that have undergone extremely stressful experiences, but none of these studies has reported clear-cut data on the co-occurrence of PTSD and somatization. The studies used somewhat different instruments to assess PTSD. With data from the ECA study, Helzer et al. (1987) found a PTSD rate of approximately 1 percent in the general population, 3.5 percent in civilians exposed to physical attack, 9.3 percent in Vietnam combat veterans, and 20 percent among wounded Vietnam veterans; because of the small numbers of subjects exposed to traumatic events, the confidence intervals of these rates were wide. In a study of Vietnam veterans, researchers from the Centers for Disease Control (CDC) found a prevalence rate of 15 percent for veterans experiencing PTSD at any time since the war, but only 2.2 percent at the time of the survey. While the CDC study revealed a substantial rate—9 to 25 percent depending on the instrument used—of somatoform complaints among Vietnam veterans, the investigators did not report a statistical association between PTSD and somatization (Centers for Disease Control Vietnam Experience Study, 1988). In a population-based study of PTSD in a random sample of young adults from an urban health maintenance organization, Breslau, Davis, Andreski, and Peterson (1991) observed a 39.1 percent lifetime exposure to traumatic events, a 23.6 percent rate of PTSD among those exposed, and an overall lifetime prevalence rate of PTSD in the sample of 9.2 percent; no association between PTSD and somatoform symptoms was addressed in this study.

Clinical studies also have assessed comorbidity of somatization and PTSD in a limited way. Escobar and colleagues found that 15 percent of Hispanic veterans with PTSD manifested somatoform complaints (Escobar, Randolph, et al., 1983). Among Asian immigrants and refugees in a primary care setting, Lin and colleagues (1985) learned that refugees experiencing severe stress showed higher rates of clinically assessed somatoform symptoms; the associations differed substantially by ethnic group. A recent study by Miranda and co-workers from a primary care academic practice in internal medicine (1991) observed that life stress was a strong predictor of somatization in a regression analysis, but PTSD was not assessed. Studies have documented increases in levels of somatic and psychological symptoms in differing proportions of subjects following exposure to military experiences and to various types of disasters that predictably would generate post-traumatic stress (Shalev, Bleich, & Ursano, 1990).

It should be noted that while PTSD is regarded as a disorder resulting from exposure to a traumatic event that is generally "outside" the range of normal experience—such as combat, torture, natural disasters, and accidental disasters—in countries such as El Salvador and Guatemala, war has become a formal practice "within" the range of normal daily experience, including both combat and torture. An example of the effect of the conditions faced by refugees on their perception and presentation of symptoms is provided by R. L., a patient in our clinic in Southern California:

> R. L. is a twenty-seven-year-old Salvadoran male. He fled his native country after finding out that his name had appeared on a death squad list for immediate execution. A white handprint with the initials E. M. (*Escuadrones de la Muerte* or Death Squads) also had appeared on the front door of his house. Nine months after his arrival in the United States, he learned that his wife had been abducted and assaulted by paramilitary forces. His two children witnessed their mother being raped and killed by a group of unidentified men during an attempt to extract information about R. L.'s whereabouts.
>
> Shortly thereafter, R. L. presented to a primary care physician at a community clinic, where he was referred from the emergency room of a local hospital. During previous weeks he had experienced multiple symptoms, including weakness (which caused him to be terminated from his temporary job), changes in sensation, abdominal pain, chest pain, insomnia, and weight loss. R. L.'s primary care physician pursued several possible organic diagnoses by ordering diagnostic studies. He also prescribed analgesics and other medications. After extensive evaluation, no physical cause was found for his somatic symptoms.
>
> Psychiatric consultation was then sought. After further psychosocial evaluation, individual therapy

became a part of the medical plan. Somatization was diagnosed. Low-dose antidepressant medication was instituted as therapy continued. The psychiatrist coordinated follow-up with the primary care internist. R. L. learned to increase awareness of emotional factors exacerbating his symptoms and developed new coping strategies. He joined a group of local Central American refugees, where he was encouraged to write and to recite poetry as a therapeutic tool. Over the course of the next six months, his somatic symptoms gradually decreased.

Conclusion

This review of the research on somatization has shown that few studies have examined the incidence, prevalence, and nature of somatization and apparently related comorbid conditions in primary care settings among minority, immigrant, and refugee populations. There is also relatively little research examining the links between somatoform symptoms and severely stressful life experiences, like those experienced by refugees. The research does clearly show, however, that several psychiatric disorders, especially depression, present as comorbid conditions along with somatization.

The currently available data suggest that the association between PTSD and somatoform symptoms deserves closer study. Clinical observations indicate that PTSD and somatization may be closely associated (Harrop-Griffiths et al., 1988; Freimer, Lu, & Chen, 1989). How traumatic life events relate to both somatization and PTSD among such patients seeking primary care remains to be determined through systematic research.

This review has also shown that many questions remain to be answered about service use. Despite the presumption that patients who somatize use services differently and in more costly ways than patients who do not, relatively little information is available about these problems in primary care settings, especially those that attract patients from culturally diverse and minority backgrounds. Such patients are at a higher risk of misdiagnosis as well as of inappropriate diagnostic or therapeutic interventions by physicians who are not sensitized to culturally based somatoform symptoms. Further research on prevalence, utilization, and costs in such settings could lead to the design of helpful interventions to address current difficulties in caring for patients with somatization.

We are currently conducting a study to examine these issues. Our research group is carrying out a longitudinal, three-year project that aims to determine how war-related premigration experiences, changes in language, and acculturation are related to the presentation of somatoform symptoms in a primary care setting. We are studying how Central American patients differ from other Latino and non-Latino patients in the expression of somatoform complaints, as well as the association between somatoform symptoms and PTSD among these patients. The research also focuses on the attitudes and behavioral responses of primary care physicians to these patients, and on the extent to which barriers to access for health care and mental health services affect the presentation of somatoform symptoms.

Our study represents only one among several that will yield new knowledge about mental disorders among immigrant, refugee, and minority populations who seek services in primary care settings. We are optimistic that the expected results of such studies will assist in the design of appropriate primary care interventions and mental health services for these target populations.

References

American Psychiatric Association. (1987). *Diagnostic and statistical manual of mental disorders* (3rd ed., rev.). Washington, DC: Author.

Angel, R., & Guarnaccia, P. J. (1989). Mind, body, and culture: Somatization among Hispanics. *Social Science and Medicine, 28,* 1229–1238.

Angel, R., & Thoits, P. (1987). The impact of culture on the cognitive structure of illness. *Culture, Medicine, & Psychiatry, 11,* 465–494.

Aron, A. (1992). Applications of psychology to the assessment of refugees seeking political asylum. *Applied Psychology: An International Review, 41*(1), 77–91.

Bach-y-Rita, G. (1982). The Mexican American: Religious and cultural influences. In R. Becerra, M. Karno, & J. I. Escobar (Eds.), *Mental health and Hispanic Americans: Clinical perspectives.* Philadelphia: Grune & Stratton.

Barker, J. B. (1992). Cultural diversity—changing the context of medical practice. *Western Journal of Medicine, 157,* 248–254.

Barsky, A. J. (1979). Patients who amplify bodily sensations. *Annals of Internal Medicine, 91,* 63–70.

Berryman, A., & Berryman, P. (1988). *In the shadows of liberty: Central American refugees in the United States.* Philadelphia: American Friends Service Committee.

Breslau, N., & Davis, G. C. (1987). Posttraumatic stress disorder: The etiologic specificity of wartime stressors. *American Journal of Psychiatry, 144,* 578–583.

Breslau, N., Davis, G. C., Andreski, P., & Peterson, E. (1991). Traumatic events and posttraumatic stress disorder in an urban population of young adults. *Archives of General Psychiatry, 48,* 216–222.

Centers for Disease Control Vietnam Experience Study. (1988). Health status of Vietnam veterans: 1. Psychosocial characteristics. *Journal of the American Medical Association, 259,* 2701–2707.

Cervantes, C. R., Salgado de Snyder, V. N., & Padilla, A. M. (1989). Posttraumatic stress in immigrants from Central America and Mexico. *Hospital and Community Psychiatry, 40,* 615–619.

Clark, M. M. (1983). Cultural context of medical practice. *Western Journal of Medicine, 139,* 806–810.

deGruy, F., Columbia, L., & Dickinson, P. (1987). Somatization disorder in a family practice. *Journal of Family Practice, 25,* 45–51.

deGruy, F., Crider, J., Hashimi, D. K., Dickinson, P., Mullins, H. C., & Troncale, J. (1987). Somatization disorder in a university hospital. *Journal of Family Practice, 25,* 579–584.

Escobar, J. I. (1987). Cross-cultural aspects of the somatization trait. *Hospital and Community Psychiatry, 38,* 174–810.

Escobar, J. I., Burnam, M. A., Karno, M., Forsythe, A., & Golding, J. M. (1987). Somatization in the community. *Archives of General Psychiatry, 44,* 713–719.

Escobar, J. I., & Canino, G. (1989). Unexplained physical complaints: Psychopathology and epidemiological correlates. *British Journal of Psychiatry. 154*(Suppl. 4), 24–27.

Escobar, J. I., Golding, J. M., Hough, R. L., Karno, M., Burnam, M. A., & Wells, K. B. (1987). Somatization in the community: Relationship to disability and use of services. *American Journal of Public Health, 77,* 837–840.

Escobar, J. I., Gomez, J., & Tuason, V. B. (1983). Depressive phenomenology in North and South American patients. *American Journal of Psychiatry, 140,* 47–51.

Escobar, J. I., Randolph, E. T., Puente, G., Spiwak, F., Asamen, J. K., Hill, M., & Hough, R. L. (1983). Post-traumatic stress disorder in Hispanic Vietnam veterans: Clinical phenomenology and sociocultural characteristics. *Journal of Nervous and Mental Disease, 171,* 585–596.

Escobar, J. I., Swartz, M., Rubio-Stipec, M., & Manu, P. (1991). Medically unexplained symptoms: Distribution, risk factors, and comorbidity. In L. J. Kirmayer & J. M. Robbins (Eds.), *Current concepts in somatization: Research and clinical perspectives.* Washington, DC: American Psychiatric Press.

Freimer, N., Lu, F., & Chen, J. (1989). Posttraumatic stress and conversion disorders in a Laotian refugee veteran: Use of amobarbital interviews. *Journal of Nervous and Mental Disease, 177,* 432–433.

Haffner, L. (1992). Translation is not enough: Interpreting in a medical setting. *Western Journal of Medicine, 157,* 255–259.

Haines, D. W. (1989). *Refugees as immigrants: Cambodians, Laotians, and Vietnamese in America.* Totowa, NJ: Rowman & Littlefield.

Hardt, E. J. (1991). *The bilingual medical interview.* Boston: Boston Department of Health and Hospitals and Boston Area Health Education Center.

Harrop-Griffiths, J., Katon, W., Walker, E., Holm, L., Russo, J., & Hickok, L. (1988). The association between chronic pelvic pain, psychiatric diagnoses, and childhood sexual abuse. *Obstetrics and Gynecology, 71,* 589–594.

Helzer, J. E., Robins, L. N., & McEvoy, L. (1987). Post-traumatic stress disorder in the general population. *New England Journal of Medicine, 317,* 1630–1634.

Hoang, G. N., & Erickson, R. V. (1982). Guidelines for providing medical care to Southeast Asian refugees. *Journal of the American Medical Association, 248,* 710–714.

Hondius, A. J., & van Willigen, L. H. (1989). Baseline health care for refugees in the Netherlands. *Social Science and Medicine, 28,* 729–733.

Kaplan, C., Lipkin, M., & Gordon, G. H. (1988). Somatization in primary care. *Journal of General Internal Medicine, 3,* 177–190.

Katon, W., Kleinman, A. M., & Rosen, G. (1982). Depression and somatization: A review. *American Journal of Medicine, 72,* 127–135.

Katon, W., Ries, R. K., & Kleinman, A. (1984a). The prevalence of somatization in primary care. *Comprehensive Psychiatry, 25,* 208–215.

Katon, W., Ries, R. K., & Kleinman, A. (1984b). Part 2: A prospective DSM-III study of 100 consecutive somatization patients. *Comprehensive Psychiatry, 25,* 305–314.

Keller, S. L. (1975). *Uprooting and social change: The role of refugees in development.* Delhi, India: Manohar Book Service.

Kirmayer, L. J. (1984). Culture, affect, and somatization. *Transcultural Psychiatry Research, 21,* 159–188.

Kleinman, A. (1982). Neurasthenia and depression: A study of somatization and culture in China. *Culture, Medicine, and Psychiatry, 6,* 117–190.

Kleinman, A. (1988). *The illness narratives.* New York: Basic Books.

Lin, E. H. B., Carter, W. B., & Kleinman, A. M. (1985). An exploration of somatization among Asian refugees and immigrants in primary care. *American Journal of Public Health, 75,* 1080–1084.

Liskow, B., Othmer, E., Penick, E. C., De Souza, C., & Gabrielli, W. (1986). Is Briquet's syndrome a heterogeneous disorder? *American Journal of Psychiatry, 143,* 666–669.

Miranda, J., Perez-Stable, E. J., Muñoz, R. F., Hargreaves, W., & Henke, C. J. (1991). Somatization, psychiatric disorder, and stress in utilization of ambulatory medical services. *Health Psychology, 10,* 46–51.

Mollica, R. F., Wyshak, G., Lavelle, J., Truong, T., Tor, S., & Yang,

T. (1990). Assessing symptom change in Southeast Asian refugee survivors of mass violence and torture. *American Journal of Psychiatry, 147,* 83–88.

Monson, R. A., & Smith, G. R., Jr. (1983). Current concepts in psychiatry: Somatization disorder in primary care. *New England Journal of Medicine, 308,* 1464–1465.

Morrison, J. (1989). Childhood sexual histories of women with somatization disorder. *American Journal of Psychiatry, 146,* 239–241.

Muecke, M. A. (1983). In search of healers—Southeast Asian refugees in the American health care system. *Western Journal of Medicine, 139,* 835–840.

Mull, J. D., & Mull, D. S. (1983). A visit with a curandero. *Western Journal of Medicine, 139,* 730–736.

Nguyen, D. (1985). Culture shock—a review of Vietnamese culture and its concepts of health and disease. *Western Journal of Medicine, 142,* 409–412.

Ortiz, K. (1985). Mental health consequences of life history method: Implications from a refugee case. *Ethos, 13,* 99–120.

Pliskin, K. L. (1987). *Silent boundaries: Cultural constraints on sickness and diagnosis of Iranians in Israel.* New Haven, CT: Yale University Press.

Putsch, R. W. (1985). Cross-cultural communication: The special case of interpreters in health care. *Journal of the American Medical Association, 254,* 3344–3348.

Rubel, A. J., O'Nell, C. W., & Collado-Ardon, R. (1984). *Susto: A folk illness.* Berkeley: University of California Press.

Shalev, A., Bleich, A., & Ursano, R. J. (1990). Posttraumatic stress disorder: Somatic comorbidity and effort tolerance. *Psychosomatics, 31,* 197–203.

Smith, G. R., Jr. (1990). *Somatization disorder in the medical setting* (DHHS Publication No. ADM 90-1631). Washington, DC: U.S. Government Printing Office.

Smith, G. R., Jr. Monson, R. A., & Livingston, R. L. (1985). Somatization disorder in men. *General Hospital Psychiatry, 7,* 4–8.

Smith, G. R., Jr., Monson, R. A., & Ray, D. C. (1986a). Patients with multiple unexplained symptoms: Their characteristics, functional health, and health care utilization. *Archives of Internal Medicine, 146,* 69–72.

Smith, G. R., Jr., Monson, R. A., & Ray, D. C. (1986b). Psychiatric consultation in somatization disorder. *New England Journal of Medicine, 314,* 1407–1413.

Smith, H. E. (1982). Doctors and society: A northern Thailand society. *Social Science and Medicine, 16,* 515–526.

Swartz, M., Landerman, R., George, L., Blazer, D., & Escobar, J. (1990). Somatization disorder. In L. N. Robins & D. Regier (Eds.), *Psychiatric disorders in America.* New York: Free Press.

U.S. Bureau of the Census. (1983). *1980 Census of the Population* (Publication No. PC 80-1-C1). Washington, DC: U.S. Department of Commerce.

U.S. Bureau of the Census. (1992). *1990 Census of Population.* Van Nuys, CA: Unpublished data from Western Region, Bureau of the Census.

Vargas, G. E. (1984). Recently arrived Central American immigrants: Mental health needs. *Research Bulletin of the Spanish Mental Health Research Center* (UCLA), Autumn, p. 5.

Westermeyer, J., Bouafuely, M., Neider, J., & Callies, A. (1989). Somatization among refugees: An epidemiologic study. *Psychosomatics, 30*(1), 34–43.

Zoccolillo, M., & Cloninger, C. R. (1986). Somatization disorder: Psychologic symptoms, social disability, and diagnosis. *Comprehensive Psychiatry, 27,* 65–73.

Zola, I. K. (1966). Culture and symptoms: An analysis of patients' presenting complaints. *American Sociological Review, 31,* 615–630.

9 *Daniel E. Ford*

Recognition and Underrecognition of Mental Disorders in Adult Primary Care

As reviewed earlier in this book, data from multiple sources and many different countries indicate that at least 50 percent of individuals with psychiatric disorders receive all or part of their care from general medical providers. From the general medical provider's point of view, between 5 and 20 percent of visits involve patients with active, ongoing mental disorders. In addition, the general medical provider is in a key position to manage patients with mental disorders, either by directly initiating treatment or by referring the patient to a specialty mental health provider. For all these reasons, the recognition of mental disorders in adult patients by general medical providers has been the subject of numerous investigations.

Before reviewing the research on physician recognition of psychiatric illness, several methodological issues should be considered. The first question that needs to be addressed is "What psychiatric symptom or disorders should the general medical provider be recognizing?" In many studies of medical patients, psychiatric illness is poorly defined. Mental disorders such as major depression may be specified, but usually the recognition of "psychiatric distress" in patients is reported. In many studies, the mental disorder to be recognized is not specified by recency of onset, when the symptoms were last active, whether the psychiatric symptoms meet criteria for a disorder-level diagnosis, whether the patient is currently being treated by a mental health specialist, whether the mental disorder has been recognized on a previous visit, or whether alcohol and drug abuse are included in the group of psychiatric disorders to be recognized. A simple phobia that began twenty years ago cannot be equated with a severe depressive disorder beginning two weeks ago in terms of the need for recognition by the general medical provider.

General medical providers and psychiatric screening instruments do not identify the same individuals as psychiatric cases. Approximately 20 percent of patients identified as psychiatric cases by general medical providers do not score positive on psychiatric screening questionnaires. General medical providers do not agree on what constitutes a psychiatric case. In one study, twenty-seven general practitioners were asked to classify the psychiatric disorders of patients after viewing identical patient visit videotapes. They differed significantly, despite having the identical clinical data on which to base diagnoses (Jenkins, Smeeton, Mainker, & Sheperd, 1985). Nonetheless, psychiatric assessments with self-administered questionnaires and occasionally structured clinical interviews are regarded as the gold standard against which the general physician's assessment is judged.

Goldberg and colleagues have developed several indices to describe the ability of a primary care physician to recognize psychiatric disease in patients (Marks, Goldberg, & Hillier, 1979). These indices were created to emphasize that accurate recognition of true cases is as important as the overall rate of patients classified as having a psychiatric disorder. In Goldberg's system, accuracy is the correlation between the number of psychiatric symptoms a patient reports and the physician's rating of psychopathology on a six-point scale. When defined this way, the problems of selecting a threshold and dichotomizing patients into cases and noncases are avoided. The identification index is the ability of the physician to identify probable psychiatric cases correctly and is equal to the observed true positives divided by the expected true positives. However, because physicians differ on the percentage of patients they correctly diagnose, a measure of each physician's bias can also be calculated (Goldberg, Jenkins, Millar, & Faragher, 1993). Bias is equal to the number of cases assigned by the physician divided by the probable prevalence of cases in the practice. Positive values for bias are found in physicians who overidentify and negative values in physicians who underidentify psychiatric cases. Not surprisingly, studies in which physicians had a high identification index also have found a positive bias toward assigning psychiatric cases.

Another methodological issue focuses on the measurement of recognition by the clinician. The reported percentage of patients recognized by their physician varies depending on the specificity of the general medical provider diagnosis required for a case to be classified as recognized. For example, in the Johns Hopkins Internal Medicine Clinic study it was reported that almost 80 percent of patients with major depression as defined by the Diagnostic Interview Schedule (DIS) were recognized as such by their physician (Von Korff et al., 1987). However, the method of measuring recognition in this study maximized the sensitivity of the physicians. Each physician was asked to indicate on a form in a yes-no format whether the patient just seen had a psychological or emotional problem and to write down the diagnosis. If physicians indicated that a patient with depression had any emotional problem—even a nervous condition or anxiety—they were considered to have "recognized" that patient's psychiatric condition.

An additional challenge relates to the selection of the method to measure physician recognition. The most nonintrusive way to measure recognition is through chart review. However, physicians may be hesitant to record a psychiatric diagnosis in the chart because of concerns related to privacy, the social stigma of mental illness, or reimbursement considerations. Alternatively, recognition could be measured by asking patients directly if their physician had told them they had a mental illness at a particular visit. Patients have been found to be reasonably good at reporting whether or not they received the results of specific tests. However, patients might not be able to clearly state whether their physician had diagnosed a psychiatric illness during a particular visit. Another method used to measure physician recognition is to have the physician complete a form at the end of a patient visit that specifically asks the physician to rate the current psychiatric status of the patient. In some ways, this research assessment tool is itself a practice intervention and may artificially inflate rates of recognition. Hoeper, Nycz, Cleary, Regier, and Goldberg (1979) demonstrated that the rate of recording mental disorders is highly dependent on the wording of the instruments and whether recording is part of the medical record. Finally, some investigators have used measures of treatment such as prescription of psychotropic medications or referral to mental health professionals as indirect measures of recognition. Although treatment rates may be reasonable measures of clinically relevant recognition, patients who refuse treatment or who are receiving mental health treatment at another health care setting would be neglected. There is probably no one optimal method of measuring physician recognition of mental disorders; each method provides one view of the process. Methodology may overshadow physician behavior in explaining differences in rates of recognition found in different settings.

One way to conceptualize the process of physician recognition of mental disorders is to look at three separate components: patient variables, physician or health care provider variables, and health system or financing variables. Although the patient and health system variables must ultimately exert their influence through the behavior of the physician, it still is useful to divide the process into three separate components.

Patient Variables

Several patient factors will be considered.

Gender

Several studies have found that general medical providers are less likely to recognize mental illness in male patients than in female patients (Hoeper, Nycz, Kessler, Burke, & Pierce, 1984; Gerber et al., 1989). Most studies did not find the gender differences to be statistically significant, but the tendency was usually for men to have lower rates of recognition. This finding may be related to prior expectations of general medical providers. Practitioners have been found to be more likely to characterize women who score in the normal range on psychiatric screens as psychiatric cases than men (Redman, Webb, Hennrikers, Gordon, & Samson-Fisher, 1991).

Most studies of recognition only report the percentage of women and men with psychiatric disorders who were detected by their physicians and not the overall accuracy of the physician's assessment. In the one study that has investigated the issue most rigorously, the correlation between physician's ratings and a standardized psychiatric assessment was higher for male patients, but the identification index was higher for female patients (Marks et al., 1979). The authors' interpretation was that psychiatric normality was more accurately identified among male patients. The higher rates of recognized psychiatric disorders in women may be due to differences in threshold, with higher sensitivity rates and lower specificity rates. One study found an interaction between gender and age (Chancellor, Mant, & Andrew, 1977). More middle-aged and elderly women, but fewer young women, were likely to be classified as disturbed by the general practitioner than would be expected by the patient's responses to the standardized psychiatric assessment.

Lower rates of recognition in male patients may also be due to differences in the way that men and women utilize the health care system and present with psychiatric distress. In several studies, men with psychiatric illness have been found to use more specialty mental health services than do women (Leaf et al., 1985; Dew, Dunn, Bromet, & Schulberg, 1988). Women with psychiatric distress are more likely to have a regular general medical provider than men and may begin in the general medical sector. In contrast, men with the most conspicuous psychiatric illness may bypass the general medical sector and go directly to specialty mental health providers.

Age

The evidence related to patient age and recognition of psychiatric illness is confusing. Several studies suggest that patients under age thirty-five and over age sixty-five with psychiatric disorders are less likely to be recognized than others. Studies that simply compare the mean age of recognized versus not recognized patients will blur these relationships. Ford and colleagues (1988) reported that even after controlling for psychiatric status, elderly patients and patients under age thirty-five were less likely than others to report discussing an emotional or psychological problem with their general medical provider. A study of ninety-one British general practitioners (Marks et al., 1979) found lower rates of recognition for fifteen- to twenty-four-year-old patients than for patients over twenty-four years of age. Perez-Stable, Miranda, Muñoz, and Ying (1990) compared physicians' ratings of depression to scores on the DIS for 265 medical outpatients. Patients positive only on the DIS were five years younger on average than patients who were positive on both the DIS and the physician rating, implying poorer recognition in the younger patients.

Recognition of depression in the elderly may be particularly hard because of uncertainty concerning the diagnosis of depression, the larger number of medical disorders present in elderly patients, and difficulties related to instituting effective treatment for patients in this age group (Barsa, Toner, Gurland, & Lantigua, 1986; Koenig & Blazer, 1992). Despite the difficulties in diagnosis, the ability of general medical providers for the elderly to recognize psychiatric illness is especially important, because elderly patients rarely use specialty mental health services (Shapiro et al., 1984). If the elderly receive any mental health care, it is overwhelmingly delivered in the general medical sector. In one study (German et al., 1987), physicians were found to benefit when receiving feedback from psychiatric screening instruments given to elderly patients; recognition of disorders improved with the feedback.

Race, Education, and Marital Status

Few studies have evaluated the impact of race, education, and marital status in physician recognition of mental disorders. Findings from the few studies addressing these issues are inconsistent. Even fewer studies have reported how these variables might interact with the patient's gender and age to influence rates of recognition. These studies do generally find that minority, poorly educated, and single or divorced patients are more likely to be judged depressed than white, educated, married patients. In one American study, patients whose physicians judged them to be depressed when a diagnostic instrument did not reveal this condition had a statistically lower level of education than those not misidentified (Perez-Stable et al., 1990). In England, Sireling, Paykel, Freeling, Rao, and Patel (1985) reported that general practitioners were more likely to miss a psychiatric illness in patients who were married and of lower social class. In contrast, Marks et al. (1979) reported that unmarried and highly educated patients with psychiatric disease were more likely to not be identified by their physician. Several studies have found no differences in recognition by marital status (Gerber et al., 1989).

The national origin of the patient was reported to impact on recognition in London general practitioner offices (Boardman, 1987). Although the number of minority patients was small, the level of recognition was lower for African and Indian patients than for patients of British and Irish origin. In an American study reporting one of the highest rates of physician recognition, over 80 percent of the patients were black (Von Korff et al., 1987). In sum, the impact of race, education, and marital status on physician recognition of mental disorders is poorly understood.

Type and Severity of Psychiatric Illness in Patients

The severity of psychiatric distress is the strongest predictor of use of mental health services. Similarly, the psychiatric status of the patient is the most powerful predictor of which patients are recognized as suffering from mental illness. Studies using various measures of severity have consistently found that general medical providers are more likely to recognize the most severe cases of psychiatric illness. General Health Questionnaire (GHQ) score (Kessler, Cleary, & Burke, 1985), HSCL-90 score (Gerber et al., 1989), independent clinical ratings of severity with the Present State Examination (Ormel et al., 1990), and Research Diagnostic Criteria psychiatric diagnoses (Gerber et al., 1989) are positively associated with physician recognition. The largest percentage of discrepancies implying nonrecognition occur for patients with fewer and less severe symptoms.

Patients who have been diagnosed with a psychiatric disorder in the past are more likely to be recognized (Kessler et al., 1985; Ormel et al., 1990). The chronic episodic nature of most psychiatric illness suggests that past history can have a large impact on recognition rates. General physicians appear to be more comfortable attributing vague symptoms to current mental illness if the patient had a documented episode of mental illness in the past.

In many studies, general medical physicians have been hesitant to assign a specific psychiatric diagnosis to their patients. Nonetheless, many of these patients go on to receive mental health treatment from the general medical provider and specialty mental health providers (Ormel et al., 1990; Jencks, 1985). Limited data are available to evaluate whether primary care physicians are better at detecting some common psychiatric disorders than others. Most studies limited to depression cannot address this issue, but Gerber et al. (1989) found that internists recognized all cases of major depression diagnosed by the research psychiatrist. In contrast, only ten of the thirty patients diagnosed with mixed anxiety-depression were identified by their internist. Studies that have assessed a broader spectrum of psychiatric disorders have produced mixed results. Goldberg and Bridges (1987) report similar rates of detection for patients with depressive or anxiety disorders. The majority of studies have found higher rates of detection for depressive disorders than for anxiety disorders. Von Korff et al. (1987) observed higher rates of detection for depressive disorders. Ormel et al. (1990) found that only 21 percent of patients in their large study of general practitioners in the Netherlands received a specific diagnosis. However, rates of recognition ranged from 100 percent for severe depression, to 62 percent for neurotic depression, to 44 percent for phobias, to only 35 percent for neurotic states using the PSE-CATEGO/ICD-8 system. Interpreting data in this area is frustrated by the fact that many patients have features of more than one psychiatric disorder.

Another aspect of the patient's psychiatric illness that has a substantial impact on rates of recognition relates to how the patient presents to the general medical provider. Both clinicians and researchers consistently comment on the fact that general medical patients with psychiatric distress frequently present with somatic symptoms and are hesitant to accept a psychiatric explanation for their symptoms. Bridges and Goldberg (1985) have stated that only 5 percent of psychiatric cases present with pure psychiatric symptoms in primary care settings. Patients with fewer somatic complaints have higher rates of recognition (Von Korff et al., 1987). Psychiatric reason for a visit, although uncommon, has been associated with increased rates of physician recognition (Kessler et al., 1985).

Several questions remain concerning the impact of patient characteristics on recognition of psychiatric disorders. From a clinical perspective, applying epidemiologic data to individual patients may create stereotypes of patients at high risk for mental illness that are more harmful than beneficial. These stereotypes could be measured by presenting case scenarios to physicians. Research concerning patients' attitudes toward mental illness and symptom presentation styles would advance the field more than exploration of relatively weak relationships with sociodemographic variables.

Physician or Health Care Provider Variables

Several characteristics of physicians are associated with higher rates of recognition of mental disorders in patients. However, data in this area were collected in studies almost exclusively where the patient, and not the physician, was the unit of analysis. In most studies, the number of patients per physician is not sufficiently large to allow inferences about each physician's individual style. To compound the problem, the scant data that are available are only for physicians who agree to participate in studies of recognition. Nonparticipating physicians may differ in their recognition rates.

In almost every study, physicians vary widely in their ability to recognize psychiatric disorders. The variation in rates of psychiatric illness reported by individual physicians is much larger than the variation in rates of psychiatric illness found in their practices when patients undergo standardized psychiatric assessments. For example, Sheperd, Cooper, Brown, and Kalton (1966) reported that general practitioners in London had almost a ninefold variation in rates of psychiatric disorders they reported in their patients. Marks et al. (1979) found that estimates of psychiatric disorders for patients in each practice varied from 3 to 77 percent. Several general medical providers have been studied who are as good as the GHQ or an observing research psychiatrist in the detection of psychiatric illness in their patients.

As was discussed earlier in this chapter, physician performance related to recognition of psychiatric disease can be measured in several ways. In general, in those studies where rates of recognition have been the highest, the physicians have also demonstrated a strong bias toward labeling many patients with a psychiatric disorder. The Von Korff et al. (1987) study provides the best example of this. In that study, over 70 percent of those with DIS anxiety and depressive disorders were detected, but the physicians also falsely identified 27.7 percent of the noncases as cases.

Demographic Characteristics

Two demographic characteristics of physicians are associated with recognition of psychiatric disorders—age and gender. Obviously, the age of the physician is highly correlated with his or her experience in practice. Marks and colleagues (1979) reported that experienced general practitioners had a higher identification index and reported more conspicuous psychiatric morbidity in their patients. Experienced general practitioners also were more likely to ask patients questions about family and home. Unfortunately, other researchers have not attempted to replicate this finding.

Several studies have explored the issue of how the gender of the physician and patient impact on recognition. Marks reported that for female physicians, a significantly greater percentage of male than female patients scored high on the GHQ. In contrast, the percentage of male and female patients with psychiatric distress was not different for male physicians (Marks et al., 1979). After accounting for psychiatric orientation and interview style, the gender of the physician was not associated with rates of recognition. Boardman (1987) attempted to replicate these findings with eighteen general practitioners in Lewisham, South East London. As in the vast majority of studies, female patients indicated higher levels of psychiatric distress. Moreover, a significantly greater percentage of patients of both genders indicated psychiatric distress for female as contrasted with male general practitioners. Female physicians had a high prevalence of probable psychiatric illness in their patients but a lower bias toward the diagnosis of psychiatric illness. Boardman suggested that symptomatic patients are attracted to women doctors in spite of their bias toward not diagnosing psychiatric illness.

There are no studies conducted in the United States that directly address whether gender of the physician is related to recognition. A recent study that analyzed the interview styles of general internists in America found that female physicians were more verbal with their patients, gave more information, and had longer patient visits. The physician participants in the study were a select sample of academic physicians connected with a medical interview interest group. Therefore, the results may not be generalizable (Roter, Lipkin, & Korsgaard, 1991).

Specialty and Certification

Only a few studies have been able to directly assess how physician specialty and certification relate to recognition of psychiatric illness. In countries other than the United States, almost all of the studies have been limited to general practitioners. In one U.S. study, general internists were more likely to correctly identify a probable psychiatric case on the GHQ than were family practitioners (Hoeper et al., 1979). However, in this study general internists also had longer office visits.

Physicians with more training and better overall knowledge have been found to have higher rates of detection of psychiatric disease in their patients (Marks et al., 1979). Family practice residents with high academic ability were found to have higher rates of recognition; this was even true of residents who expressed a relatively low level of interest in psychiatry (Goldberg et al., 1982). In another study (Moore et al., 1978), experienced third-year family practice residents were more likely to note depression in a depressed patient's chart than first-year interns.

Schulberg and colleagues (1985) specifically assessed the ability of medical practitioners and mental health clinicians to recognize depression in patients at primary care clinics and mental health centers, respectively. Depression was measured with the Center for Epidemiologic Studies–Depression Scale (CESD) and the DIS. Medical practitioners recognized only seven out of twenty-seven patients with major depression but misclassified less than 2 percent of those without major depression. Mental health professionals identified forty-two of seventy-four patients with major depression but misclassified 40 percent of those who did not meet DIS criteria for major depression. Using the kappa test as a measure of chance corrected agreement, medical practitioners had a significantly higher value than mental health clinicians (.32 versus .10). However, this was due primarily to the bias of the medical practitioners toward not diagnosing depression in their patients.

Attitudes and Psychiatric Orientation

Most general practitioners believe that they should recognize psychiatric conditions in their patients. They strongly disagree that they should treat only physical illness and leave tasks such as counseling to other professional groups. Several studies have been able to assess the effect of both physician orientation and attitudes on physicians' actual performance in the recognition of psychiatric distress. Marks et al. (1979) found that a factor "interest and concern" explained a significant amount of variance in physician performance related to recognition. The physician's interest in psychiatry as expressed in a questionnaire was included in this factor. In addition, the "conservatism" of the physician measured with a personality inventory was also negatively related to physician recognition. Conservatism was defined in this study as a tendency to prefer safe, traditional, and conventional forms of institution and behavior. The Goldberg et al. (1982) study of family practice residents in South Carolina resulted in similar findings. In this study, physicians who were aware of their own feelings, were self-confident, and scored high on Allport's Scale of Values had a higher correlation between their ratings of the patient's mental health and the patient's score on a standardized measure of psychological distress.

A study of family practitioners in Quebec found that depressed and anxious patients were more likely to be correctly recognized if their physician was more psychologically minded. Similarly, the psychologically minded physicians were less likely to blame depressed patients for causing their illness than were their less psychologically minded counterparts. Surprisingly, physicians' ability to read the facial expressions of others as assessed with videotapes was not related to recognition (Robbins, Kirmayer, & Cathebras, 1991).

Interview Style

Factors such as gender, age, personality, training, and specialty of physicians all affect the way they interact with patients and conduct medical interviews. In addition, certain interview skills may be independent of the factors just mentioned. In general, interview behaviors have been found to be the most powerful predictors of physician performance related to recognition.

The Marks et al. (1979) study utilized a single research psychiatrist, blind to the patient's score on a standardized psychological distress scale, to directly observe the general practitioner's performance related to recognition of psychiatric illness. The following factors were positively related to recognition: physician empathy (rated by a psychiatrist observer), asking patients about home and family, using open and closed psychiatric questions, using open questions in general, and not reading notes while listening and talking with patients.

Goldberg et al.'s (1982) study of family practice residents relied on evaluation of videotapes of patient encounters. A psychiatric emphasis during the interview, asking about life at home, an empathic interview style, making supportive statements, starting with an open-ended question, making eye contact, dealing well with interruptions, and not becoming buried in notes were all associated with physicians making more accurate ratings of their patient's psychiatric distress.

The medical interview is an interaction between two individuals—physician and patient. Physicians have most of the control and can directly influence the patient's behavior during an interview. One study has specifically considered this potential interaction. Davenport and colleagues (1987) explored how patients with distress interact with physicians who either had a high or a low identification index for psychiatric distress. Could physicians with a low identification index suppress cues indicating distress in their patients? After blinded ratings of videotapes of three physicians previously found to have a low identification index and three physicians with a high identification index, it was possible to draw the following conclusions. Patients with high distress seeing physicians with a high identification index were able to express almost twice as many total cues regarding their distress as high-distress patients seeing physicians with a low identification index. Patients with high distress seeing physicians with a low identification index expressed less movement and fewer vocal and verbal cues of distress. Physicians were able to suppress cues by avoiding eye contact with the patient during the initial stage of the interview, not clarifying the patient's complaint, and asking many closed questions about physical symptoms.

Others have commented that physicians may collude with patients in categorizing symptoms as being nonpsychiatric in origin (Eisenberg, 1992). Goldberg and Huxley (1992, p. 44) describe this phenomenon in the following way: "When an emotional disorder is avoided, both participants have opted for an easier path. The doctor does not have to elicit and then manage emotional distress, and the patient does not have to face up to their distress, and perhaps their own partial responsibility for their current predicament. Both take refuge in safer roles: the doctor as a fighter of supposed organic disease, and the patient as a victim. Faced with such mutual satisfaction with a professional encounter, it ill behooves an outsider to declare that anything is wrong."

Health System or Financing Variables

Characteristics of the health care system, such as reimbursement schedules and health insurance coverage, can affect physician recognition of mental health problems. In addition, physician recognition varies depending on the number of times the physician has seen the patient and whether continuity of care has been established.

The Medical Outcomes Study contrasted the ability of physicians with varied specialties practicing in several different health care systems to detect depression in patients (Wells et al., 1989). Practices in Los Angeles, Boston, and Chicago were sampled to allow assessment by type of practice (solo, health maintenance organizations, and large multispecialty group practice) as well as financing system (prepaid versus fee for service). Prepaid plans provide incentives to physicians to reduce services and thus might lead to lower rates of detection. Larger group practices might be more likely to employ mental health specialists on site and therefore might improve rates of detection. In this study, depression was measured with a screening questionnaire and the DIS. Recognition was measured by having the clinician complete a short form at the end of the visit. Appropriateness-of-care variables were developed based on recognition, counseling, and referral to a mental health specialist. Approximately 50 percent of the medical outpatients received appropriate care for their depression. Rates of recognition and appropriateness of care were slightly higher in physicians practicing in solo practices than in group sites. For type of payment, patients under a fee-for-service system were more likely to have their depression recognized and appropriately managed than patients under a prepaid system. Most of these differences only reflected an enhanced rate of detection or management of approximately 10 percent. Although these differences are still present after adjustment for site, sociodemographic factors of patients, clinician specialty, perceived general health, and severity of depression, the lower rate of participation in the study for solo versus group-practice physicians may be contributing to the reported differences by practice type. Low-quality physicians in solo sites might refuse to participate, while low-quality physicians in group practice sites would have less of a choice and so would agree to participate.

One other study investigated how rates of recognition varied by type of payment. In the Marshfield group-practice study, no differences by type of payment for services existed (Kessler et al., 1985).

The extent to which patients receive continuous, longitudinal care with a single provider may also impact on rates of recognition. Patients with depression who use the emergency room as their usual source of care are less likely to report discussing depression with their doctor than are patients who have a usual source of medical care (Bucholz & Robins, 1987). Individuals who had recently seen a general physician, who were able to name a physician as their usual source of care, or who had more than one visit in the past six months were more likely to have discussed an emotional or substance abuse problem with their physician (Ford, Kamerow, & Thompson, 1988). In the Marks et al. (1979) study, those patients who had been seen by their physician more often were more likely to be identified as having a psychiatric disorder. This result was confirmed in the Marshfield study (Kessler et al., 1985). The more that ambulatory care conforms to the model of primary care—including comprehensive, longitudinal care by a single physician—the higher the rate of recognition by the physician.

Conclusion

In comparison to many other aspects of primary care practice, the recognition of psychiatric illness in medical patients has been relatively well studied. Although recognition of psychiatric illness in only 50 percent of affected patients appears to be unacceptable, it is not clear how this compares to the diagnosis of other conditions in primary care. Primary care patients often present with less severe and more undifferentiated symptoms than patients seen by specialists. The diagnosis of psychiatric illness in medical patients is difficult because of the wide spectrum in how patients present with symptoms, the lack of consistent and practical nosology to aid diagnosis, and the difficulty in determining the etiology for symptoms with multiple potential causes. As difficult as physician recognition might be, however, some primary care physicians have been found to be very good at recognizing those patients with mental illness. Interviewing techniques of physicians appear to be the characteristics most consistently associated with recognition of psychiatric disorders. At this time, the best way to improve rates of recognition would appear to be to improve the interviewing skills of physicians. In addition, we need a better understanding of the process physicians use in evaluating patients for psychiatric illness. Do physicians ask patients about only a few key symptoms? Even after assessing patients for psychiatric symptoms, do physicians misjudge the severity of psychiatric symptoms? Do physicians ignore nonverbal behavior in their assessment of patients? How does the perception of treatability impact on efforts at recognition? A detailed assessment of physician behavior will be required to better understand the diagnostic process. At this time, use of written case scenarios and focused rating of patient-physician interactions on either audiotape or videotape would appear the best alternatives for assessing physician behavior.

Finally, future studies of physician recognition should concentrate on those psychiatric symptoms or disorders for which there are proven interventions in primary care practice. One wonders if basing physician performance on recognition alone is the best measure. Primary care patients fall on a continuum ranging from having no psychiatric symptoms to having one or two psychiatric symptoms up to the level of suffering from psychiatric disorders. It may be better to focus on management of patients rather than simply recognition. Physicians may be more consistent in referring patients to specialty mental health providers or prescribing psychotropic medications for them than in simply recognizing psychiatric disease.

References

Barsa, J., Toner, J., Gurland, B., & Lantigua, R. (1986). Ability of internists to recognize and manage depression in the elderly. *International Journal of Psychiatry, 1,* 57–62.

Boardman, A. P. (1987). The General Health Questionnaire and the detection of emotional disorder by general practitioners: A replicated study. *British Journal of Psychiatry, 151,* 373–381.

Bridges, K., & Goldberg, D. (1985). Somatic presentation of DSM-III psychiatric disorders in primary care. *Journal of Psychosomatic Research, 29,* 563–569.

Bucholz, K. K., & Robins, L. N. (1987). Who talks to a doctor about existing depressive illness? *Journal of Affective Disorders, 12,* 241–250.

Chancellor, A., Mant, A., & Andrew, G. (1977). The general practitioner's identification and management of emotional disorders. *Australian Family Physician, 6,* 1137–1143.

Davenport, S., Goldberg, D., & Millar, T. (1987). How psychiatric disorders are missed during medical consultations. *Lancet, 3,* 439–442.

Dew, M. A., Dunn, L., Bromet, E., & Schulberg, H. (1988). Factors affecting help seeking during depression in a community sample. *Journal of Affective Disorders, 14,* 223–234.

Eisenberg, L. (1992). Treating depression and anxiety in primary care: Closing the gap between knowledge and practice. *New England Journal of Medicine, 326,* 1080–1083.

Ford, D. E., Kamerow, D. B., & Thompson, J. W. (1988). Who talks to their physician about mental health and substance abuse problems? *Journal of General Internal Medicine, 3,* 363–369.

Gerber, P. D., Barrett, J., Barrett, J., Manheimer, E., Whiting, R., & Smith, R. (1989). Recognition of depression by internists in primary care. *Journal of General Internal Medicine, 4,* 7–13.

German, P. S., Shapiro, S., Skinner, E. A., Von Korff, M., Klein, L. E., Turner, R. W., Teitelbaum, M. L., Burke, J., & Burns, B. J. (1987). Detection and management of mental health problems of older patients by primary care providers. *Journal of the American Medical Association, 257,* 489–493.

Goldberg, D., & Bridges, K. (1987). Screening for psychiatric illness in general practice: The general practitioner versus the screening questionnaire. *Journal of the Royal College of General Practitioners, 37,* 15–18.

Goldberg, D., & Huxley, P. (1992). *Community mental disorders: A bio-social model.* London: Tavistock/Routledge.

Goldberg, D. P., Jenkins, L., Millar, T., & Faragher, E. B. (1993). The ability of trainee general practitioners to identify psychological distress among their patients. *Psychological Medicine, 23,* 185–193.

Goldberg, D., Steele, J. J., Jolinson, A., & Smith, C. (1982). Ability of primary care physicians to make accurate ratings of psychiatric symptoms. *Archives of General Psychiatry, 39,* 829–833.

Hoeper, E. W., Nycz, G. R., Cleary, P. D., Regier, D. A., & Goldberg, I. D. (1979). Estimated prevalence of ROC mental disorder in primary medical care. *Internal Journal of Mental Health, 6,* 6–15.

Hoeper, E. W., Nycz, G. R., Kessler, L. G., Burke, J. D., Jr., & Pierce, W. E. (1984). The usefulness of screening for mental illness. *Lancet, 1,* 33–35.

Jencks, S. F. (1985). Recognition of mental distress and diagnosis of mental disorder in primary care. *Journal of the American Medical Association, 253,* 1903–1907.

Jenkins, R., Smeeton, N., Mainker, M., & Sheperd, M. (1985). A study of the classification of mental ill-health in general practice. *Psychological Medicine, 15,* 403–409.

Kessler, L. G., Cleary, P. D., & Burke, J. D., Jr. (1985). Psychiatric disorders in primary care. *Archives of General Psychiatry, 42,* 583–587.

Koenig, H. G., & Blazer, D. G. (1992). Epidemiology of geriatric affective disorders. *Clinics in Geriatric Medicine, 8,* 235–251.

Leaf, P. J., Livingston, M. M., Tischler, G. L., Weissman, M. M., Holzer, C. E., & Myers, J. K. (1985). Contact with health professionals for the treatment of psychiatric and emotional problems. *Medical Care, 23,* 1322–1337.

Marks, J. N., Goldberg, D. P., & Hillier, V. F. (1979). Determinants of the ability of general practitioners to detect psychiatric illness. *Psychological Medicine, 9,* 337–353.

Moore, J. T., Silimperi, D. R., & Bobula, J. A. (1978). Recognition of depression by family medicine residents: The impact of screening. *Journal of Family Practice,* 7(3), 509–513.

Ormel, J., van den Brink, W., Koeter, M. W. J., Giel, R., van der Meer, K., van de Willige, G., & Wilmink, F. W. (1990). Recognition, management, and outcome of psychological disorders in primary care: A naturalistic follow-up study. *Psychological Medicine, 20,* 909–923.

Perez-Stable, E. J., Miranda, J., Muñoz, R. F., & Ying, Y.-W. (1990). Depression in medical outpatients. *Archives of Internal Medicine, 150,* 1083–1088.

Redman, S., Webb, G., Hennrikers, D., Gordon, J., & Samson-Fisher, R. (1991). Diagnosis of psychological disturbance: The effects of patient gender. *Journal of Behavioral Medicine, 14*(5), 527–540.

Robbins, J. M., Kirmayer, J. J., & Cathebras, P. (1991, September). Physician sensitivity to emotional and nonverbal expression and the recognition of depression and anxiety in primary care. *Proceedings of the Fifth Annual NIMH International Research Conference on the Classification, Recognition, and Treatment of Mental Disorders in General Medical Settings* (Abstract).

Roter, D., Lipkin, M., & Korsgaard, A. (1991). Sex differences in patients' and physicians' communications during primary care medical visits. *Medical Care, 29,* 1083–1093.

Schulberg, H. C., Saul, M., McClelland, M., Ganguli, M., Christy, W., & Frank, R. (1985). Assessing depression in primary medical and psychiatric practices. *Archives of General Psychiatry, 42,* 1164–1170.

Shapiro, S., Shanner, E. A., Kessler, L. G., Von Korff, M., German, P. S., Tischler, G. L., Leaf, P. J., Benham, L., Cottler, L., & Regier, D. A. (1984). Utilization of health and mental health services: Three Epidemiologic Catchment Area sites. *Archives of General Psychiatry, 41,* 971–978.

Shepherd, M., Cooper, B., Brown, A. B., & Kalton, G. W. (1966). *Psychiatric illness in general practice.* London: Oxford University Press.

Sireling, L. I., Paykel, E. S., Freeling, P., Rao, B. M., & Patel, S. P. (1985). Depression in general practice: Case thresholds and diagnosis. *British Journal of Psychiatry, 147,* 113–119.

Von Korff, M., Shapiro, S., Burke, J. D., Teitelbaum, M., Skinner, E. A., German, P., Turner, R. W., Klein, L., & Burns, B. (1987). Anxiety and depression in a primary care clinic. *Archives of General Psychiatry, 44,* 152–156.

Wells, K. B., Hays, R. D., Burnam, M. A., Rogers, W., Greenfield S., & Ware, J. E., Jr. (1989). Detection of depressive disorder for patients receiving prepaid or fee-for-service care. *Journal of the American Medical Association, 262,* 3298–3302.

Anne W. Riley
Lawrence S. Wissow

10

Recognition of Emotional and Behavioral Problems and Family Violence in Pediatric Primary Care

Community prevalence studies identify 18 to 20 percent of youth as having a mental disorder, with as many as 11 percent (six to eight million) experiencing sufficient impairment to warrant treatment (Anderson, Williams, McGee, & Silva, 1987; Bird et at., 1988; Cohen et al., 1987; Kashani et al., 1989; Offord et al., 1987). However, significantly less than half of these children receive any form of treatment, and much of what they do receive is inappropriate (Institute of Medicine, 1989; Saxe, Cross, & Silverman, 1988; Tuma, 1989). This inadequate response to the needs of these children and adolescents can be related to a lack of awareness that they have treatable disorders. The role of primary care medical professionals, pediatricians, family medicine specialists, and pediatric nurse practitioners is critical to any effort to improve the detection, understanding, and treatment of children and adolescents with significant emotional and behavior disorders (Tarnowski, 1991). These disorders and family violence are legitimate health concerns because they are barriers to children's development of a positive self-concept and stable mental health functioning. The purpose of this chapter is to review the research on primary care providers' recognition, management, referral, and treatment of mental health problems in their child and adolescent patients.

Many factors appear to play a role in determining which children with mental disorders will receive needed services and which will not. We will address the following aspects of the identification and management of health problems by primary care practitioners:

1. The extent to which children seeking primary health care have emotional problems, behavioral problems, and/or are experiencing family problems such as violence
2. The typical office presentation of these youth
3. The likelihood that their mental health problems will be recognized
4. The effect of detecting and not detecting disorder and family violence
5. What is known about improving the detection of mental disorder
6. Directions for future intervention and research

Current Practices

An effective primary care response to children's health problems depends on health providers' timely recognition of medical problems, mental health disturbances, and serious family dysfunction, and also on adequate use of health services by youth. Most U.S. children make a medical visit at least annually, although great variability by both age and family insurance status exists. In 1987, 93 percent of children under five years old and three-quarters of children from five to fourteen years old saw a physician at least once (National Center for Health Statistics, 1990, p. 179). However, 10 percent of the older children had not had a contact in two years or more (National Center for Health Statistics, 1990, p. 179). Although uninsured children are at much greater risk for not obtaining medical care (Lewin and Associates, 1989), a variety of programs—including school-based clinics (Lear, Gleicher, St. Germaine, & Porter, 1991) and universal coverage for children (Sheils, Spaw, &

Merritt, 1991)—are being proposed to further improve the access of all children to health care.

Children's mental health problems include syndromes that meet psychiatric diagnostic criteria as well as involving developmental delays, serious family disturbances, and other psychosocial problems. Recognition of these behavioral and developmental problems has long been a stated aim of pediatric medical care. The American Academy of Pediatrics' (1988) practice guidelines for periodic well-child visits include a major focus on assessment of children's developmental achievements, interactions with peers and parents, and, for older children, academic performance. Such efforts appear to be partially successful. For example, pediatricians were the source of a third of the referrals for those first in contact with mental health providers in Monroe County, New York over a three-year period (Griffin, Cicchetti, & Leaf, 1991). Additionally, the majority of children who have serious mental disorders are probably more likely to receive counseling from their primary care physicians and nurses than from a mental health specialist, just as is true for adults (Regier, Goldberg, & Taube, 1978; Tarnowski, 1991). Although primary care providers refer and manage mental health problems for many of their patients, recent research indicates that fewer than half the children with significant psychopathology seen in primary care receive a psychiatric diagnosis or mental health care referral (Cadman, Boyle, Szatmari, & Offord, 1987; Costello, 1986; Costello, Edelbrock, et al., 1988; Lavigne et al., 1991; Riley et al., 1993).

Definition of Mental Health Problems in Children

Prior to discussing recognition of emotional and behavioral problems, we define the classification terms. A mental, emotional, or psychiatric disorder or diagnosis can be made when an individual has symptoms that meet the minimum diagnostic criteria for a disorder required by the ICD-9 or DSM-III-R classification systems. Such diagnoses do not typically reflect the level of impairment associated with having a disorder. The term *Serious Emotional Disturbance* (SED) is widely used, particularly by the educational system, and does indicate that impairment has existed over time and interferes with educational performance (Education for All Handicapped Act, P.L. 94-142). However, SED does not indicate the specific type of disorder. Finally, the term *psychosocial problems* as used in this chapter encompasses the range of emotional, behavioral, and mental health problems that are associated with dysfunction and impairment but that do not meet strict diagnostic criteria under present guidelines. In addition to reflecting low-intensity problems or early stages of disorder, these problems may reflect responses to family and community violence, family dysfunction, and economic deprivation.

Prevalence and Physician Recognition

Prevalence studies of mental health problems among children seen in medical settings indicate that a significant proportion of children are affected. Prevalence estimates vary by the method of assessment and classification system used.

Medical Record Review

One approach to assessing prevalence is to review medical charts for mental disorder and/or psychosomatic diagnoses. This approach is likely to result in conservative prevalence estimates, given the reluctance of providers to label children with such diagnoses and the possibility that the mental health problem is overlooked or simply not the focus of the encounter. Medical record review studies indicate that about 3.5 percent of preschool children, 8 percent of the ten- to fourteen-year-olds, and 10 percent of the fifteen- to sixteen-year-olds are identified by their medical practitioner as having a DSM-level mental disorder (Goldberg, Roghmann, McInerny, & Burke, 1984). Studies of the overall rates of mental disorders and psychosocial problems yield prevalence rates of between 3 and 22 percent (Coleman, Patrick, & Baker, 1977; Jacobson et al., 1980; Starfield et al., 1980). The proportion identified varies widely by site even within a single study, reflecting differences in the definition used for the estimate (disorders versus psychosocial problems), the organization of care, the populations served, and the types of visits studied.

Screening for Psychosocial Problems

Several recent studies have had parents complete questionnaires to identify the probable presence of an emotional or behavioral problem. Although these screening questionnaires falsely identify a substantial number of children as positive for the disorder, they typically do not miss many children who do have significant problems (Campbell, 1987; Kamerow, 1987). In one study, in a health maintenance organization population, parents completed the Child Behavior Checklist (CBCL), a 113-item scale that screens for behavioral problems of children four to sixteen years of age (Achenbach & Edelbrock, 1983). Parental ratings of severity and frequency are used to distinguish those children who have a sufficient number of problems such as anxiety, depression, psychosomatic disorders, aggression, and overactivity, such that their mental health problems are likely to be clinically meaningful. According to the CBCL, 25 percent of children seven to eleven years old were in the clinical range (Costello, Edelbrock, et al., 1988).

In a younger sample drawn from nineteen different pediatric practices in New Haven, Connecticut, parents identified 17 percent of children four to eight years old as being in the clinical range on the CBCL (Horwitz, Leaf, Leventhal, Forsyth, & Speechley, 1992). In the same study, physicians identified 27 percent of the children as having a clinically significant psychosocial, developmental, and emotional problem based on a World Health Organization classification system (Burns, Burke, & Regier, 1982). Although there was poor agreement between the parents and providers on which children had a mental disorder, parent and provider agreement was good for the specific problems a child had (Horwitz et al., 1992). This finding suggests that at least some of the reported poor recognition of psychosocial problems by physicians and nurses may result from noncomparable definitions of what constitutes a psychosocial or psychiatric problem.

Two-Stage Screening and Psychiatric Assessment

A rigorous research method for identifying individuals with psychiatric disorders involves administering a mental health screening instrument to a defined sample, then administering a structured psychiatric interview to all those who score in the clinical range on the screening instrument as well as to a portion of those who do not score in the clinical range. This method permits an estimate of the prevalence of diagnosable disorder without conducting psychiatric interviews with the entire population. Costello, Edelbrock, et al. (1988) used this method to assess the prevalence of mental disorder among 789 seven- to eleven-year-old children visiting a health maintenance organization. All children who scored in the clinical range on the parent-completed CBCL and a random sample of those who scored in the normal range were given the Diagnostic Interview Schedule for Children (DISC) (Costello, Edelbrock, Dulcan, Kalas, & Klaric, 1984). This is a highly structured psychiatric interview administered by trained lay interviewers to children and their parents. The diagnostic modules generate DSM-III diagnoses applying computer algorithms. Applying stringent scoring standards, the prevalence of diagnosable mental disorder was 11.8 percent (with 95 percent confidence that the true prevalence is between 9.3 and 13.5 percent in this population). The children's pediatricians, who were surveyed separately, recognized only 17 percent of DISC-diagnosed cases, giving a "hidden morbidity rate" of 83 percent (Costello, Edelbrock, et al., 1988).

Similar results come from two-stage studies conducted in Europe and developing countries. In Britain, Garralda and Bailey (1986) used the Rutter Scale A Child Behavior Questionnaire (Rutter, Tizard, & Whitmore, 1970) to screen seven- to twelve-year-old consecutive patients at an outpatient clinic ($N = 234$). Parents of children in the clinical range and of a random sample who were apparently free of psychological problems were then given a standardized psychiatric interview about the child. The total prevalence of psychological problem cases was 23 percent. Only 8 percent of the cases, however, were identified by physicians as having a psychological problem; all the cases they identified had anxiety disorders.

In a World Health Organization study of mental disorders among children at primary health care facilities in four developing countries, rates between 12 and 29 percent were found using a two-stage screening (Giel et al., 1981). Consistent with other studies, the primary health care workers recognized only between 10 and 22 percent of the cases that ultimately met diagnostic criteria (Giel et al., 1981).

Although less is known about younger children, preliminary findings are similar to those of older children. In a recent study, pediatricians identified 6 percent of children under age six as having emotional or behavioral problems at the time of the study assessment, whereas 12 percent were identified by consensus diagnosis using a broad range of assessments (Lavigne et al., 1991). Further studies are likely to replicate the finding that pediatricians underdiagnose emotional and behavioral problems in children under age six.

In summary, pediatric health care providers vastly underdiagnose psychiatric disorders in children. When they do identify a child as having a disorder, it is often not diagnosable according to standardized psychiatric assessments. The possible reasons for and significant impact of this poor recognition are discussed later in this chapter.

Characteristics of Children Seen in Primary Care

Consistent with comparative findings from community studies, the prevalence of psychosocial problems identified in primary care is higher among certain subsamples. Boys (Costello, Edelbrock, et al., 1988; Goldberg et al., 1984), children living under lower socioeconomic conditions (Garralda & Bailey, 1986; Goldberg et al., 1984; Jacobson et al., 1980), and children whose mother or father is absent from the home (Garralda & Bailey, 1986; Goldberg et al., 1984; Riley et al., 1993) are more likely to be identified as having a psychiatric disorder than are other children. Prevalence also increases with increasing age (Costell, Edelbrock, et al., 1988; Goldberg et al., 1984; Lavigne et al., 1991), and there are peaks in prevalence as children enter elementary and middle school (Schor, 1986).

Chronic physical disorder is associated with a two- to fivefold increased risk of psychiatric disorder, and 10 percent of children experience a chronic physical disorder sometime in childhood (Pless & Douglas, 1971). Those with severe illness, sensory or neurological disorders, or significant disability are at greatest risk for mental disorder (Cadman et al., 1987; Goldberg et al., 1984; Lavigne & Faier-Routman, 1992; Rutter, Tizard, & Whitmore, 1970). Children who experience multiple acute illnesses may also be at increased risk of psychosocial problems (Starfield et al., 1984; Hankin & Starfield, 1986). Chapter Six provides a more detailed discussion of the issues associated with comorbidity in children.

Extent of Family Conflict and Violence Among Pediatric Patients

The studies reviewed above rely on diagnoses and symptom clusters to identify children. Additionally, children not meeting strict criteria for mental disorder may be exposed to situations that pose a threat to their mental health and psychosocial development. For example, exposure to violence is often a hidden risk among asymptomatic children. Interpersonal violence and maltreatment are strong predictors of children's poor psychosocial development (Browne & Finkelhor, 1986; Bryer, Nelson, Miller, & Krol, 1987; Dodge, Bates, & Pettit, 1990; Kessler & Magee, 1991). Exposure to violence is common in the United States, where homicide is the fourth leading cause of death among preschool and school-age children (National Center for Health Statistics, 1987). Conservative estimates are that over one million U.S. children annually, or 1.6 percent of the population under eighteen, meet strict criteria for having been harmed by abuse or neglect, and over 1.5 million, or 2.5 percent, are in some way harmed or endangered (U.S. Department of Health and Human Services, Office of Human Development Services, 1988). In two national population-based surveys, 2 to 4 percent of two-parent U.S. families reported severe physical violence (that is, kicking, biting, punching, threatening, or using a deadly weapon), directed by parents toward children (Gelles, 1987). Levels of violence are higher in single-parent families, probably because of the greater likelihood that these families live in poverty (Gelles, 1989). The apparent prevalence of child maltreatment increases steadily with age, so that adolescents are the group at highest risk, with estimated annual rates of maltreatment that are twice those of infants (U.S. Department of Health and Human Services, Office of Human Development Services, 1988).

One problem in identifying family violence is that some forms of parental aggression toward children are considered acceptable. Over 70 percent of U.S. parents feel that spanking or slapping are necessary disciplinary methods for childrearing, and over 50 percent report having spanked or slapped a child in the past year (Gelles, 1987). The acceptance of aggression toward children makes it difficult for health care workers to separate "acceptable" from pathological levels of violence in a home.

Violence between adults in a household may also pose risks for children; they may be injured as bystanders, struck intentionally by angry parents, or psychologically injured by witnessing assaults on loved ones (Holden & Ritchie, 1991). About 16 percent of married couples report physically violent exchanges in the past year, with 28 percent reporting physical violence at some time in their relationship (Gelles, 1987). In a national sample of two-parent families, the amount of violence between adult partners was directly correlated with violence directed toward children (Straus, Gelles, & Steinmetz, 1980).

Child abuse reporting statistics suggest that relatively little abusive violence is recognized in office-based primary care settings. In Maryland, for example, 16 percent of reports of suspected maltreatment come from hospitals (inpatient and outpatient services), while only 2 percent come from private practitioners (State of Maryland, Department of Human Resources, 1984). Much of this discrepancy may be attributable to more conservative reporting practices among office-based practitioners. In Maryland, a recent survey found that pediatricians and family practitioners in solo or group practice reported a smaller proportion of cases that they suspected of maltreatment than physicians practicing in acute care (emergency room or clinic) settings (Wissow, Wilson, & Zellman, 1991).

Similarly, spouse abuse is underrecognized in medical settings. Goldberg and Tomlanovich (1984) surveyed 492 adults coming to an urban emergency room about exposure to present and past episodes of domestic violence. Twenty-two percent of the patients reported being victims, but only 5 percent of these had been noted in the medical record. Research in the United Kingdom suggests that the majority of battered women do consult a doctor at some point, but only for a small minority of the violent incidents they suffer. According to one study (Johnson, 1985), even when battered women visit their general practitioner, only a quarter to a half disclose the violence. In most cases, physicians are willing to accept fabricated histories or fail to inquire how the injuries occurred.

Recognition of family violence in pediatric primary care settings has rarely been investigated. In a study at an inner-city hospital's pediatric continuity clinic, mothers were asked to complete the Conflict Tactics Scale (Straus, 1979) as a measure of violence within their home. Pediatricians were independently asked to predict which of their patients' mothers would report violence during their appointment. Forty percent of mothers reported abusive violence among family members within the past year, but physicians correctly identified only 27 percent of these families (Wissow, Wilson, Roter, Larson, & Berman, 1992).

Given the apparent rise of violence in communities and families and the negative impact of violence on children's development, it seems imperative that the medical community take a lead in increasing the sensitivity of practitioners to the possibility that their patients may be experiencing abuse or witnessing violence against loved ones. But obtaining such knowledge is challenging because the provider must address the issue in a way that is supportive to the child and family. Helping in an abusive situation is sometimes difficult to do, especially since child abuse must be reported when it is even suspected, and such professional responses can create a great deal of hostility in the parent. Consequently, the reluctance of providers to elicit information on abuse is understandable and points to their need to develop skills in dealing with these problems. This will require a greater commitment to the practical teaching of these skills in medical and nursing training and in continuing education and in-service training for those already in practice (U.S. Department of Health and Human Services, Office of Human Development Services, Advisory Board on Child Abuse and Neglect, 1990, p. 65).

Office Presentation of Children with Emotional and Behavioral Problems

Somatic complaints are the most frequent pediatric office presentations of children with emotional or behavioral distress (Starfield et al., 1980; Garralda and Bailey, 1986). Typical problems include abdominal pain, fatigue, headaches, and anorexia (Nikapota, 1987). In some cases, the child's bodily symptoms are truly "functional"—that is, they go away when a primary psychological problem is addressed. In many cases, however, treatable medical conditions coexist, and behavioral or emotional problems have accentuated their impact on the child and family.

No specific behavioral symptoms necessarily indicate exposure to violence in the home or community. Abused children may have a higher level of behavioral problems than are seen in the general population, but many abused children also appear normal (Jaffe, Wolfe, Wilson, & Zak, 1986). This is reflected in a survey of nearly 4,000 junior and senior high school students, which could detect no pattern of behaviors that was highly sensitive or specific for maltreatment, although eating disorders (anorexia and bulimia) and suicidal ideation were most highly associated with abuse (Hibbard, Ingersoll, & Orr, 1990). It is worth noting that in the study of inner-city pediatric patients mentioned above (Wissow, Wilson, Roter, Larson, & Berman, 1992), mothers in violent families were nearly twice as likely as those in nonviolent families to identify behavioral problems in their child, despite the fact that the physicians rated the behavior of both groups similarly.

A major difficulty in diagnosing children's emotional and behavioral problems accurately is the variation in symptoms that occurs with changes in the child's immediate environment and with the observer. In a survey of the mental health of children in Ontario, for example, teachers were more likely than parents to identify children as being hyperactive or having conduct disorders, but not more likely to label children as having emotional or somatization problems (Offord & Boyle, 1989). The social constraints of the classroom may make some children's symptoms more apparent, but teachers may also use a different standard for deviance than parents. Similar differences may occur in the physician's examining room. Children may view the encounter as frightening and react as they would to other stressful situations. Alternatively, they may respond well to the structure of the visit and appear better than they might in a disordered home environment or in a demanding academic or social situation.

The physician's task is to find the right balance between a medical and a psychosocial approach to the child's evaluation (Bridges & Goldberg, 1985). One concern is that somatic complaints will be taken at face value without inquiry into contributing psychological factors. According to national surveys and several studies, pediatric providers typically spend less than a minute in the average thirteen-minute visit inquiring about psychosocial problems and providing guidance to the child and parent (National Center for Health Statistics, 1987; Reisinger & Bires, 1980). To elicit complete and reliable information on which to base a psychosomatic, functional, or psychiatric diagnosis, pediatric providers must demonstrate interest in psychosocial problems and provide an opportunity to discuss them (Roter & Hall, 1991). This is important even if the child appears well in the office.

What Mental Health Problems Do Primary Care Providers Recognize in Children?

The most frequent psychosocial, developmental, and emotional problems that medical providers cite using the World Health Organization checklist are family problems (7.2 percent of children), behavioral problems (6 percent), and language problems (5.5 percent) (Leaf et al., 1990). Other commonly identified problems in pediatric practices include tantrums, noncompliance with parental requests, aggression, and toileting problems (enuresis, encopresis). The most common specific psychiatric diagnosis pediatric primary care physicians make is adjustment disorder, which they give to over half of those identified, perhaps because it is a convenient catchall diagnosis. Attention deficit problems, anxiety, and conduct disorders are the next most common (Lavigne et al., 1991; Costello, Edelbrock, et al., 1988; Riley et al., 1993).

Physicians identify internalizing problems such as poor self-esteem, anxiety and depression, and withdrawn behavior much less often than externalizing symptoms such as tantrums and aggression, although it is the internalizing problems that parents most often identify (Hickson, Altemeier, & O'Connor, 1983; Riley et al., 1993). School and family problems are rarely the stated subject of a primary care appointment. However, several studies have shown that these stressors are associated with high levels of medical care use (Beautrais, Fergusson, & Shannon, 1982; Schor, 1986).

Factors Influencing the Recognition of Mental Health Problems

A number of factors influence recognition of these problems in both adult and pediatric medical settings, such as the severity of the mental health problem, the interest and training of the health care provider with respect to psychosocial issues, and the reason for and time allotted to the visit. There are at least two additional factors in pediatric care. Most obviously, children often do not speak for themselves. Their parents decide when to seek health care and typically communicate on their behalf (Pantell, Stewart, Dias, Wells, & Ross, 1982). Second, the labeling of disorder presents a greater challenge in children. Mental disorder is still associated with stigma and health care providers are hesitant to make such diagnoses, relying on the possibility that the child will "outgrow" the problem. Additionally, the nomenclature for child and adolescent mental disorders is far from being firmly established as reliable and valid (Institute of Medicine, 1989), and primary care practitioners in the adult or pediatric specialties often do not accept or understand it. This last problem may be ameliorated by the availability of the Primary Care version of the *Diagnostic and Statistical Manual of Mental Disorders*. When pediatricians and nurse practitioners are encouraged to identify mental health problems and can refer to providers with whom they have a close working relationship, behavioral problems are frequently detected at early stages (Finney, Riley, & Cataldo, 1991).

Child Factors

Medical providers are most likely to make a psychiatric diagnosis if the child has a high level of symptomatology and obvious impairment in social functioning, although sensitivity is low even for these severely disturbed children (Costello, Edelbrock, et al., 1988; Lavigne et al., 1991; Riley et al., 1993). If children have a social factor believed to place them at higher risk for mental health problems, they are much more likely to receive a mental disorder diagnosis. For example, in the study by Costello, Edelbrock, et al. (1988), children independently diagnosed as having a psychiatric disorder were more likely to also be identified by their physician as having a mental disorder if they were black, male, and in the lowest third of the socioeconomic structure (Costello, 1988). Another study indicates that among children identified by parents as distressed on the CBCL, those living in single-parent households were three times more likely to receive a psychiatric diagnosis from their medical providers than children who were also distressed but living in two-parent homes (Riley et al., 1993). In contrast, the presence of poor physical health may bias physicians against making an emotional disorder diagnosis. In the study by Riley et al. (1993), children with emotional distress who also had poor physical health were four times *less* likely to receive a mental disorder diagnosis than physically healthy distressed children.

Parent Communication

Parent-expressed concerns about psychosocial or developmental problems affect the probability that primary care providers will identify children with disorders. Physicians failed to detect 87 percent of the children meeting criteria for a psychiatric disorder in a structured interview when the parents did not voice concerns about emotional problems. A smaller, though still unacceptable, proportion (67 percent) went undetected when the parents did raise an emotional or behavioral concern (Dulcan et al., 1990).

Physician Characteristics

Pediatricians and family practitioners have distinct preferences for treating some classes of problems over others; their training is predominantly in medical assessment, and so they generally see treatment and medical questions as more interesting and more appropriate than psychosocial problems (Christophersen, 1982; Hickson et al., 1983). Parents often perceive these physician priorities, which then influences the types of problems they feel comfortable raising during a visit. Between 70 and 80 percent of the questions that parents want to ask pediatricians involve psychosocial problems, although less than a third of parents actually raise these concerns (Hickson et al., 1983; McCune, Richardson, & Powell, 1984). Studies of communication between pediatricians and parents indicate that physicians dominate the interaction, providing few opportunities for parents and children to raise concerns (Pantell et al., 1982). Physicians may even actively change the subject when a parent raises a topic that the physician does not wish to discuss (Korsch, Gozzi, & Francis, 1968). However, Goldberg (1990) has also suggested that collusion between the patient (parent) and the provider is a mechanism by which significant aspects of mental disorders are not addressed in the primary care visit. Both parties often are more comfortable tacitly ignoring the mental health implications of symptoms and distress. Physicians' perceptions of parental receptivity to mental health referrals may also play a role in discouraging detection or treatment of child psychosocial problems.

Impact of Failing to Recognize Psychosocial Problems

Psychosocial problems have a potential for serious long-term sequelae (Kessler & Magee, 1991; Klein & Mannuzza, 1991; Kovacs & Goldston, 1991; Loeber, 1991; Robins, 1983) that equal or exceed the effects of medical illnesses that health care providers are preoccupied with, such as chronic otitis media (inflammation of the middle ear) and asthma. The immediate consequences of not recognizing children's emotional and behavioral problems and those of the family are threefold. First, adherence to recommended medical treatments may be compromised by concerns or impairments associated with the unaddressed mental health problem (Ormel & Giel, 1990), thus increasing the risk of poor-quality medical care (Bensing, 1991). At best, the patient's problems are incompletely addressed; at worst, the wrong problem is treated.

Second, an obvious consequence of overlooking mental health problems is continued distress for the child and family. A number of studies have found that children who have emotional problems according to their mothers or physicians are more likely to be high users of care (Jacobson et al., 1980; Riley et al., 1993). It should be noted, though, that in two population-based studies in which the presence of an emotional or behavioral disorder was identified independent of a health provider, the rates of ambulatory medical care were not different between those with and without the disorder (Costello, Burns, et al., 1988; Offord et al., 1987). But those with mental disorders used more mental health care and, therefore, more health care overall (Woodward et al., 1988).

Third, and perhaps most important, while many children do "outgrow" their problems and many psychological problems are self-limiting, fully 50 percent of children with significant emotional or behavioral problems will continue to experience similar problems into adolescence and adulthood (Robins, 1983; Rutter, Tizard, Yule, Graham, & Whitmore, 1976). Significant behavioral problems in young children have been shown to persist and develop into disorders in a high proportion of cases. In one study, 67 percent of children who were hard to manage at ages three and six met criteria for conduct or hyperactivity disorders when they were nine (Campbell and Ewing, 1990).

Conduct disorders are well known to persist into adult life. Half the youth with this disorder subsequently manifest such adult antisocial behavior as alcohol abuse, criminal activity, and poor occupational outcomes (Loeber, 1991; Robins, 1966; Rutter et al., 1976). Longitudinal research has more recently demonstrated that hyperactive behavior disorders persist, especially among boys, resulting in a heightened risk of continued hyperactivity, antisocial personality disorder, and substance use disorder (Klein & Mannuzza, 1991; McGee, Partridge, Williams, & Silva, 1991).

Prospective research has recently begun to demonstrate that depression in childhood and adolescence is associated with a high likelihood of experiencing an affective disturbance in adult life (Harrington, Fudge, Rutter, Pickles, & Hill, 1990; Kovacs, Feinberg, Crouse-Novak, Paulauskas, & Finkelstein, 1984; Kovacs & Goldston, 1991). Additionally, child abuse has been shown to result in a significantly heightened risk of depression throughout life (Kessler & Magee, 1991). There is also a growing consensus that many children suffer for years from psychological and social difficulties associated with divorce (Wallerstein, 1991).

These problems probably exert their influence by interfering with the ways children process social cues and develop a sense of self. Even a short-lived problem may cause major disruption if it occurs at a crucial time in a child's social or academic development. Aggressive behavior is particularly maladaptive, since it tends to make children unpopular and unable to adapt to the school environment (Ensminger and Slusarcick, 1992). Early social and school failure is difficult to overcome, since those who fail are often removed from mainstream interactions rather than treated for their problems in the regular environments. This replicates the pattern of negative and rejecting interactions that cause or contribute to serious emotional disturbance.

What Is the Evidence That Childhood Mental Health Problems Can Be Treated?

Detection of a disorder is most important when it can be shown that an available intervention will favorably influence the course of the disorder (Campbell, 1987; Goldberg, 1990). Preliminary evidence suggests the value of detection of emotional and behavior problems in pediatric primary care—a topic fully discussed in Chapter Six.

Treatment of child mental disorder by mental health clinicians applying specific interventions has been shown to be effective in two meta-analyses of well-designed treatment studies. The results of seventy-five studies indicate that the treated children function two-thirds of a standard deviation better on a range of measures than untreated children (Casey & Berman, 1985). A review of 108 therapy studies with children and adolescents (four to sixteen years old) indicates that the average treated child was better adjusted after treatment than 79 percent of those not treated (Weisz, Weiss, Alicke, & Klotz, 1987). Both studies found that behavioral treatments performed better than nonbehavioral treatments, possibly because behavioral treatments are typically applied to well-specified problems with defined treatment goals. Childhood problems such as fears, specific types of anxiety, noncompliance with adult requests, enuresis, encopresis, impulsivity, aggression, and self-control can be effectively modified using behavioral treatments (Casey & Berman, 1985; Weisz et al., 1987). More generalized goals such as improvement in self-concept and attitudes are difficult to achieve by any treatment method (Barnett, Docherty, & Frommelt, 1991).

These research outcomes may be fundamentally different from those of children treated routinely in local mental health clinics and practices. An indication that it may not be valid to generalize from well-controlled therapy outcome research to everyday mental health practice comes from a study of therapy routinely delivered in nine clinics. Ninety-three youth who completed treatment were compared with sixty who dropped out after intake. There was no significant effect of therapy at the six- and twelve-month follow-up (Weisz & Weiss, 1989). This result is consistent with a longitudinal study of childhood depression in which routine community mental health treatment was not associated with improved outcomes (Kovacs et al., 1984). These "naturalistic" outcome studies suggest that optimal outcomes are unlikely when mental health problems are not well defined and treatment is not standardized and systematic.

Evaluations of programs to treat severely dysfunctional families—those that have already been referred for child maltreatment—yield somewhat discouraging results. The National Clinical Evaluation Study (Daro, 1988), which compiled data from nineteen treatment programs, found that a substantial percentage of families either refuse to enter treatment or drop out along the way. Among those who complete treatment, 60 percent are rated by program staff as having improved. Recidivism rates are high, ranging from 19 percent of cases involving sexual abuse to 75 percent for emotional maltreatment. More encouraging are the results from secondary prevention trials. Programs that provide support to mothers and information about child behavior and normal parenting dilemmas have shown some ability to decrease the rate of abuse in at-risk families (Olds, Henderson, Chamberlin, & Tatelbaum, 1986). Self-help programs such as Parents Anonymous, while not rigorously evaluated, also appear capable of stabilizing families at risk for abuse.

Improving the Detection and Management of Emotional and Behavioral Problems

Time constraints and the inconsistent opportunities for assessing psychosocial needs are often seen as barriers to improving recognition of psychosocial problems in primary care. One solution is self- or parent-report screening instruments (Simonian, Tarnowski, Stancin, Friman, & Atkins, 1991). Such screens are inexpensive, take only a short time to complete, and can be applied uniformly to most children. Despite the potential value of screening instruments, they should not be used without a thorough understanding of their inherent limitations (Campbell, 1987; Kamerow, 1987). When imperfect instruments are used to screen for rare disorders, errors are made in the false positive direction. Often, approximately half of the individuals they identify as having a disturbance will not actually have the problem on further assessment (Campbell, 1987; Shrout, Skodol, & Dohrenwend, 1986). The large proportion of children falsely identified as having a mental health problem makes it incumbent on practitioners to perform a second stage of screening designed to distinguish between the children who are truly disturbed and those who are not.

While this need to follow up on the information provided by a screening instrument is critical, both anecdotal and research evidence indicates that practitioners frequently fail to make use of the information obtained from mental health screening questionnaires. In a randomized trial of mental health screening, 1,045 parents reported on their child's behavioral problems and social functioning on the CBCL. Feedback on the presence of behavioral and social problems was given to the pediatric provider for one-half of the children. Children were followed for six months to determine the effect of health care provider knowledge about serious behavioral problems on patient management. Among children who were in the clinical range on the CBCL, some mental health care was obtained by 28 percent of those whose providers received no CBCL information about them and by 24 percent of those whose providers were notified (Hankin, Goodman, & Starfield, 1987). One reason for the lack of an effect in this study may have been the timing of feedback to the physicians: parents completed the CBCL after the visit and feedback was given to the provider within twenty-four hours. To manage the identified problem, the child would have had to return for another visit within the six month follow-up or the provider would have had to contact the parent by phone. Better results may have been obtained if the screening information was available at the start of the index visit. Although the results from similar studies with adults are inconsistent, at least two well-controlled studies do demonstrate some positive effect of informing providers about screening results (Johnstone & Goldberg, 1976; Shapiro et al., 1987).

Approaches that facilitate the communication of patients' psychosocial concerns are likely to improve the accurate identification of problems (Dulcan et al., 1990; Goldberg, 1990). One study conducted in pediatric waiting rooms prior to well-clinic visits helped parents of very young children clarify their concerns. Parents who received this brief intervention initiated more communications about child health topics during the pediatric visit. Moreover, 100 percent of the initial parental concerns of the prompted group were discussed in the visit, compared to only 83 percent of the concerns of the control-group parents (Finney et al., 1990). These results are similar to previous patient-provider communication studies that encouraged adult patients (Greenfield, Kaplan, & Ware, 1985; Roter, 1977) and parents of developmentally delayed or young children (Delgado & Lutzker, 1988; Kohr, Parrish, Neef, Driessen, & Hallinan, 1988) to be more active during health care visits.

Preliminary work with adult patients indicates that training in communication skills can have a positive effect on outcomes of patients' emotional problems. In one study, Roter and Hall (1991) trained internists and family medicine practitioners in communication skills in a two-session Continuing Medical Education course. Using a control group design, they demonstrated that among patients who were in the clinical range on the General Health Questionnaire (GHQ-28; Goldberg, 1972), those who were seen by a physician trained in communication skills showed significant improvement on their GHQ scores three and six months later compared to those seen by untrained physicians.

Improving the reimbursement for mental health services is sometimes suggested as an approach to improving detection and treatment of psychosocial problems in primary care. Two studies, however, suggest that improving reimbursement does not, in itself, improve these practices. During 1987 and 1988 in Canada, where health insurance is universal and physician payment is guaranteed, pediatricians were paid 34 percent more for mental health services than for other office visits. But Canadian pediatricians averaged eight mental health service visits every five weeks, not significantly different from the typical pediatrician in the United States (Richman, 1991). In the United States, the RAND Health Insurance Experiment found that a guarantee of reimbursement to the patient and provider did not ensure that the majority of adults with significant psychological distress would receive mental health treatment (Ware, Manning, Duan, Wells, & Newhouse, 1984).

Conclusion

Mental health and psychosocial problems are prevalent, are associated with negative health and developmental impacts, and are more likely to persist over time than to remit entirely. Despite their obvious effects, these problems most often go untreated or are treated inappropriately. Although primary health care providers should be able to identify and treat children's mental health problems more successfully, primary care doctors and nurses currently recognize and manage these problems poorly. This is likely to be especially true for those treating children with chronic physical disorders. Although there are many possible explanations for the poor performance of medical providers in managing these important threats to children's health and development, the main point is that increased efforts to improve management are critical.

First, enhanced education of primary care providers is needed regarding the prevalence of mental disorders and their persistent effects on later life functioning. Second, primary care and specialty residency training should provide more opportunities for formal and informal communication skill building (Gask, Goldberg, Lesser, & Millar, 1987; Goldberg, Steele, Smith, & Spivey, 1983). Third, students' experiences with severely disturbed psychiatric inpatients in both medical and nursing schools must be balanced with greater exposure to patients in ambulatory mental health care who have the relatively common emotional and behavioral problems encountered in general medical practice. Finally, practitioners should be trained in discriminating which problems they can treat and which should be referred. They also require training in methods of treating children's emotional and behavioral problems themselves and in ongoing management of the cases referred to mental health specialists.

The mental health research and treatment community has obligations as well. The need for a classification system acceptable in primary care has been addressed through the development of a Primary Care version of the DSM-IV manual. Further research and collaborations between mental health and medical providers are required to determine the cost-effectiveness, treatment utility, and negative effects of screening for mental health problems in the waiting rooms of primary care providers. Additional efforts are necessary to ensure the effectiveness of mental health treatments, especially in routine community practice. This is perhaps most critical, since without assurance that routine referrals are likely to produce improvements in child and family well-being, medical providers are justified in not making referrals for mental health care.

A potential approach that institutions can implement is to increase the accountability for identifying emotional or behavioral problems through existing quality assurance mechanisms. Documentation that psychosocial problems were assessed in the visit is an appropriate aspect of quality-of-care review, especially for groups of patients who are at highest risk for undetected problems. These include chronically ill children, youth with multiple acute recurring illnesses, children with high levels of utilization without significant medical problems, children with high levels of injuries, young adolescents with sexually transmitted disease, and those whose families are experiencing disruption. Giving feedback to providers on the adequacy of their attention to psychosocial issues may prove effective in increasing their communication with parents and children.

Perhaps the most important future work will be investigations of the outcomes of children with psychosocial problems who are and who are not identified and actively managed within the primary care setting. Apart from simply determining if providers recognize, treat, and refer mental health problems, we need to know whether this effort makes a difference in the lives of children and their families. This will require information about how the patient functioned at the time of problem identification and how functioning changed from the point at which the problem was identified in primary care, through mental health treatment, and for some time afterward.

As Ormel and Giel (1989) suggest, only when providers are effective at eliciting concerns about psychosocial problems, trained in handling information about the presence of an emotional or behavioral problem, and have effective mental health interventions available and opportunities to implement them will their patients show significant improvement. The current national interest in improving the lives of children and enhancing their development may provide the impetus needed to refine communication and detection techniques and disseminate these skills so that providers of primary health care can more effectively manage these common threats to healthy child development.

References

Achenbach, T., & Edelbrock, C. (1983). *Manual for the child behavior checklist and revised child behavior profile*. Burlington, VT: Queen City Printers.

American Academy of Pediatrics. (1988). *Guidelines for health supervision*. Elk Grove Village, IL: American Academy of Pediatrics.

Anderson, J. C., Williams, S., McGee, R., & Silva, P. A. (1987). DSM-III disorders in preadolescent children. *Archives of General Psychiatry, 44,* 69–80.

Barnett, R. J., Docherty, J. P., & Frommelt, G. M. (1991). A review of child psychotherapy research since 1963. *Journal of the American Academy of Child and Adolescent Psychiatry, 30,* 1–14.

Beautrais, A. L., Fergusson, D. M., & Shannon, F. T. (1982). Life events and childhood morbidity: A prospective study. *Pediatrics, 70,* 935–940.

Bensing, J. (1991). *Doctor-patient communication and the quality of care*. The Hague, the Netherlands: Gegeven Koninklijke Bibliotheek.

Bird, H. R., Canino, G., Rubio-Stipec, M., Gould, M. S., Ribera, J., Sesman, M., Woodbury, M., Huertas-Goldman, S., Pagan, A., Sanchez-Lacay, A., & Moscoso, M. (1988). Estimates of the prevalence of childhood maladjustment in a community survey in

Puerto Rico: The use of combined measures. *Archives of General Psychiatry, 45*(12), 1120–1126.

Bridges, K. W., & Goldberg, D. P. (1985). Somatic presentations of DSM-III psychiatric disorders in primary care. *Journal of Psychosomatic Research, 29,* 563–569.

Browne, A., & Finkelhor, D. (1986). Impact of child sexual abuse: A review of the research. *Psychological Bulletin, 99,* 66–77.

Bryer, J. B., Nelson, B. A., Miller, J. B., & Krol, P. A. (1987). Childhood sexual and physical abuse as factors in adult psychiatric illness. *American Journal of Psychiatry, 144,* 1426–1430.

Burns, B. J., Burke, J. D., Jr., & Regier, D. A. (1982). A child oriented psychosocial classification for primary care. In M. Lipkin & K. Kupka (Eds.), *Psychosocial factors affecting health* (pp. 185–208). New York: Praeger.

Cadman, D., Boyle, M., Szatmari, P., & Offord, D. (1987). Chronic illness, disability, and mental and social well-being: Findings from the Ontario Child Health Study. *Pediatrics, 79,* 805–813.

Campbell, S. B., & Ewing, L. J. (1990). Follow-up of hard-to-manage preschoolers: Adjustment at age 9 and predictors of continuing symptoms. *Journal of Child Psychology, Psychiatry, and Allied Disciplines, 31,* 871–889.

Campbell, T. L. (1987). Is screening for mental health problems worthwhile in family practice? An opposing view. *Journal of Family Practice, 25,* 184–187.

Casey, R. J., & Berman, J. S. (1985). The outcome of psychotherapy with children. *Psychological Bulletin, 98,* 388–400.

Christophersen, E. (1982). Incorporating behavioral pediatrics into primary care. *Pediatric Clinics of North America, 29,* 261–296.

Cohen, P., Velez, C. N., Kohn, M., Schwab-Stone, M., & Johnson, J. (1987). Child psychiatric diagnosis by computer algorithms. *Journal of the American Academy of Child and Adolescent Psychiatry, 26,* 631–638.

Coleman, J. V., Patrick, D. L., & Baker, S. M. (1977). The mental health of children in an HMO program. *Behavioral Pediatrics, 91*(1), 150–153.

Costello, E. J. (1986). Primary care pediatrics and child psychopathology: A review of diagnostic, treatment, and referral practices. *Pediatrics, 78,* 1044–1051.

Costello, E. J. (1988, October). *Who gets treated?* Paper presented at the American Academy of Child and Adolescent Psychiatry meeting, Seattle, WA.

Costello, E. J., Burns, B. J., Costello, A., Edelbrock, C., Dulcan, M., & Brent, D. (1988). Service utilization and psychiatric diagnosis in pediatric primary care: The role of the gatekeeper. *Pediatrics, 82,* 435–441.

Costello, E. J., Edelbrock, C., Costello, A., Dulcan, M., Burns, B., & Brent, D. (1988). Psychopathology in pediatric primary care: The new hidden morbidity. *Pediatrics, 82,* 415–424.

Costello, E. J., Edelbrock, C. S., Dulcan, M. K., Kalas, R., & Klaric, S. H. (1984). *Development and testing of the NIMH Diagnostic Interview Schedule for Children (DISC) in a clinical population: Final report* (National Institute of Mental Health Contract No. RFP-DB-81-0027). Rockville, MD: Center for Epidemiological Studies.

Daro, D. (1988). *Confronting child abuse: Research for effective program design.* New York: Free Press.

Delgado, L. E., & Lutzker, J. R. (1988). Training young parents to identify and report their children's illnesses. *Journal of Applied Behavior Analysis, 21,* 311–319.

Dodge, K. A., Bates, J. E., & Pettit, G. S. (1990). Mechanisms in the cycle of violence. *Science, 250,* 1678–1683.

Dulcan, M. K., Costello, E. J., Costello, A. J., Edelbrock, C. S., Brent, D., & Janiszewski, S. (1990). The pediatrician as gatekeeper to mental health care for children: Do parents' concerns open the gate? *Journal of the American Academy of Child and Adolescent Psychiatry, 29,* 453–458.

Ensminger, M. E., & Slusarcick, A. L. (1992). Paths to high school graduation or dropout: A longitudinal study of a first grade cohort. *Sociology of Education, 65*(2), 95–113.

Finney, J. W., Brophy, C. J., Friman, P. C., Golden, A. S., Richman, G. S., & Ross, A. F. (1990). Promoting parent-provider interaction during young children's health supervision visits. *Journal of Applied Behavior Analysis, 23,* 207–213.

Finney, J. W., Riley, A. W., & Cataldo, M. F. (1991). Psychology in primary health care: Effects of brief targeted therapy on children's medical care utilization. *Journal of Pediatric Psychology, 16,* 447-461.

Garralda, M. E., & Bailey, D. (1986). Children with psychiatric disorders in primary care. *Journal of Child Psychology and Psychiatry, 27,* 611-624.

Gask, L., Goldberg, D., Lesser, A. T., & Millar, T. (1987). Improving the psychiatric skills of the general practice trainee: An evaluation of a group training course. *Medical Education, 21,* 362-368.

Gelles, R. J. (1987). *Family violence* (2nd ed.). Newbury Park, CA: Sage.

Gelles, R. J. (1989). Child abuse and violence in single-parent families: Parent absence and economic deprivation. *American Journal of Orthopsychiatry, 59,* 492-501.

Giel, R., de Arango, M. V., Climent, C. E., Harding, T. W., Ibrahim, H. H. A., Ladrido-Ignacio, L., Srinivasa-Murthy, R., Salazar, M. C., Wig, N. N., & Younis, Y. O. A. (1981). Childhood mental disorders in primary health care: Results of observations in four developing countries. *Pediatrics, 68,* 677-683.

Goldberg, D. (1972). *The detection of psychiatric illness by questionnaire.* London: Oxford University Press.

Goldberg, D. (1990). Reasons for misdiagnosis. In N. Sartorius, D. Goldberg, G. de Girolamo, J. A. Costa e Silva, Y. Lecrubier, & H.-U. Wittchen (Eds.), *Psychological disorders in general medical settings.* Toronto: Hogrefe & Huber.

Goldberg, D., Roghmann, K. J., McInerny, T. K., & Burke, J. D. (1984). Mental health problems among children seen in pediatric practice: Prevalence and management. *Pediatrics, 73,* 278-293.

Goldberg, D., Steele, J., Smith, C., & Spivey, L. (1983). *Training family practice residents to recognize psychiatric disturbances.* Rockville, MD.: National Institute of Mental Health. Also available from National Technical Information Service, U.S. Department of Commerce, 5285 Port Royal Road, Springfield, VA 22161.

Goldberg, D., & Tomlanovich, M. C. (1984). Domestic violence victims in the emergency department. *Journal of the American Medical Association, 251,* 3259-3264.

Greenfield, S., Kaplan, S., & Ware, J. E. (1985). Expanding patient involvement in care. *Annals of Internal Medicine, 102,* 520–528.

Griffin, J. A., Cicchetti, D., & Leaf, P. (1991, November). *Case register analysis of child mental health service utilization.* Paper presented at the 119th annual meeting of the American Public Health Association, Atlanta, GA.

Hankin, J. R., Goodman, A., & Starfield, B. (1987, June). *The impact of sharing the results of psychosocial screening on the psychosocial management of the child.* Paper presented at the first annual NIMH Conference on Mental Health in General Medical Settings, Seattle, WA.

Hankin, J. R., & Starfield, B. (1986). Epidemiologic perspectives on psychosocial problems in children. In N. A. Krasnegor, J. D. Arasteh, & M. F. Cataldo (Eds.), *Child health behavior: A behavioral pediatrics perspective.* New York: Wiley.

Harrington, R., Fudge, H., Rutter, M., Pickles, A., & Hill, J. (1990). Adult outcomes of childhood and adolescent depression: 1. Psychiatric status. *Archives of General Psychiatry, 47,* 465–473.

Hibbard, R. A., Ingersoll, G. M., & Orr, D. P. (1990). Behavioral risk, emotional risk, and child abuse among adolescents in a nonclinical setting. *Pediatrics, 86,* 896–901.

Hickson, G., Altemeier, W., & O'Connor, S. (1983). Concerns of mothers seeking care in private pediatric offices: Opportunities for expanding services. *Pediatrics, 72,* 619–624.

Holden, G. W., & Ritchie, K. L. (1991). Linking extreme marital discord, child rearing, and child behavior: Evidence from battered women. *Child Development, 62,* 311–327.

Horwitz, S. M., Leaf, P. J., Leventhal, J. M., Forsyth, B., & Speechley, K. N. (1992). The identification and management of psychosocial and developmental problems in community-based, primary care pediatric practices. *Pediatrics, 89,* 480–485.

Institute of Medicine. (1989). *Research on children and adolescents with mental, behavioral, and developmental disorders.* Washington, DC: National Academy Press.

Jacobson, A. M., Goldberg, I. D., Burns, B. J., Hoeper, E. W., Hankin, J. R., & Hewitt, K. (1980). Diagnosed mental disorder in children and use of health services in four organized health care settings. *American Journal of Psychiatry, 137,* 559–565.

Jaffe, P., Wolfe, D., Wilson, S. K., & Zak, L. (1986). Family violence and child adjustment: A comparative analysis of girls' and boys' behavioral symptoms. *American Journal of Psychiatry, 143,* 74–77.

Johnson, N. (1985). Police, social work, and medical responses to battered women. In N. Johnson (Ed.), *Marital violence* (Sociological Review Monograph No. 31) (pp. 109–123). London: Routledge & Kegan Paul.

Johnstone, A., & Goldberg, D. P. (1976, March 20). Psychiatric screening in general practice. *Lancet, 1,* 605–608.

Kamerow, D. B. (1987). Is screening for mental health problems worthwhile in family practice? An affirmative view. *Journal of Family Practice, 25*(2), 181–183.

Kashani, J. H., Ovaschel, H., Rosenberg, T. K., & Reid, J. C. (1989). Psychopathology in a community sample of children and adolescents: A developmental perspective. *Journal of the American Academy of Child and Adolescent Psychiatry, 28,* 701–706.

Kessler, R. C., & Magee, W. J. (1991, November). Childhood adversity and adult depression: Basic patterns of association in a U.S. national survey. Paper presented at the annual meeting of the American Public Health Association, Atlanta, GA.

Klein, R. G., & Mannuzza, S. (1991). Long-term outcome of hyperactive children: A review. *Journal of the American Academy of Child and Adolescent Psychiatry, 30,* 383–387.

Kohr, M. A., Parrish, J. M., Neef, N. A., Driessen, J. R., & Hallinan, P. C. (1988). Communication skills training for parents: Experimental and social validation. *Journal of Applied Behavior Analysis, 21,* 21–30.

Korsch, B. M., Gozzi, E. K., & Francis, V. (1968). Gaps in doctor-patient communication: Doctor-patient interaction and patient satisfaction. *Pediatrics, 48,* 855–871.

Kovacs, M., Feinberg, T. L., Crouse-Novak, M. A., Paulauskas, S. L., & Finkelstein, R. (1984). Depressive disorders in childhood: 1. A longitudinal prospective study of characteristics and recovery. *Archives of General Psychiatry, 41,* 229–237.

Kovacs, M., & Goldston, D. (1991). Cognitive and social cognitive development of depressed children and adolescents. *Journal of the American Academy of Child and Adolescent Psychiatry, 30,* 388–392.

Lavigne, J. V., Christoffel, D. K., Binns, H. J., Rosenbaum, D., Arend, R., Smith, K., & Hayford, J. R. (1991, September). *Psychopathology among preschoolers in pediatric primary care: Prevalence and pediatric recognition.* Paper presented at the fifth annual NIMH International Research Conference on the Classification, Recognition, and Treatment of Mental Disorders in General Medical Settings, Bethesda, MD.

Lavigne, J. V., & Faier-Routman, J. (1992). Psychological adjustment to pediatric physical disorders: A meta-analytic review. *Pediatric Psychology, 17*(2), 133–158.

Leaf, P. J., Horwitz, S., Leventhal, J., Speechley, K., Forsyth, B., Schwab-Stone, M., & Pakes, J. (1990, October). *Primary care pediatrics: What is detected, what is done.* Paper presented at the American Academy of Child and Adolescent Psychiatry, Chicago.

Lear, J. G., Gleicher, H. B., St. Germaine, A., & Porter, P. J. (1991). Reorganizing health care for adolescents: The experience of the school based adolescent health care program. *Journal of Adolescent Health Care, 12,* 450–458.

Lewin and Associates. (1989, June). *Health care for the medically indigent in Pennsylvania.* Report prepared for the Pennsylvania Health Care Cost Containment Council.

Loeber, R. (1991). Antisocial behavior: More enduring than changeable? *Journal of the American Academy of Child and Adolescent Psychiatry, 30,* 393–397.

McCune, J. D., Richardson, M., & Powell, J. (1984). Psychosocial health issues in pediatric practices: Parents' knowledge and concerns. *Pediatrics, 74,* 183–190.

McGee, R., Partridge, F., Williams, S., & Silva, P. A. (1991). A twelve-year follow-up of preschool hyperactive children. *Journal of the American Academy of Child and Adolescent Psychiatry, 30,* 224–232.

National Center for Health Statistics. (1987). *Advance report of final mortality statistics, 1985. Monthly Vital Statistics Report,* 1–48. (DHHS Publication No. (PHS) 87-1120).

National Center for Health Statistics. (1990). *Health, United States,*

1989 (DHHS Publication No. (PHS) 90-1232). Hyattsville, MD: Public Health Service.

Nikapota, A. D. (1987). *Recognition and management of children with functional complaints: A training package for the primary care physician.* New Delhi, India: World Health Organization, Regional Office for Southeast Asia.

Offord, D. R., & Boyle, M. H. (1989). Correlates of disorder. *Journal of the American Academy of Child and Adolescent Psychiatry, 28,* 856–860.

Offord, D. R., Boyle, M. H., Szatmari, P., Rae-Grant, N. I., Links, P. S., Cadman, D. T., Byles, J. A., Crawford, J. W., Munroe Blum, H., Byrne, C., Thomas, H., & Woodward, C. A. (1987). Ontario Child Health Study: Six month prevalence of disorder and rates of service utilization. *Archives of General Psychiatry, 44,* 832–836.

Olds, D. L., Henderson, C. R., Chamberlin, R., & Tatelbaum, R. (1986). Preventing child abuse and neglect: A randomized trial of nurse home visitation. *Pediatrics, 78,* 65–78.

Ormel, J., & Giel, R. (1990). Medical effects of non-recognition of affective disorders in general medical settings. In N. Sartorius, D. Goldberg, G. de Girolamo, J. A. Costa e Silva, V. Lecrubier, & H.-U. Wittchen (Eds.) *Psychological disorders in general medical settings* (pp. 146–158). Lewiston, NY: Hogrefe & Huber.

Pantell, R. H., Stewart, T. J., Dias, J. K., Wells, P., & Ross, A. W. (1982). Physician communication with children and parents. *Pediatrics, 70,* 396–402.

Pless, I. B., & Douglas, J. W. B. (1971). Chronic illness in childhood: 1. Epidemiological and clinical characteristics. *Pediatrics, 47,* 405–414.

Regier, D. A., Goldberg, D., & Taube, C. A. (1978). The de facto U.S. mental health services system. *Archives of General Psychiatry, 35,* 685–693.

Reisinger, K. S., & Bires, J. A. (1980). Anticipatory guidance in pediatric practice. *Pediatrics, 66,* 889–892.

Richman, A. (1991, November). *Does National Health Insurance increase children's accessibility to mental health service from primary physicians?* Paper presented at the annual meeting of the American Public Health Association, Atlanta, GA.

Riley, A. W., Finney, J. W., Mellits, E. D., Starfield, B., Kidwell, S., Quaskey, S., Cataldo, M. F., Filipp, L., & Shematek, J. (1993). Determinants of children's health care use: An investigation of psychosocial factors. *Medical Care, 31,* 767–783.

Robins, L. N. (1966). *Deviant children grown up.* Baltimore, MD: Williams & Wilkins.

Robins, L. N. (1983). Continuities and discontinuities in the psychiatric disorders of children. In D. Mechanic (Ed.), *Handbook of health, health care, and the health professions.* New York: Free Press.

Roter, D. L. (1977). Patient participation in the patient-provider interaction: The effects of patient question asking on the quality of interaction, satisfaction, and compliance. *Health Education Monographs, 5,* 281–315.

Roter, D., & Hall, J. (1991, September). *Recruitment and training of primary care physicians in interviewing skills to identify and address patients' psychosocial distress.* Paper presented at the fifth annual NIMH International Research Conference on the Classification, Recognition, and Treatment of Mental Disorders in General Medical Settings, Bethesda, MD.

Rutter, M., Tizard, J., & Whitmore, K. (Eds.). (1970). *Education, health, and behaviour.* London: Longmans, Green.

Rutter, M., Tizard, J., Yule, W., Graham, P., & Whitmore, K. (1976). Isle of Wight Studies 1964–1974. *Psychological Medicine, 6,* 313–332.

Saxe, L., Cross, T., & Silverman, N. (1988) Childrens' mental health: The gap between what we know and what we do. *American Psychologist, 43,* 800–807.

Schor, E. L. (1986). Use of health care services by children and diagnoses received during presumably stressful life transitions. *Pediatrics, 77,* 834–841.

Shapiro, S., German, P. S., Skinner, E. A., Von Korff, M., Turner, R. W., Klein, L. E., Teitelbaum, M. L., Kramer, M., Burke, J. D., & Burns, B. J. (1987). An experiment to change detection and management of mental morbidity in primary care. *Medical Care, 25,* 327–339.

Sheils, J., Spaw, N., & Merritt, K. (1991). *An illustrative universal coverage program for children and pregnant women in Mary-*

land. Draft final report. (Prepared for the Maryland Governor's Commission on Health Care Policy and Financing.)

Shrout, P. E., Skodol, A. E., & Dohrenwend, B. P. (1986). A two-stage approach for case identification and diagnosis. In J. E. Barrett & R. M. Rose (Eds.), *Mental disorders in the community* (pp. 286–303). New York: Guilford Press.

Simonian, S. J., Tarnowski, K. J., Stancin, T., Friman, P. C., & Atkins, M. S. (1991). Disadvantaged children and families in pediatric primary care settings: 2. Screening for behavior disturbance. *Journal of Clinical Child Psychology, 20,* 360–371.

Starfield, B., Gross, E., Wood, M., Pantell, R., Allen, C., Gordon, I. B., Moffatt, P., Drachman, R., & Katz, H. (1980). Psychosocial and psychosomatic diagnoses in primary care for children. *Pediatrics, 66,* 159–163.

Starfield, B., Katz, H., Gabriel, A., Livingston, G., Benson, P., Hankin, J., Horn, S., & Steinwachs, D. (1984). Morbidity in childhood—A longitudinal view. *New England Journal of Medicine, 310,* 824–829.

State of Maryland, Department of Human Resources. (1984). *Child abuse in Maryland: The Central Registry Report* (DHR Publication No. SSA 1058 3/86). Baltimore, MD: Social Services Administration, Office of Child Welfare, Protective Services to Children and Families.

Straus, M. A. (1979). Measuring intrafamily conflict and violence: The Conflict Tactics (CT) scales. *Journal of Marriage and Family, 41,* 75–88.

Straus, M. A., Gelles, R. J., & Steinmetz, S. K. (1980). *Behind closed doors.* Garden City, NY: Anchor Books.

Tarnowski, K. J. (1991). Disadvantaged children and families in pediatric primary care settings: 1. Broadening the scope of integrated mental health service. *Journal of Clinical Child Psychology, 20,* 351–359.

Tuma, J. M. (1989). Mental health services for children: The state of the art. *American Psychologist, 44,* 188–199.

U.S. Department of Health and Human Services, Office of Human Development Services. (1988). *Study findings: Study of national incidence and prevalence of child abuse and neglect.* Washington, DC: U.S. Government Printing Office.

U.S. Department of Health and Human Services, Office of Human Development Services, Advisory Board on Child Abuse and Neglect. (1990). *Child abuse and neglect: Critical first steps in response to a national emergency*. Washington, DC: U.S. Government Printing Office.

Wallerstein, J. S. (1991). The long-term effects of divorce on children: A review. *Journal of the American Academy of Child and Adolescent Psychiatry, 30,* 349–360.

Ware, J. E., Manning, W. G., Duan, N., Wells, K. B., & Newhouse, J. P. (1984). Health status and the use of outpatient mental health services. *American Psychologist, 39,* 1090–1100.

Weisz, J. R., & Weiss, B. (1989). Assessing the effects of clinic-based psychotherapy with children and adolescents. *Journal of Consulting and Clinical Psychology, 57,* 741–746.

Weisz, J. R., Weiss, B., Alicke, M. D., & Klotz, M. L. (1987). Effectiveness of psychotherapy with children and adolescents: A meta-analysis for clinicians. *Journal of Consulting and Clinical Psychology, 55,* 542–549.

Wissow, L. S., Wilson, M. E. H., Roter, D., Larson, S., & Berman, H. (1992). Family violence and the evaluation of behavioral concerns in a pediatric primary care setting. *Medical Care, 30* (Suppl.), 150–165.

Wissow, L. S., Wilson, M. E. H., & Zellman, G. (1991). Physician decisions to report and label suspected child maltreatment. *American Journal of Diseases of Children, 145,* 385.

Woodward, C. A., Boyle, M. H., Offord, D. R., Cadman, D. T., Links, P. S., Monroe-Blum, H., Byrne, C., & Thomas, H. (1988). Ontario Child Health Study: Patterns of ambulatory medical care utilization and their correlates. *Pediatrics, 82,* 425–434.

11

Linda Gask

Improvement of Recognition of Psychiatric Disorders in Primary Care

Accurate recognition of psychiatric disorders in primary care settings depends on the skills of general practitioners as medical interviewers (Marks, Goldberg, & Hillier, 1979). But general practitioners and other key members of the primary health care team are still not being given the necessary training in this area (Burns, Scott, Burke, & Kessler, 1983). Too often, psychiatrists in the United Kingdom relate to general practitioners either by lecturing to them or by carrying out clinics (Strathdee & Williams, 1985). Unfortunately, neither of these methods is likely to alter the way general practitioners interview patients or, therefore, the rate at which they are able to detect psychiatric illness among patients.

After discussing why improved recognition of psychiatric disorders is needed and speculating on the factors that make some doctors better at this task than others, this chapter sketches two methods for improving recognition: (1) the use of screening questionnaires by the primary care physician, and (2) training that involves video and/or audio feedback on consultations. The chapter also touches on the teaching of specific skills and briefly summarizes research evaluating various approaches to improving recognition.

What Makes Improved Recognition Worthwhile?

The research tends to show that general practitioners who detect psychiatric disorders favorably influence the treatment outcome. For example, Johnstone and Goldberg (1976) carried out a small project in a solo general practice in the United Kingdom. Patients with high scores on the General Health Questionnaire (GHQ) were randomly assigned to either an index group, about whose mental state the general practitioner was informed, or a control group, where this information was not available. After three months, the index group had a much better outcome than the control group, indicating that recognition did in fact improve clinical outcome. This project has since been replicated in different ways by Zung, Magill, Moore, & George (1983) and Rand, Badger, and Coggins (1988) in the United States. But two other research groups in the United States were unable to replicate the original findings (Hoeper, Nycz, Kessler, Burke, & Pierce, 1984; Shapiro et al., 1987). In the original study, patients were helped by what the doctor did as a result of the information provided. In the two U.S. studies with negative findings, the practitioners did nothing different for the index and control groups and seemed to play a passive role in the research projects. To achieve positive results, general practitioners probably need to be willing and active participants who are skillful enough to discuss the findings of the screening questionnaire with their patients. I will return to this point later in discussing the routine use of screening questionnaires in primary care.

Two further naturalistic studies, using independent research assessment of depressive illness, have shown that cases of depression that are recognized by the general practitioner have a better outcome than those that are not (Tylee & Freeling, 1989 [United Kingdom]; Ormel, Koeter, van den Brink, & van de Willige, 1990 [the Netherlands]. Ormel and colleagues compared 106 patients whose depression was detected by the general practitioner with eighty patients whose illnesses were not detected and showed that the former group had a significantly better outcome after six months. As in the earlier study by Johnstone and Goldberg (1976), improvement was not confined to patients receiving a particular form of treatment. Although in both studies severely depressed patients were prescribed antidepressants, the doctor-patient transaction was modified in other ways: patients were encouraged to discuss their problems and were given counseling. Two controlled studies (Thompson et al., 1982; Hollyman, Freeling, Paykel, Bhat, & Sedgewick, 1988) have shown that depressed patients in primary care do significantly better on antidepressants than on placebos. The evidence suggests that detection of depression in general practice does improve outcome.

Why Are Some Doctors Better at Recognition Than Others?

The ability of a doctor to identify mental disorder has been quantified by Marks, Goldberg, and Hillier (1979) as an *identification index* (if a two-stage screening procedure is used, this is given by the number of detected true positives divided by the expected number of true positives). Marks and colleagues found the mean identification index among ninety-one Manchester general practitioners to be 54 percent (on average, they were missing about 46 percent of the psychiatric cases among their patients). An independent observer rated doctors with high identification indices as having greater interest in and concern for the patient, being more interested in psychiatry, and being more interested in patient management. They were also somewhat older than average. The following list—based on Goldberg & Huxley (1980)—summarizes their behavior in the interview situation:

Start of Interview

Makes good eye contact
Clarifies the nature of the patient's complaint

General Interview Skills

Picks up verbal cues
Picks up nonverbal cues
Deals well with interruptions

Does not get buried in case notes
Makes supportive comments

Types of Questions Posed

Asks directive "psychiatric" questions
Asks closed "psychiatric" questions
Asks questions about family and home situation

Davenport, Goldberg, and Millar (1987) have demonstrated that the nature of the interaction between patient and doctor can vary. Patients interviewed by a doctor with a high identification index will tend to provide more verbal cues, to allow more distress to appear in their voices, and to move more restlessly than those interviewed by a doctor with a low identification index. In other words, patients interviewed by doctors good at detecting psychiatric disorders seem to make the diagnosis easier for them by giving more cues indicating psychological distress. On the other hand, certain patients do not show any evidence of psychological problems during an interview despite high scores on the GHQ.

Another study—by Millar, Goldberg, and Jenkins (1991)—showed that practitioners who were successful at recognizing psychiatric disorders tended to make more eye contact with their patients throughout the interviews. They also encouraged the patients' responses more often and asked more questions with a social content. All these differences between the doctors were present irrespective of the patients' GHQ scores; the only finding specific to patients with high GHQ scores was that the more able doctors tended to ask them directive social questions about their home life early in the interview. Doctors with high identification indices were significantly better not only at detection but also at management of psychological disorders and gave explanatory information, advice, and treatment instructions in a clear and negotiated way. The ability to make accurate assessment of psychological distress is not a specific skill, but part of a generally superior ability to communicate with patients. Training in recognition of psychological disorders is similarly difficult to separate from training in management skills, because management also to a certain degree depends on good communication (although specific strategies may need to be learned and practiced).

Methods for Improving Recognition

I first consider the use of screening questionnaires, then turn to training in psychiatric interviewing skills.

Use of Screening Questionnaires

A number of different instruments have been used to formally screen for mental disorder in primary and general medical settings. The twenty-eight-item version of the GHQ (Goldberg & Hillier, 1979) and the Hospital Anxiety and Depression (HAD) Inventory (Zigmond & Snaith, 1983) have been tested extensively in general practice in the United Kingdom. For the GHQ, a cutoff score of 4/5 has been widely used for research purposes, because at that threshold the positive predictive value is 77 percent and the specificity is 85 percent. However, Wright and Perini (1987) have argued that a higher cutoff score is more clinically useful. In general medical settings, a higher cutoff score is also recommended (for example, see Bridges & Goldberg, 1986).

In theory, screening questionnaires could be employed in three ways in the primary care setting: (1) *universally*—that is, given to all patients—which would be time consuming but would identify the extent of hidden morbidity in a practice (and could be specifically useful when teaching detection skills); (2) with *high-risk categories* only, by screening only those known to be "at risk" because of life-style, physical illness, adverse circumstances, or family history of psychiatric illness, which would decrease the false positive rate but might mean that some cases are missed; and (3) *postinterview,* to screen those for whom there is a suspicion of a problem hidden by presentation of somatic complaints, which would again result in fewer false positives but might not end up being particularly useful clinically.

In practice, problems exist in the screening process. Although improving recognition of psychiatric disorders results in better treatment outcome, introducing routine screening may or may not contribute to a better outcome. As Goldberg and Williams (1988, p. 29) have stated in response to the negative studies cited earlier, "Mere feedback of the GHQ-score to a doctor is not, by itself, of any value. It is certainly necessary for the doctor to be interested in the information, and probably necessary for the doctor to discuss social and psychological problems with the patient as a result of seeing the GHQ if the patient is to benefit from a case-finding procedure."

To be able to discuss these matters, the doctor must clearly possess good communication skills, In the next section, we will focus on attempts to improve the skills of primary care physicians so that they feel confident and able to raise such matters in the consultation regardless of whether this is in response to a screening questionnaire.

Training in Psychiatric Interviewing Skills

Training, based on audio or video feedback of real or role-played consultations, can be carried out one to one or in a group setting. The latter has three distinct advantages. First, it is more efficient; several doctors are being trained rather than one. Second, a group is more likely to generate a range of suggestions for alternative behavior when the tape stops. Third, a group can provide a great deal of support for a trainee *if facilitated effectively*. But much teaching of consultation skills in general practice in the United Kingdom takes place on a one-to-one basis between trainer and trainee, and all the skills that will be described can be taught this way. Teaching for doctors that employs methods other than video or audio feedback (for example, role-playing, demonstration, lectures) has not so far been demonstrated to improve recognition, unless combined with some form of feedback teaching.

The problem-based approach to teaching psychiatric interviewing skills in primary care (Lesser, 1981, 1985; Gask, Boardman, & Standart, 1991) has now been extensively researched and will be described in some detail, although it is not the only such model to be employed and evaluated. The key difference between the problem-based approach to teaching with video or audiotape and others previously described is that tapes are used specifically for the *rehearsal of new skills*—not to assess the performance of the doctor, rate the consultation, or interpret the patient's behavior. The tape is stopped throughout to discuss how particular cues given by the patient might have been responded to differently and to highlight skills useful for detection, assessment, and management of patient problems. Audiotapes of consultations can be particularly useful for obtaining repeated recordings of a single patient, especially if the practice does not possess its own video camera.

In general, we ask members of the group to try to select material before the session and to bring patients with whom they are experiencing some difficulty. However, if members of the group *always* select patients to be discussed during the session, they are unlikely to choose patients with hidden psychiatric morbidity, since they cannot be expected to select such patients if they are unaware of their disorders. A way around this is to ask a member of the group to make videotapes of an entire clinic. Each patient seen completes a psychiatric screening questionnaire such as the GHQ, and the teacher is presented with a list showing the names of the patients in the order in which they appear, the questionnaires, and the videotape. The teacher views the tape before the teaching session, looking only at the interviews between the trainee and patients who score high on the screening questionnaire. Teaching can then focus on consultations where the practitioner is likely to have missed emotional disorders and can bring to light both missed "cues" and behaviors demonstrated by the doctor that may have discouraged the patients from discussing problems.

Group participants should always be asked how they felt about being taped so that particular anxieties can be addressed. Older participants may never have observed themselves on video before, while trainees may have had negative experiences with video feedback in their medical school teaching.

The key step in improving skills is stopping the tape and rehearsing what could have been done or said differently at a given point in the interview. This is almost impossible to do from memory at the end of the consultation and even more difficult to do when working from case notes rather than a video presentation. Facilitators should always try, however hard it is, to say something positive about what has happened in the interview before making any negative comments (as in Pendleton, Schofield, Tate, & Havelock, 1983).

Group members should be responsible for their own learning (Lesser, 1985). If the facilitator constantly stops the tape and points out everything to the group, they will never improve their own powers of observation or skills. Trainers employ a hierarchy of prompts, such as the following: "Why do you think I stopped the tape?" "Did you notice anything happening at that point?" "What did you notice about the patient's voice?" "Did you notice how her voice changed when she started talking about her husband?" "How did it change?" If necessary, the tape can be rewound to listen to or watch the relevant section a second time. New ways of phrasing statements or different strategies can be handled in a similar way. Possible questions include the following: "How would you have done it?" "What would you have said?" (The emphasis is on what can be said, because phrases that have been rehearsed will be remembered.) Then, and only then, should the trainer demonstrate how he or she would do it.

Teaching focuses on three important sources of information, which Lesser (1985) has described in detail. These are:

1. What the patient tells the doctor—the events, symptoms, and feelings that the patient talks about. Taking the patient's formal medical history really only emphasizes this source of information, and then only in a limited way, since the importance of attending to verbal cues given by the patient is not taught.
2. What the doctor "sees"—in other words, the appearance and nonverbal behavior of the patient (note that tone of voice can be a key "nonverbal" cue).
3. How the doctor feels. Doctors are often discouraged from identifying their own feelings in consultations, yet these feelings are in themselves a useful source of information and may say something about how other key people in the patient's life might react to him or her.

The beginning of the interview provides many opportunities for teaching recognition skills. Especially with trainees, stopping the tape may be desirable at this point. Comments can be invited about whether the doctor makes good eye contact, begins with an open-ended question, and puts the patient at ease. Discussion might include whether to ask the patient's permission if the doctor has decided to take extensive notes or examine the records in detail. The beginning of the interview is a crucial time. Group members can often identify the point at which difficulties arise in the practitioner-patient interaction, causing the interview to change course.

Throughout the interview, opportunities exist for teaching the basic skills of picking up *verbal cues* (words or phrases patients use that are important clues to how they are feeling or what their concerns are). Opportunities also exist for detecting *nonverbal cues* (such as posture, eye contact, change of gaze, and expression) and *vocal cues* (such as vocal pitch and tone). Teaching then focuses on how these cues can be responded to in a variety of ways:

1. By asking *open questions*—for instance, "Tell me about how you've been feeling lately . . . "
2. By asking for *clarification*—for example, "Tell me what you mean when you say you're feeling out of sorts . . . "
3. By asking for an *example*—for instance, "Tell me what happened the last time you felt panicky . . . " (this is a useful way of getting a lot of relevant information quickly)
4. By asking questions that *gently follow up on nonverbal cues*—for example, "You seem to look upset right now . . . I wonder . . . would you like to talk about it?" (this can be a powerful technique for changing the interview from one that has been superficial to one where the patient suddenly plunges into feelings and anxieties; it may form the basis for a *supportive statement* such as "I can see this is really getting on top of you at the moment")

To recognize somatization, we teach how to explore *health beliefs and concerns.* Trainees can also be taught how to demonstrate *empathy* by making explicit statements that are supportive with a clear link between the "I" of the doctor and the "you" of the patient—for example, "I can see that it's hard for you to talk about this." Warmth and encouragement are important, but they are not enough to convey to patients that practitioners understand their feelings.

Many doctors (not just trainees) find it difficult to get the right degree of control in an interview, and tapes provide excellent opportunities for teaching how to *set a clear agenda, summarize* what has been said so far, *clarify* the main tasks for the present interview, and politely *negotiate* with the patient what areas to cover next in order to *bring the patient back to the point.*

The teaching of management skills is beyond the scope of this chapter, but when a group meets over a period of time, the teaching of these skills becomes important. Primary care physicians resent being asked to "open up a can of worms" without being given the skills to help the patient. Recognition of psychiatric disorders in itself may be a crucial part of management; simply allowing patients to ventilate feelings can be therapeutic. Thus, recognition and management are in practice inseparable. When a group has begun to master recognition skills, they can devote several sessions to the management of particular "commonly occurring problems." Participants are encouraged to obtain consecutive interviews (audio or video) recorded with patients they are discussing in the group. By reviewing progress with patients discussed earlier, the group can discover whether the new interventions suggested by members had the expected outcome. Thus, a course of training sessions has a considerable advantage over a single session. Particular management skills may be taught in this setting (Lesser, 1981; Gask et al., 1991). However, the group discussion may also be a focus for teaching the correct use of psychotropic medication and the indications for psychiatric referral.

Teaching Specific Skills

Recent developments in the United Kingdom have attempted to address particular needs of primary care physicians in detecting and managing particular problems. In Manchester, a training package has been developed to help general practitioners recognize and manage patients with emotional disorders that present as somatic problems (Goldberg, Gask, & O'Dowd, 1989). The package comprises a videotape demonstrating a model for such an interview and the skills required to allow patients who present with somatic complaints yet suffer from psychological illness to grasp the psychological rather than physical basis of their symptoms. To treat such patients successfully, doctors must be able to change the agenda of the interview to include the psychological symptoms they have elicited and should be able to explain to the patients how their physical and psychological symptoms are linked. A second videotape gives practitioners the opportunity to practice the specific microskills of the model by stopping the tape and responding to cues delivered by "patients" on the videotape. After they have practiced their response (by role-playing in pairs), the tape is restarted and one possible correct response is demonstrated. This is best combined with an opportunity for doctors to then observe their own performance on video with a role-player or real patients in a small-group setting. These skills are perceived as desirable by a larger number of general practitioners than would be prepared to attend an intensive group course on interview skills training. The tapes allow the opportunity to bring such teaching to a wider audience by attempting to evaluate and meet consumer demand.

Evaluating Training

Only a few primary care training courses seem to have evaluated the changes that have actually occurred in the interviewing skills of their participants. This evaluation is best done by assessing pre- and posttraining videotaped interviews with real or role-played patients (Verby, Holden, & Davis, 1979; Goldberg, Smith, Steele, & Spivey, 1980; Goldberg, Steele, & Smith, 1980; Bensing & Sluijs, 1985; Gask, McGrath, Goldberg, & Millar, 1987; Gask, Goldberg, Lesser, & Millar, 1988; Gask, Goldberg, Porter, & Creed, 1989; Whewell, Gore, & Leach, 1988). A change in patient outcome should also be demonstrated and linked to the training process (Cohen-Cole, 1980).

The studies by Gask et al. (1988) and Whewell et al. (1988) confirmed the earlier finding of Goldberg, Smith, et al. (1980) and Goldberg, Steele, et al. (1980) that video feedback (provided one to one) can improve recognition of psychiatric disorder. Both these studies also demonstrated that feedback can be provided as effectively in a group setting as on an individual basis. We have further demonstrated that training has a significant impact on the behavior of both trainees and experienced practitioners (Gask et al., 1987, 1988, 1989), is maintained over time (Bowman, Goldberg, Millar, Gask, & McGrath, 1991), and has an impact on patient care (Gask and Goldberg, in press). The two longer-term outcome studies call for further discussion.

The first outcome study (Gask and Goldberg, in press) attempted to evaluate the impact of training—as described above—on patient care. Patients presenting with new psychological symptoms to two groups of family physicians were followed up over six months. One group of physicians had received group video feedback training to improve psychiatric interviewing skills. The other group had not received this training. Patients were assessed to evaluate the impact of training on the care they received, their satisfaction, and clinical outcome.

The index group of eight trained family physicians were recruited from a group of fourteen who had undergone video feedback training in psychiatric interviewing skills during their training. They were personally trained by Lesser during his stay in Manchester in 1985 over eighteen weekly sessions, each lasting two hours. Evaluation of this training (Gask et al., 1988) has demonstrated its effectiveness in significantly improving both the accuracy in detection and psychiatric skills of the trainees. Correlations (Spearman's rho) between physicians' ratings and patients' scores on the GHQ-28 increased from 0.38 before training to 0.52 post-training (ANOVA $p < 0.005$). After training, the doctors were better at sensing the patients' distress, better at defining their problems, missed fewer verbal cues, asked more psychological and social questions, gave more psychosocial advice, and gave advice that was more immediately relevant to the patients' problems.

The control group consisted of a closely matched group of doctors who had otherwise undergone similar training and were of the same age and experience. Fifty index and fifty-one control patients scoring seven or more on the GHQ-28 were recruited. No significant differences between the groups for age, gender, social class, duration of presenting symptoms, baseline Present State Examination (PSE) symptom scores, or consultation rates for the previous year were demonstrated.

Significantly more references to patients' psychological state and patients' problems were found in the case notes in the index group. Physicians in the index group who prescribed new medication in the first month were significantly more likely to tell the patient about its side effects. Index patients were significantly more likely to believe that the practitioner understood their problems. Analyses of variance and covariance revealed that total PSE symptom change scores were nonsignificantly greater in the index group. However, when baseline GHQ score was introduced as a covariate, there was a significantly better outcome in the index group. When specific diagnostic groups were examined, it became apparent that most of the difference in outcome resulted from the impact of the trained doctors on those patients in the index group who were both anxious and depressed. For patients who met diagnostic criteria for both case anxiety and case depression, significant differences in outcome were demonstrated. GHQ-28 change scores over the six-month follow-up were also significantly greater in the index group for patients with both case anxiety and case depression. Regression analysis further confirmed the important role that training played in outcome for this group of patients, though for the whole group, clinical and social factors were more important.

This study suggested that training family physicians to improve their psychiatric interviewing skills significantly improves clinical outcome, particularly for patients with mixed anxiety and depression. The latter finding is of particular interest, since these patients are often poorly managed in general medical settings.

A group of ten experienced and older practitioners in the Northwest of England were found to be similarly receptive to such training (Gask et al., 1987). The skills of this group of experienced general practitioners have been maintained over a two-year follow-up period. Bowman et al. (1991) followed up these experienced practitioners and found that they had maintained their tendency to ask fewer closed questions and more social and psychological questions. The training initially resulted in more questions that responded to verbal cues given by the patient (rather than medical "checklist" questions from the physician's agenda); this was also maintained at follow-up. Some of these findings—for example, asking more socially oriented questions and fewer "checklist" questions—were not significant at initial follow-up but achieved significance after two years. Thus, the training seemed to have a longer-term educational impact on the physicians' style than was at first apparent.

This study prompted a much larger study in both London and Manchester in which trainers have been successfully taught how to teach skills to their trainees (Gask, Boardman, & Standart, 1991). Research is now being carried out in the Department of General Practice at Newcastle University on the cost-benefit aspects of training.

Recent work has focused on teaching key skills in both the detection and management of psychological disorders presenting as somatic complaints. Using the videotaped teaching package described above (Goldberg, Gask, & O'Dowd, 1989), trainers have been able to teach the basic skills that are crucially important in recognizing emotional disorders in the presence of somatization and engaging patients in conversation about the emotional symptoms (as well as helping them to *feel understood,* which is the name given to the first part of the model). The second and third parts of the model then go on to demonstrate how to *change the agenda* from one that is purely physical to one in which both somatic and emotional symptoms can be acknowledged and how to *make the link* between emotional and somatic symptoms.

Training Other Members of the Primary Care Team

In this review, I have concentrated on the training of doctors, because primary care physicians play a central role in recognizing psychiatric disorders. However, recent work in the United Kingdom has demonstrated the role that health visitors can play in the recognition and management of postpartum depression, for which a training approach has been devised (Holden, Sagovsky, & Cox, 1989). The practice nurse is also likely to become an increasingly important person in screening for disorders, and we are currently adapting our training approach to provide similar skills training for nurses attached to primary care teams.

Conclusion

The recognition of psychiatric disorders in primary care can be most effectively improved by video or audio feedback training, possibly in combination with screening questionnaires. Changes persist over time, and improved recognition results in improved outcome. However, if training in the skills required to improve recognition is to be widely disseminated in primary care, psychiatrists and psychologists must collaborate with primary care teachers in order to reach the widest possible audience.

References

Bensing, J. M., & Sluijs, E. M. (1985). Evaluation of an interview training course for general practitioners. *Social Science and Medicine, 20,* 737–744.

Bowman, F., Goldberg, D., Millar, T., Gask, L., & McGrath, G. (1991). Improving the psychological skills of experienced general practitioners: Do effects of training persist? *Medical Education.*

Bridges, K. W., & Goldberg, D. P. (1986). The validation of the GHQ-28 and the use of the MMSE in neurological in-patients. *British Journal of Psychiatry, 148,* 548–553.

Burns, B. J., Scott, E., Burke, J. D., & Kessler, L. G. (1983). Mental health training of primary care residents: A review of recent literature (1974–1981). *General Hospital Psychiatry, 5,* 157–169.

Cohen-Cole, S. A. (1980). Training outcomes in liaison psychiatry: Literature review and methodological proposals. *General Hospital Psychiatry, 2,* 282–288.

Davenport, S., Goldberg, D., & Millar, T. (1987). How psychiatric disorders are missed during medical consultations. *Lancet, 2,* 139–140.

Gask, L., Boardman, J., & Standart, S. (1991). Teaching communication skills: A problem-based approach. *Postgraduate Education for General Practice, 2,* 7–15.

Gask, L., & Goldberg, D. (in press). The impact on patient care, clinical outcome, and satisfaction of improving the psychiatric interviewing skills of general practitioners.

Gask, L., Goldberg, D., Boardman, J., Craig, T., Goddard, C., Jones, O., Kiseley, S., McGrath, G., & Millar, T. (1991). Training general practitioners to teach psychiatric interviewing skills: An evaluation of group training. *Medical Education, 25*(5), 444-451.

Gask, L., Goldberg, D., Lesser, A. L., & Millar, T. (1988). Improving the psychiatric skills of the general practice trainee: An evaluation of a group training course. *Medical Education, 22,* 132-138.

Gask, L., Goldberg, D., Porter, R., & Creed, F. (1989). The treatment of somatization: Evaluation of a teaching package with general practice trainees. *Journal of Psychosomatic Research, 33,* 697-703.

Gask, L., McGrath, G., Goldberg, D., & Millar, T. (1987). Improving the psychiatric skills of established general practitioners. *Medical Education, 21,* 362-368.

Gask, L., Scott, J., & Standart, S. (1991). *Managing depression* [Film].

Goldberg, D., Gask, L., & O'Dowd, T. (1989). The treatment of somatization: Teaching the techniques of Retribution. *Journal of Psychosomatic Research, 33,* 689-695.

Goldberg, D., & Hillier, V. (1979). A scaled version of the General Health Questionnaire. *Psychological Medicine, 9,* 138-145.

Goldberg, D., & Huxley, P. (1980). *Mental illness in the community.* London: Tavistock.

Goldberg, D., Smith, C., Steele, J. J., & Spivey, L. (1980). Training family doctors to recognize psychiatric illness with increased accuracy. *Lancet, 2,* 521-523.

Goldberg, D., Steele, J. J., & Smith, C. (1980). Teaching psychiatric interview techniques to family doctors. *Acta Psychiatrica Scandinavica, 62,* 41-47.

Goldberg, D., & Williams, P. (1988). *A users guide to the General Health Questionnaire.* Windsor, Berkshire, England: NFER-Nelson.

Hoeper, E., Nycz, G., Kessler, L., Burke, J., & Pierce, W. (1984). The usefulness of screening for mental illness. *Lancet, 1,* 33-35.

Holden, J. M., Sagovsky, R., & Cox, J. L. (1989). Counselling in general practice settings: A controlled study of health visitor intervention in the treatment of post-natal depression. *British Medical Journal, 298,* 223–226.

Hollyman, J., Freeling, P., Paykel, E., Bhat, A., & Sedgewick, P. (1988). Double-blind controlled trial among depressed patients in general practice. *Journal of the Royal College of General Practitioners, 38,* 393–397.

Johnstone, A., & Goldberg, D. (1976). Psychiatric screening in general practice. *Lancet, 1,* 605–608.

Lesser, A. L. (1981). The psychiatrist and family medicine: A different training approach. *Medical Education, 15,* 398–406.

Lesser, A. L. (1985). Problem-based interviewing in general practice: A model. *Medical Education, 19,* 299–304.

Marks, J. N., Goldberg, D. P., & Hillier, V. F. (1979). Determinants of the ability of general practitioners to detect psychiatric illness. *Psychological Medicine, 9,* 337–353.

Millar, T., Goldberg, D., & Jenkins, L. (1991). *Determinants of the psychological skills of family doctors.* Manuscript submitted for publication.

Ormel, J., Koeter, H., van den Brink, W., & van de Willige, G. (1990). The extent of non-recognition of mental health problems in primary care and its effect on management and outcome. In D. Goldberg & D. J. Tantam (Eds.), *The public health impact of mental disorder.* Basel, Switzerland: Hogrefe & Huber.

Pendleton, D., Schofield, T., Tate, P., & Hevelock, J. (1983). *The consultation: An approach to learning and teaching.* Oxford, England: Oxford University Press.

Rand, E., Badger, L., & Coggins, D. (1988). Towards a resolution of contradictions: Utility of feedback from the GHQ. *Hospital Psychiatry, 10,* 189–196.

Shapiro, S., German, P., Skinner, E. A., Von Korff, M., Turner, R., Klein, L., Teitelbaum, M., Kramer, M., Burke, J., & Burns, B. (1987). An experiment to change detection and management of mental morbidity in primary care. *Medical Care, 25,* 327–339.

Strathdee, G., & Williams, P. (1985). Patterns of collaboration. In P. Williams & G. Wilkinson (Eds.), *Mental illness in primary care setting.* London: Tavistock.

Thompson, J., Rankin, H., Ashcroft, G. W., Yates, C. M., McQueen, J. K., & Cummings, S. W. (1982). The treatment of depression in general practice: A comparison of L-tryptophan, amitriptyline, and a combination of L-tryptophan and amitriptyline with placebo. *Psychological Medicine, 12,* 741–751.

Tylee, A., & Freeling, P. (1989). The recognition, diagnosis, and acknowledgment of depressive disorders by general practitioners. In E. Paykel & K. Herbst (Eds.), *Depression: An integrative approach.* London: Heinemann.

Verby, J. E., Holden, P., & Davis, R. H. (1979). Peer review of consultations in primary care: The use of audio-visual recordings. *British Medical Journal, 1,* 1686–1688.

Whewell, P., Gore, V., & Leach, C. (1988). Training general practitioners to improve their recognition of emotional disturbance in the consultation. *Journal of the Royal College of General Practitioners, 38,* 259–262.

Wright, A., & Perini, A. (1987). Hidden psychiatric illness: Use of the General Health Questionnaire in general practice. *Journal of the Royal College of General Practitioners, 37,* 164–167.

Zigmond, A. S., & Snaith, R. P. (1983). The Hospital Anxiety and Depression Scale. *Acta Psychiatrica Scandinavica, 67,* 361–370.

Zung, W. W. K., Magill, M., Moore, J., & George, D. T. (1983). Recognition and treatment of depression in a family practice. *Journal of Clinical Psychiatry, 44,* 3–6.

Part Four

Treatment of Mental Disorders in Primary Care

12

Herbert C. Schulberg
Kathleen A. Pajer

Treatment of Depression in Primary Care

Depression in primary care patients has been described in an extensive literature, much of which is presented in earlier chapters of this volume. As these chapters indicate, affective disturbance among ambulatory medical patients can range from major depression (whose prevalence approximates 6 to 8 percent) to subsyndromal but nevertheless distressing dysphoria. In addition to diverse severity levels, the clinical presentation of depressed medical patients can vary as well. Symptoms of either the mood or neurovegetative types may predominate, often depending on whether psychiatric and medical morbidity coexist. Of growing interest are syndromes characterized by both anxiety and depression.

In contrast to the earlier emphasis on the epidemiology and assessment of depression in primary care practice, we believe that in the future, clinicians and investigators will focus increasingly on treatment-related concerns. This shifting agenda reflects the clear documentation of high rates of depression in primary care patients, as well as an awareness of the few studies investigating the efficacy of treatments in reducing symptoms (Schulberg, 1990) or the functional disability associated with depressive disorder (Von Korff, Ormel, Katon, & Lin, 1992). The gap in knowledge about treatment efficacy was highlighted by the concerted efforts of the National Institute of Mental Health (NIMH) and professional organizations to train generalist physicians in state-of-the-art techniques for managing their affectively disturbed patients. For example, curricula developed for local Detection Awareness Research and Training (D/Art) programs (Regier et al., 1988) typically urged primary care physicians to utilize pharmacological and psychotherapeutic treatment standards developed with depressed psychiatric patients. Implementation of these guidelines is questionable, however, given: (1) concerns as to whether the etiology, severity, and natural course of depression in medical patients resemble those found with psychiatric patients, and (2) the lack of data regarding the validity of transferring treatment standards from the specialist to the generalist sector (Schulberg et al., 1991). The Depression Treatment Panel was established by the U.S. Public Health Service's Agency for Health Care Policy and Research (AHCPR) to formulate guidelines for managing depressive disorder in primary care practice. After reviewing published randomized controlled clinical trials for findings about the treatment of mood disorders, the panel has concluded that few pertinent studies investigating outcome among depressed ambulatory medical patients exist and, therefore, a high priority should be set for such future research (Rush, Trivedi, Schriger, & Petty, 1992).

This chapter analyzes what is known and remains to be known about treating depression in primary care practice. First, we consider how the need for treatment is assessed by physicians and factors influencing their decision to initiate an active intervention. Second, we review the extant knowledge base regarding the efficacy of somatic and/or psychosocial treatments and emphasize areas in which it must be refined for guideline development purposes. Third, we analyze which interventions appear most effective at the acute, continuation, and/or maintenance phases of treatment. Thus, our chapter offers a framework for selecting clinical strategies and/or research priorities for those seeking to optimize the care of depressed medical patients.

Assessing the Need for Treatment

The initial step in a primary care physician's decision on how to treat a depressed patient is determining whether an active intervention is warranted. A sizable literature has concluded that the majority of ambulatory medical patients experiencing a current major depression are untreated and thus presumably improperly managed (for example, Blacker & Clare, 1987), but one should not automatically assume that all diagnosed depressions require treatment. An ambiguous relationship between diagnosis and treatment exists in daily practice, even within academic psychiatric centers. This is problematic for those who consider the two clinical tasks closely intertwined (Keller et al., 1986). Schulberg, Block, and Coulehan (1989) concluded that primary care physicians determine whether to treat a medical patient's depression by considering the depression's severity, the extent of social and vocational dysfunction associated with it, the presence of medical and psychiatric comorbidity, and/or the patient's probability of complying with a prescribed treatment or referral to the specialist sector. While few physicians perform such explicit analytical tasks as calculating probabilities at each chance node of the decision tree or the risks of morbidity/mortality resulting from an incorrect assessment, they make these implicit judgments routinely. For this reason, we consider what is known about the facts contributing to the assessment process in the following sections.

Clinical Severity

The DSM-III-R diagnosis of major depression requires that at least five symptoms be experienced over a two-week duration. Within this framework, however, the depression's severity may be wide ranging. Individuals at the highly symptomatic end of the continuum typically are judged to need treatment, particularly when suicidal ideation is evident. When the major depression is of the moderate or milder types, though, the episode may remit either spontaneously or with minimal professional support.

Few primary care studies directly address the relationship between severity, treatment, and outcome, however. The study conducted by Paykel, Hollyman, Freeling, and Sedgwick (1988) randomized general practice patients experiencing a major depression to amitriptyline or a placebo. They found the active treatment to be superior when the patient's initial severity on the Hamilton Rating Scale–Depression (HRS-D) exceeded 12. For patients with an initial HRS-D between 6 and 12 (13 percent of those experiencing a current major depression), the active drug and placebo produced equally beneficial outcomes.

A different outcome pattern was reported by the NIMH Treatment of Depression Collaborative Research Program (TDCRP), which also analyzed the relationship of major depression's initial clinical severity to treatment type but in a study of ambulatory psychiatric patients (Elkin et al., 1989). These investigators determined that active treatment (imipramine, interpersonal psychotherapy, or cognitive behavioral therapy) produced superior outcomes compared to a drug placebo for patients whose screening HRS-D score was 20 or greater but not for patients with an initial HRS-D in the range of 14 to 19.

Severity of depression thus needs to be considered when choosing between an active therapeutic agent and watchful supportive waiting. Patients with an initial HRS-D above 19 clearly require the former, but those with severity scores below 13 can likely be followed with the latter. Randomized trials that initially stratify on severity are needed, however, to determine which intervention is most clinically effective and cost efficient for the sizable number of primary care patients whose major depression is of moderate severity—that is, their treatment HRS-D score ranges from 13 to 19.

Social and Vocational Dysfunction

While closely related to the severity of affective and neurovegetative symptomatology, degree of social and vocational dysfunction warrants a distinct assessment, since it reveals how harmful the depression is to the person's daily life (Wells et al., 1989). Little research has been carried out on the severity of such dysfunction, which may require active intervention rather than supportive watchful waiting. No such study could be found in the primary care literature, although it is urgently needed (Von Korff et al., 1992). It may be helpful, therefore, to again turn to the findings of the NIMH TDCRP, which did investigate this issue.

Elkin et al. (1989) administered the Global Assessment Scale (GAS)—a widely used unidimensional measure of general functioning—to the TDCRP's psychiatric outpatient subjects and found a significant interaction between initial GAS score, mode of intervention, and treatment outcome. Patients with less severe initial dysfunction (GAS scores of 51 or higher) exhibited similar degrees of improvement on follow-up, regardless of mode of intervention. However, patients whose initial general functioning was more impaired (GAS scores of 50 or lower) fared much better with active treatment than with a drug placebo. Imipramine was particularly effective in raising daily functioning to a satisfactory level. If these results are generalizable to primary care patients, physicians should choose an active pharmacological or psychotherapeutic intervention for depressed patients presenting with severely impaired social and vocational functioning. However, generalized dysfunction of more moderate severity may improve without active treatment. As noted previously, research investigating the impact of treatment on social and vocational functioning should be undertaken.

Medical Comorbidity

One of the most difficult issues in diagnosing major depression in primary care practice concerns how to interpret the signs and symptoms of medically ill patients. Studies investigating the prevalence of depressive symptoms in such cohorts have reported that approximately 20 percent of inpatients have significant dysphoria (for example, Cavanaugh, Clark, & Gibbons, 1983; Fava, Pilowsky, Pierfederici, Bernardi, & Pathak, 1982; Moffic & Paykel, 1975; Schwab, Bialow, Brown, & Holzer, 1967). The prevalence of depressive symptoms in medical outpatients is typically lower, although the reported range of 5 to 32 percent (Glass, Allan, Uhlenhuth, Kimball, & Borinstein, 1978; Neilson & Williams, 1980; Porter, 1970) is affected by the instrument and criteria used for case identification. Specific medical diagnoses are associated with particularly high depression rates—for example, end-stage renal disease (Kutner, Fair, & Kutner, 1985; Lowry, 1979), cancer (Bukberg, Penman, & Holland, 1984; Derogatis et al., 1983), and spinal cord injury (Frank, Kashani, Wonderlich, Lising, & Visot, 1985).

Given that depression and medical illness frequently coexist, what can be said about their relationship? The first question to be answered in clinical practice is whether the depressive symptoms are caused by, or are secondary to, a medical illness. We cannot delineate the extensive list of medical disorders and their treatments that are depressogenic here. However, hypothyroidism and Parkinson's disease exemplify the former, and propranolol and oral contraceptives are examples of the latter. Hall (1980) and Fava, Sonino, and Wise (1988) provide full reviews of this relationship. With regard to secondary depression, the initial intervention is to treat the medical disorder or to discontinue the depression-causing medication. If this strategy is unsuccessful or unfeasible (for instance, in a liver transplant patient dependent on steroids for immunosuppression), directly treating the depression with psychiatric interventions has been found useful (Ban, Guy, & Wilson, 1984; Larcombe & Wilson, 1984; Shader, Weinberger, & Greenblatt, 1978; Steinmuller, 1978).

If the medical patient's mood and neurovegetative symptoms are not secondary to a medical illness, the clinician must determine whether the depressive signs and symptoms are due to the organic illness (for example, cancer, end-stage renal disease), or reflect a stress-related or biological depression that will respond to psychiatric interventions. The assessment task is complex, since many depressive symptoms—such as lethargy, decreased concentration, insomnia, and anorexia—resemble those of organic illnesses. Several studies have addressed this problem by trying to identify clinical features differentiating depression from organic illness. However, patients diagnosed only with depression have a higher number of or more severe symptoms than nondepressed, medically ill patients (Kathol & Petty, 1981). Cognitive-affective symptoms and suicidal ideation distinguish between the two groups, but somatic and neuropsychological symptoms do not (Cavanaugh, Clark, & Gibbons, 1983; Fava & Molnar, 1987). A significant methodological problem with most of these studies is that patients are diagnosed as depressed only if their symptoms are severe and persistent, thus possibly biasing the findings. Further research is needed to identify symptom clusters typical of depressed medically ill patients who will or will not respond to psychiatric treatment (Gregory, Jimerson, Walton, Daley, & Paulsen, 1992). At this point, the best clinical approach to primary care patients reporting somatic symptoms is to maintain a high index of suspicion for depression and a low threshold for treatment when symptoms are severe or persist for longer than a few weeks.

A difficult differential diagnosis in the ambulatory medical sector is "normal" self-limiting dysphoria associated with severe physical suffering versus clinical depression requiring psychiatric intervention. No empirical data exist to guide this determination. The primary care physician or consultation-liaison psychiatrist often must resort to an empirical trial of an antidepressant or psychotherapy and then be guided by the clinical outcome.

Referral Compliance

When the primary care physician decides that the patient's depression warrants treatment, the physician must judge whether to treat the patient personally or refer the person to a mental health specialist. The frequency and circumstances under which each option is selected have been studied in English and other European general practices, as well as in American primary care practices. With regard to the latter settings, a questionnaire study by Fauman (1983) determined that internists refer 38 percent of their depressed patients to a psychiatrist. Using a similar methodology, Mitchell and Thompson (1988) found that family practitioners and internists refer 62 percent of their patients with a mood disorder to such a mental health specialist.

Given that possibly equal numbers of primary care patients diagnosed as depressed are treated by generalists and specialists, does outcome of the episode vary in relation to the treating clinician's discipline? Balestrieri, Williams, and Wilkinson (1988) performed a meta-analysis of studies comparing treatment provided by mental health specialists and by general practitioners and estimated that specialists achieve a 10 percent greater success rate. However, in estimating the clinical utility of the referral option, Schulberg et al. (1989) cautioned that a proportion of depressed patients do not comply with the referral. For example, Knesper (1982) found that even among moderately to extremely suicidal patients in a university hospital's emergency room, 24 percent did not follow through when referred within the university health system and 33 percent did not comply when referred outside this system. Referrals from one mental health specialist to another produced a 45 percent noncompliance rate at a general hospital's outpatient psychiatric clinic (Krulee & Hales, 1988). Thus, in establishing guidelines for treating depression in primary care practice, one must weigh the possibly greater effectiveness of mental health specialists against the unwillingness of at least some medical patients to receive treatment from such clinicians.

Treatment Approaches

The effectiveness of particular treatments for depression has not yet been definitely established with depressed primary care patients. Nevertheless, there is an emerging consensus that the present body of scientific findings is sufficiently valid to formulate guidelines for use by generalist physicians and mental health specialists. The U.S. Public Health Service's treatment guidelines urge that clinician and patient consider both the benefits and costs of available interventions before selecting among them (U.S. Department of Health and Human Services, Public Health Service, Agency for Health Care Policy and Research, 1993). With regard to the benefits, treatment is typically aimed at eliminating the dysphoric mood and neurovegetative symptoms and at minimizing the social and vocational dysfunction resulting from the disorder. However, achieving these benefits entails such costs as personal or third-party payments to the clinician (and for medication when it is prescribed), the risks or side effects associated with the treatment, and possible stigma from being assigned a psychiatric diagnosis.

Precise analyses are still needed of the benefits and costs of any particular treatment. Until they are performed, the cost-benefit perspective must remain suggestive rather than definitive. This section considers the present state of knowledge regarding five treatment approaches for depression: watchful waiting, psychosocial treatments, pharmacological treatments, combined treatments, and electroconvulsive therapy.

Watchful Waiting

As discussed previously, one of the most difficult diagnostic issues in primary care settings is the case definition of mood disorder. Even with improvements in a physician's ability to recognize major depression, many ambulatory medical patients present with a combination of depression and anxiety, or with symptoms not conforming to DSM-III-R criteria for major depression (Barrett, Barrett, Oxman, & Gerber, 1988). These symptom profiles may represent transient distressed states, subclinical presentations of major depression, or even a distinct syndrome not routinely seen in psychiatric settings. When the primary care physician establishes the diagnosis of major depression within DSM-III-R criteria, this formulation has clear implications for treatment. However, with patients whose clinical symptoms do not meet the syndrome, we have few data on which to base clinical treatment guidelines. In this latter case, is the relatively nonintrusive intervention of watchful waiting appropriate?

We may obtain a partial answer to this question by reviewing studies of the natural course of mental disorders in general practice (Abrahamson, 1969; Cooper, Fry, & Kalton, 1969; Kessler, Cleary, & Burke, 1985; Mann, Jenkins, & Belsey, 1981). The proportion of patients with persisting symptoms at follow-up points of six to thirty-six months ranged from 21 to 68 percent. Since the samples were diagnostically heterogeneous, these rates may not accurately portray the outcomes of patients described by Barrett et al. (1988). Nevertheless, the rates signal the possibility that some primary care practice patients with psychiatric symptoms experience self-limiting distress. Further evidence in support of watchful waiting is provided by Moffic and Paykel (1975), who found that in 28 percent of medical inpatients significantly depressed on admission, the depression had spontaneously cleared up by the time of discharge. In summarizing the few investigations that have analyzed outcomes of treated and untreated patients in primary care practice, Schulberg et al. (1989) concluded that 65 to 86 percent of depressed patients improve with antidepressant medication and 18 to 70 percent improve without it. Controlled clinical trials are clearly indicated, therefore, to further evaluate the need for aggressive intervention in patients with minor or intermittent depression. Since some patients receive medications even though they fail to meet criteria for a formal psychiatric diagnosis (Broadhead, Clapp-Channing, Finch, & Copeland, 1989), risk-benefit analyses should be conducted with this subgroup as well.

Since rigorous scientific evidence from studies with primary care patients is lacking, the following general clinical guidelines can be implemented and validated as soon as possible. If the patient clearly meets DSM-III-R criteria for major depression and is dysfunctional, active depression-specific treatment is indicated. The same strategy pertains to patients with particularly dangerous symptoms (for example, suicidal ideation, severe anorexia, severe insomnia, psychosis) even when all criteria for major depression are not met. On the other hand, patients who do not meet criteria for this disorder or whose depressive symptoms produce only mild levels of suffering or disability could be managed with watchful waiting. This approach is not to be confused with ignoring the patient and the symptoms. The patient should be scheduled for weekly phone or office appointments over the course of several weeks; symptoms should be monitored closely in a supportive fashion. This monitoring may suffice for symptoms that are transient or related to external stressors. However, if the symptoms have not subsided or have worsened after several weeks, a more aggressive intervention is warranted.

Psychosocial Treatments

Over 200 psychosocial treatments are described in the literature, but only a few aim specifically to: (1) reduce the mood and neurovegetative symptoms characterizing a depressive episode; and (2) improve the social and vocational dysfunction associated with it. Descriptions of the theoretical orientation, goals, major strategies, and mechanisms of change underlying psychodynamic, cognitive, and interpersonal psychotherapy are provided by Karasu (1990). With regard to empirical evidence about the efficacy of these psychotherapies, the available knowledge base is much smaller than that pertaining to pharmacotherapy. Moreover, few of the randomized clinical trials of psychotherapy's efficacy have been conducted with depressed ambulatory medical patients, even though this treatment is commonly provided within health maintenance organizations and other ambulatory health care settings (Austad & Berman, 1991). Among the limited number of such methodologically rigorous investigations conducted in primary care settings are the studies by Blackburn, Bishop, Glen, Whalley, and Christie (1981) and Teasdale, Fennell, Hibbert, and Amies (1984), which investigated the efficacy of cognitive therapy, and the study by Catalan et al. (1991), which focused on the usefulness of brief problem-oriented psychological treatment. Additionally, Corney (1984) gave depressed female general practice patients a "social work" intervention that included elements of both counseling and practical assistance, thus making it difficult to specify the psychotherapy's unique effect.

This limited body of primary care research forces those concerned with the efficacy of psychosocial interventions in resolving a depression to analyze the larger body of evidence derived from studies with affectively disturbed psychiatric patients. Investigators who do this consistently arrive at the conclusion that several types of psychotherapies are effective. Robinson, Berman, and Meimeyer (1990) reviewed the literature comparing psychotherapy with no treatment and found that the effect of therapy is both statistically reliable and substantial in magnitude. Despite the typically brief duration of treatment, the average client on termination was functioning approximately three-fourths of a standard deviation better than untreated control subjects.

On the other hand, evidence regarding the superiority of any particular psychotherapy over others is inconsistent regardless of whether symptomatic or functional criteria are used to assess outcome. Robinson et al. suggest that when significant differences are reported among depression-specific psychotherapies, they may be an artifact of the theoretical allegiances of researchers conducting these studies. When an investigator preferred a particular type of psychotherapy, it tended to produce more favorable results than the intervention with which it was being compared. A regression analysis performed by Robinson et al. to predict outcome under the condition of "no investigator allegiance" found no reliable differences in the effectiveness of treatments.

A review of the research literature on psychotherapies of depression also led Beckham (1990) to conclude that while these interventions are effective, none is clearly superior to any other. Familiar explanations for their equal outcomes include the possibility that the treatments contain common elements such as a caring "doctor-patient" relationship, the strengthening of hope, emotional arousal, and overcoming of social alienation. A more complex perspective on this pattern of therapeutic equivalence is presented by Beckham, who conceptualizes major depression as a relatively unstable homeostasis that can be disrupted in various ways. This model suggests that different psychotherapies may be effective for different reasons; each undermines the depressive homeostasis at different points within the complex web of factors sustaining it.

In light of the consistent finding that psychotherapy can effectively resolve a depression, we agree with Robinson et al. (1990) that additional comparisons between therapies are likely to be less informative than studies of the processes and mechanisms unique to each. Beckham offers two rather different approaches to process research. The first uses experimental designs to manipulate key elements of the therapy and analyzes immediate and delayed effects of manipulated factors. The second allows the therapeutic approach to evolve naturalistically with minimal interference by the investigator. Since each approach has advantages and disadvantages, the researcher's theoretical predilections and practical considerations should be accommodated in selecting a methodology for more thoroughly investigating therapeutic processes used in resolving a depressive episode.

Pharmacological Treatments

The other common treatment for major depression is medication, with or without psychotherapy. The polycyclic agents and monoamine oxidase (MAO) inhibitors formed the mainstay of the pharmacological approach until recently, when agents such as fluoxetine and buproprion were introduced. A comprehensive review of antidepressant medications is beyond the scope of this chapter, but we will present the important clinical features of each drug category in the context of primary care use. Lithium and psychostimulants have also been used in treating depressed patients, but we will not discuss them here since they typically are not prescribed by primary care physicians.

Efficacy. Patients experiencing an initial episode of major depression who are treated with an antidepressant drug at appropriate dosages and for an adequate duration have a 70 percent chance of full remission. All antidepressants have been shown to be equally efficacious in randomized controlled trials with depressed psychiatric patients (Baldessarini, 1989). Clinical evidence suggests, however, that some patient subgroups respond better to one type of antidepressant than another (that is, to either the drug blocking the reuptake of norepinephrine or the drug blocking the reuptake of serotonin). A previous positive response to a particular antidepressant usually predicts success with the same type again, as does a family history of successful treatment with this particular type of antidepressant. However, most patients exhibit few specific signs or symptoms to guide the physician in an initial drug choice. The clinical exception is atypical depression (hypersomnia, hyperphagia, lethargy, anxiety, and somatic complaints), where outcome is better with MAO inhibitors than polycyclics (Quitkin et al., 1988).

The known efficacy of antidepressant drugs is based on trials with psychiatric patients. Given ambiguities of case definition in primary care practice, it is reasonable to question whether outcome data from psychiatric patients generalize to the medical population. Seven primary care studies have provided pertinent data. Three (Blashki, Mowbray, & Davies 1971; Rickels et al., 1973; Thompson et al., 1982) clearly showed that amitriptyline or imipramine were superior to placebo in treating depression in primary care practice. However, all studied severely depressed subjects or samples that were not well defined. None specified the severity of the medical illness in their cohorts.

Paykel et al. (1988) treated a heterogeneous group of 141 depressed primary care patients with amitriptyline or placebo and, as noted earlier, found a significant improvement in patients with moderate or severe symptom levels given the active drug. Predictors of response to medication were severity, presence of endogenous symptoms of depression, recent stressors, and selected demographic and history variables. Preliminary data suggest that pharmacological treatment also benefits depressed patients with major medical illnesses (Lipsey, Robinson, Pearlson, Rao, & Price, 1984; Rifkin et al., 1985). However, Popkin, Callies, and MacKenzie (1985) found that severe medical comorbidity in medically hospitalized patients reduces the antidepressant's efficacy to a rate of only 45 percent.

Side Effects. The most problematic aspect of using antidepressants is their side effect profiles. This is of particular concern in primary care practice where many patients are already distressed by symptomatic comorbid medical illnesses. Each of these drugs produces its antidepressant effect by increasing synaptic serotonin, norepinephrine, or both. However, the drugs also interact with various other receptors, thus producing weight gain and sedation (antihistaminic effects); confusion, delirium, dry mouth, and constipation (anticholinergic effects); and orthostatic hypotension and reflex tachycardia (alpha-adrenergic blockade). While newer agents such as fluoxetine and buproprion interact negligibly with these receptors, they produce equally problematic side effects—for example, nausea, headaches, anxiety, and insomnia.

Side effects may be intolerable and even dangerous in select groups such as the elderly; possible problems include delirium or orthostatic hypotension resulting in hip fracture from a fall. The cardiac effects of the tricyclics are of particular concern. However, the earlier assumption that tricyclics are unsafe with cardiac patients has not been supported (Glassman, Pardell, & Woodring, 1988). Antidepressants should be chosen, therefore, either to minimize side effects or to capitalize on a desired side effect (for instance, producing nighttime sedation in a patient with severe insomnia).

Dosage and Length of Treatment. Primary care physicians prescribing psychotropic medications typically err on the side of underdosing (Broadhead et al., 1989; Katon, Von Korff, Lin, Bush, & Ormel, 1992; Magruder-Habib et al., 1989). This practice is rationalized with two beliefs: primary care patients respond to lower doses of antidepressants, and they are less tolerant of side effects. However, clinical trials do not support either assumption (Blacker, Shanks, Chapman, & Davey, 1988; Robertson & Trimble, 1985).

Patients prescribed antidepressant drugs usually receive initial relief from somatic symptoms such as insomnia or anorexia, at which point general practitioners stop increasing the dose, thinking the depression has resolved. Even when dosages are increased, it is often done so quickly that the patient lacks time to adjust to side effects. Thus, antidepressant medication should be initiated at low doses and gradually increased every three or four days until the standard therapeutic dose range is reached. If side effects are severe, the dosage should be decreased slightly and held at that level to allow the patient to tolerate the symptoms. When the patient is stabilized, the dosage should be increased again.

Once a therapeutic dosage of antidepressant is reached, the patient may take as long as four weeks to achieve relief from the mood disturbance. When combined with the initiation phase of one to three weeks, the total duration of an adequate trial of an antidepressant medication approximates six to eight weeks. If the patient remains unimproved after this period on a therapeutic dosage, drug monitoring or switching to another antidepressant should be considered.

Therapeutic Drug Monitoring. Therapeutic drug monitoring (TDM) is of great value to the primary care physician when implemented properly, but the lack of a validated relationship between dosage, plasma concentrations, and clinical effect precludes its routine use in pharmacotherapy. TDM has been most thoroughly investigated for the tricyclic antidepressants, and nortriptyline is the only drug with a clearly defined therapeutic window (50–150 ng/ml). Available data on TDM suggest that it can be a cost-effective tool to check compliance, maximize clinical response, and avoid toxicity (Preskorn, Dorey, & Jerkovich, 1988). Its usefulness in the primary care setting, where response to a medication may be more difficult to monitor, has yet to be tested.

Combined Treatments

Since psychosocial and pharmacological treatments for depression have been found effective when each is provided alone, clinicians and researchers have investigated whether a treatment's individual benefits are additive or even synergistic when provided jointly. Rush and Hollon (1991) think that the rationale for potentially enhanced benefits of combined treatment in reducing acute depressive distress includes one or more of the following elements: (1) the magnitude of symptom relief is increased, (2) the probability of improvement is heightened, and (3) the breadth of therapeutic response is extended. The combining of treatments has many analogues in other realms of clinical practice—for example, the control of malignant tumors with both surgery and chemotherapy. However, a strategy of joint interventions with regard to depression provoked intense ideological conflict between the various schools of psychiatry in the 1960s and 1970s (Klerman, 1991). Pharmacotherapy proponents, who conceived depression's etiology in terms of biochemical imbalance theories, considered the addition of psychotherapy potentially harmful since its probing and uncovering of defenses would intensify depressive symptoms. At best, pharmacotherapists viewed psychotherapy as costly and irrelevant. Proponents of psychotherapy, conceiving of depression in terms of psychodynamic conflicts, argued that adding antidepressant drugs would harm their intervention by raising a patient's desire for quick symptomatic relief alone, by placing therapists in an authoritarian prescribing role, and by possibly producing symptom substitution. Klerman (1991) observes that demands from empirical evidence have replaced ideologically driven treatment strategies. Consequently, the efficacy of combined treatments is now judged from a pragmatic rather than a personal value-based perspective.

Accepting this pragmatic perspective and given that combined treatments are more expensive for the patient in terms of time, money, and the medication's possible side effects, can it be demonstrated that psychotherapy plus pharmacotherapy are superior to either of the modalities provided alone? The reviews by Rush and Hollon (1991) and Wexler and Cicchetti (1992) of pertinent randomized controlled trials (conducted almost totally with psychiatric outpatients) conclude that this is not the case. Thus, routine combined treatment of major depression does not appear indicated. On the other hand, combined treatment has not been found more harmful than either intervention alone, and clinical indications for this practice exist despite the lack of scientific support for it. More specifically, the option of combined treatment should be considered for patients displaying the following: only a partial response to either treatment alone, a more chronic current episode, a prior history of poor interepisode recovery, a coexisting personality disorder, and interpersonal problems producing social and vocational dysfunction.

Electroconvulsive Therapy

Since electroconvulsive therapy (ECT) was first introduced (Cerletti & Bini, 1938), it has consistently been found a safe and relatively rapid treatment for depression (Frankel, 1984; Martin, 1986). Nevertheless, its use remains highly controversial because of the rather barbaric reputation it received when initially administered without general anesthesia. Segments of the media continue to portray the treatment as primitive despite significant clinical advances in seizure control, anesthesiology, and unilateral application (d'Elia, 1970), which markedly reduce posttreatment delirium and memory deficits. ECT is now an easier procedure to administer than most same-day surgeries.

The currently accepted indications for ECT are: severe depression with significant neurovegetative features; inability to take antidepressant medication; antidepressant-resistant depression; and life-threatening crises such as severe wasting due to anorexia, severe psychotic depression, or manic excitement unresponsive to medication (Rich, Spiker, Jewell, & Neil, 1984; Whitlock, 1982). Clinicians have expressed concerns regarding ECT's safety with medically ill patients, but research data strongly indicate that as currently practiced, ECT can be safely administered even to medical patients such as pregnant women (Repke & Berger, 1984; Wise, Ward, Townsend-Parchman, Gillstrap, & Hauth, 1984) and those with cardiac disease and seizure disorders (Bidder, 1981).

Treatment Phases

The preceding overview of approaches to treating depression will now be extended by considering whether particular therapies are more effective than others at specific points in the course of a depressive episode. The growing scientific evidence available for this analysis reflects the understanding that (1) depressive symptoms progress through a continuum ranging from normalcy to syndrome to disorder, and (2) a complete remission may be interrupted—that is, relapse can occur before the present episode runs its course or can recur at some future point in time (Frank et al., 1991; Rush & Hollon, 1991).

Within these dimensions for defining the nature of depression, clinicians classify treatment as being of the acute, continuation, or maintenance types. *Acute* treatment aims to relieve the intense mood or neurovegetative symptoms characterizing the disorder. When accomplished successfully, the depression is deemed in remission. *Continuation* treatment seeks to prevent the return of affective symptoms once remission is achieved. If this clinical improvement persists beyond approximately six months, the patient is considered recovered. The reappearance of earlier depressive symptoms during the continuation treatment phase is thought to signal a relapse of the prior episode. Finally, longer-term *maintenance* treatment aims to prevent the onset of new depressive episodes. This intervention is thought particularly vital for individuals with two or more prior episodes and a significant family history of depression. The following paragraphs consider evidence of treatment efficacy with respect to these three intervention phases.

Acute Phase

Once a physician has determined that the patient is experiencing a clinically significant depression, treatment should be undertaken within the following framework: (1) the physician and patient should collaborate whenever possible in selecting the initial treatment, (2) the treatment should be provided in an optimal manner and for sufficient duration to judge whether it is effective, (3) the patient's clinical state should be assessed regularly and systematically, (4) alternative treatments should be considered when depressive symptoms do not disappear within the time period established for the initial intervention, and (5) the diagnosis should be reevaluated when the patient remains nonresponsive to two or more medications.

The prevailing thinking is that medication should be prescribed for patients experiencing a moderate to severe depression. This treatment has the advantage of being relatively easy to administer, and it produces symptomatic relief within four to eight weeks. An established psychotherapy may or may not be combined with the drug, but the pharmacotherapist always should provide clinical management to ensure patient compliance and cooperation with the treatment plan.

A variety of depression-specific psychotherapies have been found effective for the acute treatment of nonpsychotic depressions in the mild-to-moderate range of severity. Such a psychotherapy has the advantage of not producing physiological side effects, and it directly focuses on the psychosocial stressors or cognitive beliefs presumed associated with the episode's onset. Typically, however, an intervention such as interpersonal psychotherapy requires four weeks longer to produce symptomatic relief than medication does.

Regardless of severity level, other idiosyncratic factors such as family history, number of earlier episodes, and response to prior interventions can influence a patient's responsiveness to acute treatment of the depression. Thus, currently it is not possible, despite the previously stated severity-related guideline, to predict with absolute certainty that a given patient will benefit more from one acute treatment than another (Sotsky et al., 1991). Further studies are needed to clarify how biological, psychological, and social factors interact with a given treatment's therapeutic properties.

Continuation Phase

Clinicians increasingly are aware that a depressive episode requires continued treatment to prevent relapse. Patients whose symptoms have remitted in response to acute-phase pharmacotherapy are thought to require an additional six to nine months of the medication at the dosage level that resolved the acute episode (Prien & Kupfer, 1986). If depressive symptoms reappear when the medication is tapered, the clinical relapse should be treated again with a full course of pharmacotherapy.

In contrast to the various clinical trials that have investigated the efficacy of an antidepressant drug in preventing relapse, only a few studies have considered psychotherapy's efficacy as a continuation-phase treatment (Blackburn et al., 1981; Weissman et al., 1979). Thus, extended psychotherapy whose objective is to resolve residual or persistent depression-related psychosocial problems currently lacks a clear scientific basis. Still, it should be considered when the patient is motivated to work on these problems and appears to benefit from continued psychological treatment.

Maintenance Phase

Depression is a chronic disabling condition for many individuals; thus, for clinical and public health purposes, it is vital to refine interventions that prevent or delay recurrence. Only a small number of investigators have accepted this challenge, however, and most of their research has compared the efficacy of medications (NIMH/NIH Consensus Development Conference Statement, 1985). As an example, Frank et al. (1990) determined that imipramine prescribed for up to three years significantly reduced the recurrence of depression in persons with at least three prior episodes and that monthly interpersonal psychotherapy also served to lengthen the time between episodes in those not receiving the medication.

Clinicians should prescribe antidepressant drugs with minimal side effects and at the dosage level that resolved the acute episode indefinitely for persons whose depression is likely to recur—that is, for individuals with at least three prior episodes or two prior episodes and a family history of mood disorder. The efficacy of psychotherapy alone as a maintenance phase treatment needs further exploration. Given that Frank et al.'s (1990) maintenance phase protocol provided interpersonal psychotherapy only on a monthly basis, Klerman (1990) suggests that a future dose-response study compare the efficacy of weekly, biweekly, and monthly psychotherapy sessions.

Conclusion

Clinical interventions for depression have been extensively researched during the past three decades, and knowledge has progressed to the point where treatment guidelines are being offered practitioners through the AHCPR and such professional bodies as the American Psychiatric Association and the American Psychological Association. The management of major depression in primary care practice has special importance, given the disorder's prevalence of 6 to 8 percent and the complex ways in which medical comorbidity affects diagnostic and treatment decisions. This chapter has reviewed existing knowledge that can help in selecting appropriate interventions, and we emphasize once again that the scientific evidence is drawn mainly from research conducted with psychiatric rather than medical patients. The propriety of transferring treatments from one caregiving setting to another remains to be determined, even though the AHCPR guidelines accept the validity of this practice. An additional research priority in this age of managed care and cost containment is the cost-benefit ratio of various pharmacological and psychosocial treatments of depression. Virtually no data exist regarding the economic premises influencing acute, continuation, and maintenance treatment choices. Thus, outcome studies focused on the costs of achieving symptom relief and improved social/vocational functioning would be invaluable.

References

Abrahamson, D. (1969). Untreated psychiatric morbidity: A general practice study. *Social Psychiatry, 4,* 5–11.

Austad, C., & Berman, W. (Eds.). (1991). *Psychotherapy in managed health care.* Washington, DC: American Psychological Association.

Baldessarini, R. (1989). Current status of antidepressants: Clinical pharmacology and therapy. *Journal of Clinical Psychiatry, 50,* 117–126.

Balestrieri, M., Williams, P., & Wilkinson, G. (1988). Specialist mental health treatment in general practice: A meta-analysis. *Psychological Medicine, 18,* 711–717.

Ban, T., Guy, W., & Wilson, W. (1984). The psychopharmacological treatment of depression in the medically ill patient. *Canadian Journal of Psychiatry, 29,* 461–465.

Barrett, J. E., Barrett, J. T., Oxman, T., & Gerber, P. (1988). The prevalence of psychiatric disorders in primary care practice. *Archives of General Psychiatry, 45,* 1100–1106.

Beckham, E. (1990). Psychotherapy of depression research at a crossroads: Directions for the 1990s. *Clinical Psychology Review, 10,* 207–228.

Bidder, T. (1981). Electroconvulsive therapy in the medically ill patient. *Psychiatric Clinics of North America, 4,* 391–405.

Blackburn, I., Bishop, S., Glen, A., Whalley, L., & Christie, J. (1981). The efficacy of cognitive therapy in depression: A treatment trial using cognitive therapy and pharmacotherapy, each alone and in combination. *British Journal of Psychiatry, 139,* 181–189.

Blacker, C., & Clare, A. (1987). Depressive disorder in primary care. *British Journal of Psychiatry, 150,* 737–751.

Blacker, C., Shanks, N., Chapman, N., & Davey, A. (1988). The drug treatment of depression in general practice: A comparison of nocte administration of trazodone with mianserin, dothiepin, and amitriptyline. *Psychopharmacology, 95*(Suppl.), S18–S24.

Blashki, T., Mowbray, R., & Davies, B. (1971). Controlled trial of amitriptyline in general practice. *British Medical Journal, 1,* 133–138.

Broadhead, W., Clapp-Channing, N., Finch, J., & Copeland, J. (1989). Effects of medical illness and somatic symptoms on treatment of depression in a family practice residency practice. *General Hospital Psychiatry, 11,* 194–200.

Bukberg, J., Penman, D., and Holland, J. (1984). Depression in hospitalized cancer patients. *Psychosomatics, 46,* 199–212.

Catalan, J., Gath, D., Anastasiades, P., Bond, S., Day, A., & Hall, L. (1991). Evaluation of a brief psychological treatment for emotional disorders in primary care. *Psychological Medicine, 21,* 1013–1018.

Cavanaugh, S., Clark, D., & Gibbons, R. (1983). Diagnosing depression in the hospitalized medically ill. *Psychosomatics, 24,* 809–815.

Cerletti, V., & Bini, L. (1938). Un nuevo metodo di shockterapie l'Ettroshock. *Bollo Academica Medica Roma, 64,* 136–138.

Cooper, B., Fry, J., & Kalton, G. (1969). A longitudinal study of psychiatric morbidity in a general practice population. *British Journal of Preventive and Social Medicine, 23,* 210–217.

Corney, R. (1984). The effectiveness of attached social workers in the management of depressed female patients in general practice. *Psychological Medicine, 6*(Suppl.), 47.

d'Elia, G. (1970). Unilateral electroconvulsive therapy. *Acta Psychiatrica Scandinavica, 215,* 1–98.

Derogatis, L., Morrow, G., Fetting, J., Penman, D., Piasetsky, S., Schmale, A., Henrichs, M., & Carnicke, C. (1983). The prevalence of psychiatric disorders among cancer patients. *Journal of the American Medical Association, 249,* 751–757.

Elkin, I., Shea, T., Watkins, J., Imber, S., Sotsky, S., Collins, J., Glass, D., Pilkonis, P., Leber, W., Docherty, J., Fiester, S., & Parloff, M. (1989). National Institute of Mental Health Treatment of Depression Collaborative Research Program: General effectiveness of treatments. *Archives of General Psychiatry, 46,* 971–983.

Fauman, M. (1983). Psychiatric components of medical and surgical practice: 2. Referral and treatment of psychiatric disorders. *American Journal of Psychiatry, 140,* 760–763.

Fava, G., & Molnar, G. (1987). Criteria for diagnosing depression in the setting of medical disease. *Psychotherapeutic Psychosomatics, 48,* 21–25.

Fava, G., Pilowsky, I., Pierfederici, A., Bernardi, M., & Pathak, D. (1982). Depressive symptoms and abnormal illness behavior in general hospital patients. *General Hospital Psychiatry, 4,* 171–178.

Fava, G., Sonino, N., & Wise, T. (1988). Management of depression in medical patients. *Psychotherapeutic Psychosomatics, 49,* 81–102.

Frank, R., Kashani, J., Wonderlich, S., Lising, A., & Visot, L. (1985). Depression and adrenal functioning in spinal cord injury. *American Journal of Psychiatry, 142,* 252–253.

Frank, E., Kupfer, D., Perel, J., Cornes, C., Jarrett, D., Mallinger, A., Thase, M., McEachran, A., & Grochocinski, V. (1990). Three-year outcomes for maintenance therapies in recurrent depression. *Archives of General Psychiatry, 47,* 1093–1099.

Frank, E., Prien, R., Jarrett, R., Keller, M., Kupfer, D., Lavori, P., Rush, A., & Weissman, M. (1991). Conceptualization and rationale for consensus definitions of terms in major depressive disorder. *Archives of General Psychiatry, 48,* 851–855.

Frankel, F. (1984). Electroconvulsive therapy. In T. Karasu (Ed.), *The psychiatric therapies.* Washington, DC: American Psychiatric Press.

Glass, R., Allan, A., Uhlenhuth, E., Kimball C., & Borinstein, D. (1978). Psychiatric screening in a medical clinic: An evaluation of a self-report inventory. *Archives of General Psychiatry, 35,* 1189–1195.

Glassman, A., Pardell, R., & Woodring, S. (1988). Cardiovascular effects of the standard tricyclic antidepressants. *Clinical Chemistry, 34,* 856–858.

Gregory, R., Jimerson, D., Walton, B., Daley, J., & Paulsen, R. (1992). Pharmacotherapy of depression in the medically ill: Directions for future research. *General Hospital Psychiatry, 14,* 36–42.

Hall, R. (Ed.). (1980). *Psychiatric presentations of medical illness: Somatopsychic disorders.* New York: SP Medical and Scientific Books.

Karasu, T. (1990). Toward a clinical model of psychotherapy for depression: 1. Systematic comparison of three psychotherapies. *American Journal of Psychiatry, 147,* 133–147.

Kathol, R., & Petty, F. (1981). Relationship of depression to medical illness. *Journal of Affective Disorders, 3,* 111–121.

Katon, W., Von Korff, M., Lin, E., Bush, T., & Ormel, J. (1992). Adequacy and duration of antidepressant treatment in primary care. *Medical Care, 30,* 67–76.

Keller, M., Lavori, P., Klerman, G., Andreason, N., Endicott, J., Coryell, W., Fawcett, J., Rice, J., & Hirschfeld, R. (1986). Low levels and lack of predictors of somatotherapy and psychotherapy received by depressed patients. *Archives of General Psychiatry, 43,* 458–466.

Kessler, L., Cleary, P., & Burke, J. (1985). Psychiatric disorders in primary care. *Archives of General Psychiatry, 42,* 583–587.

Klerman, G. (1990). Treatment of recurrent unipolar major depressive disorder. *Archives of General Psychiatry, 47,* 1158–1162.

Klerman, G. (1991). Ideological conflicts in integrating pharmacotherapy and psychotherapy. In B. Beitman & G. Klerman (Eds.), *Integrating pharmacotherapy and psychotherapy* (pp. 3–19). Washington, DC: American Psychiatric Press.

Knesper, D. (1982). A study of referral failures for potentially suicidal patients: A method of medical care evaluation. *Hospital and Community Psychiatry, 33,* 45–52.

Krulee, D., & Hales, R. (1988). Compliance with psychiatric referrals from a general hospital psychiatry outpatient clinic. *General Hospital Psychiatry, 10,* 339–345.

Kutner, M., Fair, P., & Kutner, M. (1985). Assessing depression and anxiety in chronic dialysis patients. *Journal of Psychosomatic Research, 29,* 23–31.

Larcombe, N., & Wilson, P. (1984). An evaluation of cognitive-behavior therapy for depression in patients with multiple sclerosis. *British Journal of Psychiatry, 145,* 366–371.

Lipsey, J., Robinson, R., Pearlson, G., Rao, K., & Price, T. (1984). Nortriptyline treatment of post-stroke depression. *Lancet, 1,* 297–300.

Lowry, M. (1979). Frequency of depressive disorder in patients entering home dialysis. *Journal of Nervous and Mental Disease, 167,* 199–204.

Magruder-Habib, K., Zung, W., Feussner, J., Alling, W., Saunders, W., & Stevens, H. (1989). Management of general medical patients with symptoms of depression. *General Hospital Psychiatry, 11,* 201–206.

Mann, A., Jenkins, R., & Belsey, E. (1981). The twelve-month outcome of patients with neurotic illness in general practice. *Psychological Medicine, 11,* 535–550.

Martin, B. (1986). Electroconvulsive therapy: Contemporary standards of practice. *Canadian Journal of Psychiatry, 31,* 759–771.

Mitchell, W., & Thompson, T. (1988). Primary care physicians' perceptions of psychiatric disorders and treatment approaches in young and middle-aged adult patients. *Psychosomatics, 29,* 85–93.

Moffic, H., & Paykel, E. (1975). Depression in medical inpatients. *British Journal of Psychiatry, 126,* 346–353.

Neilson, A., & Williams, T. (1980). Depression in ambulatory medical patients: Prevalence by self-report questionnaire and recognition by nonpsychiatric physicians. *Archives of General Psychiatry, 37,* 999–1004.

NIMH/NIH Consensus Development Conference Statement. (1985).

Mood disorders: Pharmacologic prevention of recurrences. *American Journal of Psychiatry, 142,* 469–476.

Paykel, E., Hollyman, J., Freeling, P., & Sedgwick, P. (1988). Predictors of therapeutic benefit from amitriptyline in mild depression: A general practice placebo controlled trial. *Journal Affective Disorders, 14,* 83–95.

Pincus, H., Francis, A., Wakefield, W., First, M., & Widiger, T. (1992). DSM-IV and new diagnostic categories: Holding the line on proliferation. *American Journal of Psychiatry, 149,* 112–117.

Popkin, M., Callies, A., & MacKenzie, T. (1985). The outcome of antidepressant use in the medically ill. *Archives of General Psychiatry, 42,* 1160–1163.

Porter, A. (1970). Depressive illness in a general practice: A demographic study and controlled trial of imipramine. *British Medical Journal, 1,* 773–778.

Preskorn, S., Dorey, R., & Jerkovich, G. (1988). Therapeutic drug monitoring of tricyclic antidepressants. *Clinical Chemistry, 34,* 822–828.

Prien, R., & Kupfer, D. (1986). Continuation drug therapy for major depressive episodes: How long should it be maintained? *American Journal of Psychiatry, 143,* 18–23.

Quitkin, F., Stewart, J., McGrath, P., Liebowitz, M., Harrison, W., Tricamo, E., Klein, D., Rabkin, J., Markowitz, J., & Wager, S. (1988). Phenelzine versus imipramine in the treatment of probably atypical depression: Defining syndrome boundaries of selective MAOI responders. *American Journal of Psychiatry, 145,* 306–311.

Regier, D., Hirschfeld, R., Goodwin, F., Burke, J., Lazar, J., & Judd, L. (1988). The NIMH Depression Awareness, Recognition, and Treatment Program: Structure, aims, and scientific basis. *American Journal of Psychiatry, 145,* 1351–1357.

Repke, J., & Berger, N. (1984). Electroconvulsive therapy in pregnancy. *Obstetrics and Gynecology, 63,* 395–415.

Rich, C., Spiker, D., Jewell, S., & Neil, J. (1984). DSM-III, RDC, and ECT. *Journal of Clinical Psychiatry, 45,* 14–18.

Rickels, K., Gordon, P., Jenkins, W., Perloff, M., Sachs, T., & Stepansky, W. (1973). Drug treatment of depressive illness (amitriptyline and chlordiazepoxide in two neurotic populations). *Diseases of the Nervous System, 31,* 30–42.

Rifkin, A., Reardon, G., Siris, S., Karagji, B., Kim, Y., Hackstaff, L., & Endicott, N. (1985). Trimipramine in physical illness with depression. *Journal of Clinical Psychiatry, 46,* 4–8.

Robertson, M., & Trimble, M. (1985). The treatment of depression in patients with epilepsy. *Journal of Affective Disorders, 9,* 127–136.

Robinson, L., Berman, J., & Meimeyer, R. (1990). Psychotherapy for the treatment of depression: A comprehensive review of controlled outcome research. *Psychological Bulletin, 108,* 30–49.

Rush, J., & Hollon, S. (1991). Depression. In B. Beitman & G. Klerman (Eds.), *Integrating pharmacotherapy and psychotherapy* (pp. 121–142). Washington, DC: American Psychiatric Press.

Rush, J., Trivedi, M.., Schriger, D., & Petty, F. (1992). The development of clinical practice guidelines for the diagnosis and treatment of depression. *General Hospital Psychiatry, 14,* 230–236.

Schulberg, H. (1990). Mental disorders in the primary care setting: Research priorities for the 1990s. *General Hospital Psychiatry, 13,* 156–164.

Schulberg, H., Block, M., & Coulehan, J. (1989). Treating depression in primary care practice: An application of decision analysis. *General Hospital Psychiatry, 11,* 208–215.

Schulberg, H., Coulehan, J., Block, M., Scott, C., Imber, S., & Perel, J. (1991). Strategies for evaluating treatments for major depression in primary care patients. *General Hospital Psychiatry, 13,* 9–18.

Schwab, J., Bialow, M., Brown, J., & Holzer, C. (1967). Diagnosing depression in medical inpatients. *Annals of Internal Medicine, 67,* 695–707.

Shader, R., Weinberger, D., & Greenblatt, D. (1978). Psychopharmacological approaches to the medically ill. In B. Karasau & R. Steinmuller (Eds.), *Psychotherapeutics in medicine.* Philadelphia: Grune & Stratton.

Sotsky, S., Glass, D., Shea, T., Pilkonis, P., Collins, J., Elkin, I., Watkins, J., Imber, S., Leber, W., Mayer, J., & Oliveri, M. (1991). Patient predictors of response to psychotherapy: Findings in the

NIMH Treatment of Depression Collaborative Research Program. *American Journal of Psychiatry, 148,* 997–1008.

Steinmuller, R. (1978). Psychotherapeutic planning in the medically ill. In B. Karasu & R. Steinmuller (Eds.), *Psychotherapeutics in medicine.* Philadelphia: Grune & Stratton.

Teasdale, J., Fennell, M., Hibbert, G., & Amies, P. (1984). Cognitive therapy for major depressive disorder in primary care. *British Journal of Psychiatry, 144,* 400–406.

Thompson, J., Rankin, H., Ashcroft, G., Yates, C., McQueen, J., & Cummings, S. (1982). The treatment of depression in general practice: A comparison of L-tryptophan, amitriptyline, and a combination of L-tryptophan and amitriptyline with placebo. *Psychological Medicine, 12,* 741–751.

U.S. Department of Health and Human Services, Public Health Service, Agency for Health Care Policy and Research. (1993). *Clinical Practice Guidelines: Depression in Primary Care: Treatment of Major Depression* (Publication No. 93-0551). Rockville, MD: Author.

Von Korff, M., Ormel, J., Katon, W., & Lin, E. (1992). Disability and depression among high utilizers of health care: A longitudinal analysis. *Archives of General Psychiatry, 49,* 91–100.

Weissman, M., Prusoff, B., DiMascio, A., Neu, C., Goklaney, M., & Klerman, G. (1979). The efficacy of drugs and psychotherapy in the treatment of acute depressive episodes. *American Journal of Psychiatry, 136,* 555–558.

Wells, K., Stewart, A., Hays, R., Burnam, A., Rogers, W., Daniels, M., Berry J., Greenfield, S., & Ware, J. (1989). The functioning and well-being of depressed patients: Results from the Medical Outcomes Study. *Journal of the American Medical Association, 262,* 914–919.

Wexler, B., and Cicchetti, D. (1992). The outpatient treatment of depression: Implications of outcome research for clinical practice. *Journal of Nervous and Mental Disease, 180,* 277–286.

Whitlock, F. (1982). *Symptomatic affective disorders.* San Diego, CA: Academic Press.

Wise, M., Ward, S., Townsend-Parchman, G., Gillstrap, L., & Hauth, J. (1984). Case report of ECT during high risk pregnancy. *American Journal of Psychiatry, 141,* 99–101.

13

Frank V. deGruy

Treatment of Anxiety in Primary Care

The presence of anxiety does not necessarily signify a problem. Anxiety is a universal human emotion that appears as a normal response to certain situations, such as imminent physical harm or the threat of significant loss. In fact, anxiety can and often does serve a constructive purpose in healthy individuals. For example, one may be scheduled to speak in public but not be prepared. Anxiety at the prospect of standing before several hundred people and making a fool of oneself may be motivation to prepare the speech. Many a medical house officer has been motivated, late at night when the bed was calling, to read about the newly admitted patient, for fear of being found ignorant on rounds the next morning. Anxiety may motivate people to accomplish unpleasant but necessary tasks, to work on improving interpersonal relationships, and to otherwise devote energy to important things that would be left undone if apathy prevailed.

But anxiety is not always functional. It may be so intense as to be disabling or so global and nonspecific as to interfere with everyday life. Furthermore, the anxious person may have developed means of dealing with the anxiety that are ineffective or counterproductive, such as alcohol abuse.

When encountering an anxious patient, the clinician must first assess whether the anxiety is itself disabling, and if so, how much reduction or transformation will be necessary to remove the disabling and dysfunctional components of anxiety and yet leave the patient with optimum capacities. In other words, the end point in the management of anxiety is not the removal of all anxiety, but titration or modulation into a "therapeutic window," in which the anxiety serves rather than disables the patient.

Of course, an anxious person is part of a context or a system (for example, the family), which may be functioning in a way that produces anxiety in the presenting patient. Alternatively, the patient's role in the system—though it provokes anxiety—may be so important for other reasons that the patient or other family members may resist changing. Therefore, the most sensible interventions must always take into account and sometimes operate directly on the system as a whole or other members of the system, rather than maintaining an exclusive focus on the patient.

Many of the interventions discussed in this chapter are condition specific. Nevertheless, several therapeutic modalities have a general, nonspecific effect of reducing anxiety irrespective of the diagnostic manifestation and will be mentioned before we turn to specific entities.

The first of these—supportive psychotherapy—involves actively listening to and empathizing with the patient; offering acceptance, reassurance, and clarification. Most patients respond with a reduction in anxiety to being heard, understood, reassured, and encouraged. Active listening and empathy with the patient's condition can legitimately be considered part of the diagnostic process. Engel (1988) has made an eloquent argument that accurate clinical data can only be acquired under conditions of trust and empathy; I strongly agree. *The clinician must understand the patient's predicament in detail before even beginning the formulation of a therapeutic plan, and therefore must develop the interviewing skills necessary to create the conditions of trust under which that understanding can come about.* Although the therapeutic value of a supportive approach has not been evaluated rigorously and probably never will be, the prevailing standard of care in most primary care medical settings requires a supportive approach for anxious patients. In fact, supportive psychotherapy should be a component of most clinician-patient encounters, whether or not the patient shows anxiety.

The second general modality for anxiety reduction is physical exercise. Petruzzello, Landers, and Hatfield (1991) performed a detailed meta-analysis of over 100 papers on the relationship between anxiety and exercise; among their conclusions are the following:

1. Irrespective of how anxiety is assessed, or in whom (that is, age, health status, diagnosis), exercise is associated with a reduction in anxiety.
2. Aerobic exercise is the form of exercise most consistently shown to reduce anxiety.
3. Exercise duration of greater than twenty minutes seems necessary to accomplish reductions in state and trait anxiety. Most studies had confounding variables associated with this finding, so that further research is needed to corroborate it.
4. The efficacy of exercise in reducing anxiety is both statistically and clinically significant. Aerobic exercise reduces anxiety by about .24 standard deviations when using any of a large number of instruments.
5. Although people with high cardiovascular fitness tend to have lower levels of anxiety and depression, as well as less physical illness following stressful life events, the anxiety-reducing benefits of aerobic exercise are equally apparent in both fit and unfit subjects.
6. Even a single bout of aerobic activity in physically fit or unfit subjects reduces state anxiety, but trait anxiety is not consistently reduced until a regular program has been followed for greater than sixteen weeks.
7. Anxiety reduction is equally apparent irrespective of the form of aerobic exercise.
8. Anxiety reduction achieved through aerobic exercise is similar to the reduction achieved through meditation or relaxation.

The above findings provide a compelling argument for prescribing aerobic physical exercise for anxiety reduction in any patient capable of undertaking it.

Secondary Conditions

Anxiety states can be secondary to medical diseases. These would include thyroid disease (hyper- and even hypothyroidism), hypoglycemia, pheochromocytoma, mitral valve prolapse, cardiac arrhythmias, angina pectoris, myocardial infarction, chronic and acute obstructive lung disease, and temporal lobe epilepsy, to name several of the most important ones. The treatment of anxiety in the presence of these conditions involves treatment of the primary disorder. Resolution of the anxiety with resolution of the medical condition suggests that the anxiety was in fact secondary, and usually no further management is necessary. If at the time of presentation the anxiety is disabling, the clinician should resort to specific antianxiety measures, such as an anxiolytic medication, until the primary condition is brought under control. In general, this is a safe and effective approach. Despite the widespread proscription against the use of anxiolytics in patients with obstructive lung disease, benzodiazepines in moderate doses—especially those with short half-lives—have been used in this setting without significant deterioration in respiratory function (Man, Hsu, & Sproule, 1986; Midgren, Hansson, Skeidsvoll, & Elmquist, 1989; Wedzicha, Wallis, Ingram, & Empey, 1988). Of course, the anxiety may persist after the primary condition has been treated; in this case, the two conditions should be considered comorbid, and each treated.

Anxiety may also be secondary to drug abuse. The drugs most commonly implicated are ethanol, cocaine, decongestants, caffeine, and amphetamines, although withdrawal syndromes from almost any habituating substance may provoke acute anxiety. As with the medical conditions described above, treatment consists of removal of the primary offending agent. Short-term treatment with a psychoactive anxiolytic is highly effective in reducing anxiety but is fraught with hazard in substance abusers because of the potential for abuse. This is particularly true of the benzodiazepines. Therefore, either these medications must be avoided altogether or used as a last resort under close supervision and for short duration (Landry, Smith, McDuff, & Baughman, 1991). Other modalities of anxiety reduction, such as relaxation therapy, biofeedback, or aerobic exercise, may be useful (Landry et al., 1991; Weiss & Billings, 1988), but their efficacy has not been convincingly demonstrated.

Subthreshold Disorders

Subthreshold anxiety disorders are common in the primary care setting (see Chapter Seven). These are conditions of insufficient intensity or duration to qualify as a DSM-III-R diagnosis. The most common is undoubtedly acute situational anxiety. This is a condition in which the anxiety is symptomatic, perhaps even disabling, and is the result of a discrete event or circumstance that would be expected to generate anxiety. In other words, the anxiety response stirred up by a problematic situation is appropriate. This type of anxiety is one of the great understudied areas in primary medical care. We need standardized diagnostic criteria, demographic and clinical descriptions, and therapeutic trials. The following recommendations are offered in the absence of these data and are based on both personal clinical experience and the available literature.

1. Situational anxiety is an acute problem, so short-term rather than long-term strategies make the most sense.
2. Because by definition situational anxiety is appropriate for the situation, the principal focus should be on coping with the event or circumstance rather than dealing with the anxiety as a symptom.
3. Supportive psychotherapy, with a strong emphasis on empathy, calm reassurance, and the development of coping strategies, should be the backbone of management.
4. Other therapies, such as relaxation therapy, biofeedback, aerobic exercise, and hypnosis, may be useful, but their efficacy has not been documented.
5. Pharmacotherapy, such as prescribing benzodiazepines, should not be instituted except in special circumstances. The clinician should initially consider this a circumscribed disorder that will

respond to straightforward, primarily supportive work—that is, talking with the patient. If possible, the situation should be viewed as an opportunity for the patient to develop more effective coping skills. The early or aggressive use of anxiolytics may militate against this coping work.

6. Anxiolytics may serve a useful role if the above strategies are ineffective, if the anxiety has incapacitated the patient, or if secondary symptoms such as insomnia are aggravating the condition. In such a case, the diagnosis should be reevaluated and the drug should be used at a low-to-moderate dose for a week or two at most before attempting to taper the patient off the drug.
7. Generally, the primary care provider can manage acute situational anxiety. If the patient's symptoms persist or worsen despite the above interventions, the diagnosis may need to be revised (usually to adjustment disorder with anxious mood, or, if the symtomatic episode extends beyond six months, generalized anxiety disorder) and the management modified accordingly. Consultation with a mental health specialist is occasionally necessary for dealing with severe or complex anxiety syndromes precipitated by a disturbing life event.

Other Mental Disorders

Mental disorders other than the primary anxiety disorders may have anxiety as a prominent feature. Nearly every mental disorder can present with anxiety as a feature, but two disorders are worth discussing because of their frequency and importance in the primary care setting.

Adjustment Disorder with Anxious Mood

Adjustment disorder with anxious mood is the most frequent psychiatric diagnosis among seriously physically ill patients (Andreasen & Wasek, 1980; Derogatis, Morrow, & Fetting, 1983). Although treatment recommendations are available in the literature, they are based on clinical experience and expert opinion rather than controlled clinical trials. For example, Schatzberg (1990) suggests a nonpharmacological approach unless the anxiety is severe and incapacitating; then a drug should be added to the regimen. In outlining the nonpharmacological approach, he follows the recommendations of Diamond and Grauer (1987), who recommend offering interpersonal support and reassurance and dealing with the anxiety openly, directly, and immediately. If pharmacotherapy is necessary, one to three weeks of low-dose treatment with a short-acting benzodiazepine (for example, alprazolam 0.25 mg three times a day), with a two-week taper off the medication, has been recommended (McGlynn & Metcalf, 1989). If the anxious state persists beyond six months, or becomes more incapacitating, the diagnosis should be revised (often to generalized anxiety disorder) and clinical management adjusted accordingly. Consultation with a mental health professional may also be indicated at this point.

Mixed Anxiety-Depression

While there is some evidence for the existence of a discrete anxiety-depression syndrome (Coplan & Gorman, 1990), a large and heterogeneous group of patients will display symptoms of both anxiety and depression as part of their clinical presentation, particularly in the primary care setting (Barrett, Barrett, & Oxman, 1988). These patients should be taken seriously, because they have been shown to have a graver prognosis—for example, a higher rate of suicide—than patients who have no symptoms of anxiety (McGlynn & Metcalf, 1989). This is particularly true if the manifestation of anxiety involves panic symptoms (Fawcett, 1988).

The clinician's first task is to assess whether substance abuse or medical conditions could be causing or contributing to the anxiety. Psychosocial assessment is also important at this juncture, to assess factors that may be contributing to the onset or maintenance of the symptoms. These potential contributing factors should be reevaluated if the planned therapy is not having its intended effect. Any cognitive or behavioral techniques planned or currently in use for the treatment of depression can be modified for application to the specific manifestations of the anxiety disorder.

There are two schools of thought concerning the pharmacotherapy of mixed anxiety-depression. The first is to use a single drug that is effective for both of these disorders (Dubovsky, 1990). This approach has the advantage of parsimony and a more manageable side effect profile. Several drugs are useful in this approach: the cyclic antidepressants (Liebowitz, Fyer, & Gorman, 1988), monoamine oxidase (MAO) inhibitors (Liebowitz, Quitkin, & Stewart, 1984), buspirone at high doses (Robinson, Alms, & Shrotriya, 1989), and fluoxetine (Gorman, Liebowitz, & Fyer, 1987). All these drugs have demonstrated efficacy in anxiety and depression alone. The benzodiazepines are likewise effective in both anxiety and depression and would be a particularly attractive choice if the depression were considered secondary to the anxiety syndrome. Depression is a frequent comorbid factor in panic disorder (Aden, 1987).

The second approach is to use two drugs: one principally for the depression, and one for the anxiety (Fawcett, 1990). The advantages of this approach include controlling the symptoms of anxiety more rapidly than with an antidepressant alone and taking advantage of the synergistic effect produced by the concurrent use of both agents. In fact, sometimes a combination of a benzodiazepine and an antidepressant will facilitate improvement not seen with either drug alone. This regimen may be indicated if the symptoms of either syndrome are particularly severe, if the patient manifests suicidal ideation, or if treatment with one or more single-agent regimens has not been effective.

Primary Anxiety Disorders

Seven DSM-III-R disorders in which anxiety is the primary or exclusive symptom will be discussed below.

Panic Disorder

Because of its frequent occurrence in the primary care medical setting and the consequences of misdiagnosis or mismanagement, panic disorder is one of the most important disorders for primary care practitioners to diagnose accurately and manage properly. Fortunately, the literature has become quite active in this area—particularly concerning the etiology and early evolution of panic disorder—and a number of effective treatments are being developed.

The long-term natural history is less well understood. The treatment literature reflects this pattern: much attention has recently focused on the acute treatment of panic disorder, with recommendations for acute treatment usually based on evidence from controlled clinical trials. But uncertainty remains concerning long-term management, and recommendations tend to be less securely grounded in replicated clinical trials. Many authorities are now conceptualizing panic disorder as a chronic illness (Ballenger, 1991; Schatzberg & Ballenger, 1991), principally on the basis of clinical experience and indirect evidence from clinical trials—most subjects enrolled in studies have been symptomatic for many years. This chronic disease model, which may change as our knowledge of panic disorder evolves, has profound long-term treatment implications. These will be outlined below.

Once physicians make the diagnosis of panic disorder, they must follow through with at least the following steps:

1. Determine whether the attacks are primary or secondary. Panic may be caused by medical conditions, such as hyperthyroidism, or ingested substances (for example, amphetamines, cocaine, caffeine). Moreover, panic attacks may occur in the context of other mental disorders (for instance, agitated depression, acute schizophrenia, adjustment disorder with anxious mood), which might take treatment precedence. Primary medical conditions should be identified and managed; this approach to differential diagnosis may rule out a suspected panic disorder.

2. Determine whether the patient's condition is sufficiently severe to justify acute treatment. Although the patient's symptoms may meet the diagnostic criteria for panic disorder, the individual circumstances may suggest that treatment is unnecessary. For example, the attacks may have occurred in anticipation of a high-stress event, such as a courtroom appearance, or in the temporary absence of a key support person, such as a spouse. The symptoms may resolve spontaneously when the event is over or the support is restored. The full regimen described below would be inappropriate in this case. Schatzberg and Ballenger (1991) suggest acute treatment of panic attacks if any one of the following criteria is met: (a) severity or frequency sufficient to disable the patient; (b) clear morbidity such as functional impairment, phobic avoidance, or suicidal ideation; (c)

a comorbid disorder such as depression or alcohol abuse present; and (d) perhaps a family history of suicide or alcohol abuse.

3. Once the decision to treat panic disorder has been made, the clinician must then decide which treatment modalities to institute. At this point, the chronic disease perspective becomes important, and, particularly if pharmacotherapy is contemplated, the clinician should consider a treatment plan that will most likely continue for at least six months and perhaps much longer, even permanently. Ballenger (1991) has formulated a four-phase long-term treatment model for the pharmacotherapy of this disorder, consisting of an acute stage (one to three months), a stabilization stage (two to six months), a maintenance stage (three to twelve months), and a discontinuation stage (after twelve months). Any of the pharmacotherapeutic agents available for panic disorder can be used within this model. Nonpharmacological interventions, which may be the sole therapy or may be used in combination with antipanic medication, can also be instituted as long-term measures.

At least three classes of drugs and several nonpharmacological psychotherapeutic modalities have been shown to be effective in the treatment of panic disorder.

Benzodiazepines. The benzodiazepines, and particularly alprazolam, have been thoroughly studied in a number of controlled clinical trials; they have consistently been shown to be efficacious, even when used without adjunctive psychotherapy. For example, alprazolam was compared to placebo in Phase I of the Cross-National Collaborative Panic Study (Ballenger, Burrows, & Dupont, 1988). This study was a large multinational controlled trial of over 500 subjects with panic disorder and agoraphobia who were recruited from community settings. Alprazolam was used for eight weeks in doses up to 10 mg a day (mean daily dose = 5.7 mg a day) and was found to be significantly more efficacious than placebo beginning in the first week of therapy. Dramatic improvement was noted in all outcome measures, including lowered number of attacks, anticipatory anxiety, and phobic fear and avoidance. In addition, 92 percent of the alprazolam patients showed moderately or markedly improved global ratings, as compared with 63 percent of placebo-treated patients. Global anxiety ratings, somatization scores, and work and social disability ratings were also improved. The low dropout rate of patients in the alprazolam group (16 versus 50 percent dropout of the placebo group) suggests that this drug is well tolerated, even at the relatively high doses used in this trial. At least 60 percent of patients reported sedation, but this complaint generally subsided within a week, even without reduction of dosage. Thus, alprazolam has the advantages of a rapid onset of action, a dramatic effectiveness, and an acceptable side effect profile. Patients can be started at 0.25 to 0.50 mg three times a day and increased by 0.25 to 0.50 mg every three days until the panic attacks, anticipatory anxiety, and phobic avoidance subside. Clinical remissions may occur at dosages of less than 4 mg a day (in one-third of patients), but in another one-third, the dose will need to exceed 6 mg a day. The panic attacks themselves tend to subside at lower doses, with the phobic symptoms abating more slowly and in the higher dosage ranges. Sedation may require that the dosage be increased more slowly. Ballenger (1991) recommends that the physician be "assertive in pushing the dose upward" during this phase of treatment and that a relatively high dose be maintained for at least a month. During the next two or three months, the dose is adjusted to minimize side effects while the patient consolidates initial clinical gains and resolves residual phobic behavior. Discontinuation of the drug either too early or too quickly can result in high relapse rates (Fyer, Liebowitz, & Gorman, 1987).

The next three to nine months constitute the maintenance phase, during which the drug is tapered gently downward to the minimum effective dose while the patient resumes and consolidates the premorbid life-style. Several studies have documented that alprazolam maintains its effectiveness with long-term use, and most patients on maintenance therapy use significantly less of the drug than during their acute treatment (Nagy, Krystal, & Woods, 1989; Pollack, Tesar, & Rosenbaum, 1986; Sheehan, 1987).

After eight to twelve months, discontinuation should be considered. One of the principal drawbacks of the benzodiazepines is the potential for withdrawal symptoms. These symptoms will occur in about one-third of patients if too rapid a taper (that is, one month) is attempted, even after only two months of treatment with alprazolam (Pecknold, Swinson, Kuch, & Lewis, 1988). These symptoms are less problematic when the drug is tapered more slowly, over three to six months (Fyer et al., 1987), but a substantial fraction of patients will relapse and require reinstitution of therapy (Ballenger, 1991; Sheehan, 1987).

The potential for abuse of benzodiazepines has been investigated closely (Griffiths & Roache, 1985). In the absence of a history of alcohol or other drug abuse, patients rarely, if ever, use escalating doses of benzodiazepines. In fact, given control over the dosing, patients will tend to use less over time. Drug and alcohol abusers, however, appear to experience a "reinforcing" or "drug-liking" effect and may utilize benzodiazepines as drugs of abuse (Griffiths & Roache, 1985; Woods, Katz, & Winger, 1988).

Other benzodiazepines, though less exhaustively studied, have been shown to be as effective as alprazolam in the treatment of panic disorder. In one controlled trial, clonazepam at a mean dose of 2.5 mg a day was as effective as alprazolam and significantly more effective than placebo (Tesar et al., 1991).

Teboul and Chouinard (1991) consider clonazepam the benzodiazepine of choice for panic disorder, because the longer half-life prevents nocturnal breakthrough and allows less frequent dosing. Because nocturnal attacks occur in the majority of patients (Mellman & Uhde, 1989), clonazepam is often most effective if administered twice daily.

Diazepam has likewise been shown to be as effective as alprazolam if used in sufficient doses (mean daily dose = 44 mg a day) (Dunner, Ishiki, Avery, Wilson, & Hyde, 1986; Noyes et al., 1984). Lorazepam has also been shown effective in controlled clinical trials (Charney & Woods, 1989; Charney et al., 1987). The notion that many benzodiazepines are ineffective in the treatment of panic disorder probably arose from trials in which inadequate doses were used. All the benzodiazepines share the advantages of rapid effectiveness and acceptable side effect profile, and all share the potential for a withdrawal reaction. Evidence that some patients may respond to one benzodiazepine but not another (Spier, Tesar, Rosenbaum, & Woods, 1986) should encourage clinicians to try another drug in this class if the first one attempted is not effective.

About two-thirds of patients with panic disorder either have or have had major depression. The benzodiazepines are equally effective in patients with and without depression, and depression scores improve significantly in the course of treatment of panic disorder with benzodiazepines (Deltito, Argyle, & Klerman, 1991; Klerman, 1990).

Tricyclic Antidepressants. Several members of this class of drugs have been shown to be as effective in the treatment of panic disorder as the benzodiazepines. Imipramine is the most extensively studied and was used in Phase II of the Cross-National Collaborative Panic Study (Deltito et al., 1991). In this well-designed clinical trial, alprazolam, imipramine, and placebo were compared in 1,168 outpatients. Both imipramine and alprazolam were significantly superior to placebo on most outcome measures and roughly equal to one another in efficacy. Both were well tolerated during the eight weeks of treatment, but there were more complaints of side effects with imipramine. Although alprazolam has a faster onset of efficacy (one week versus four weeks for imipramine), imipramine has the advantage of once-daily dosing, is relatively inexpensive, and has low abuse potential. However, many patients (up to 20 percent) will drop out of initial therapy with this medication because of the delayed onset of efficacy and the troublesome side effects: about one-fourth of patients will experience an amphetamine-like reaction (Noyes, Garvey, Cook, & Samuelson, 1989). Other patients will be bothered by the anticholinergic side effects, postural hypotension, sexual dysfunction, or weight gain. Tricyclic antidepressants must be used with caution in patients with heart disease: they prolong the PR, QRS, and QT intervals, have type I anti-arrhythmic effects at therapeutic doses, and at higher doses have been implicated in a number of dangerous disturbances of cardiac rhythm. Some tricyclic side effects, particularly the anticholinergic and hyperstimulatory effects, can be minimized by starting with a very low dose (for example, 10 mg a day) and increasing slowly, by 10 mg every three days. Some patients will respond to doses as low as 25 mg, but most will require at least 150 mg and others will require up to 300 mg a day.

The same principles of long-term management that were detailed above for the benzodiazepines also apply to drugs of this class.

During the discontinuation phase, imipramine should be tapered slowly, by about 25 mg every month (Noyes & Perry, 1990).

Most other antidepressants appear to be effective, although their effectiveness is less thoroughly documented than imipramine's (Lydiard & Ballenger, 1987). Some patients may respond to one antidepressant over another, and drug selection may be influenced for a particular patient by desired or undesired incidental effects (for example, sedating versus nonsedating antidepressants).

Monamine Oxidase Inhibitors. These drugs, particularly phenelzine, have been shown to be effective in the treatment of panic disorder. Phenelzine may be the most effective drug available for panic disorder, particularly in patients with atypical depressive features (Liebowitz et al., 1984). It may work when other drugs have failed. This drug has the disadvantage of a slow onset of action, generally requiring six to eight weeks to reach maximum efficacy, and a high side effect profile. Most physicians are aware that MAO inhibitors can precipitate a dangerous hypertensive crisis in patients who ingest substances containing tyramine; these drugs can also cause hyperpyrexic reactions, orthostatic hypotension, sexual dysfunction, and weight gain (Bryant & Brown, 1988). Primary care physicians who choose to use MAO inhibitors should carefully study the side effect and interaction profile of these drugs and should be certain patients have done the same; they should insist that the patient know the dietary restrictions that apply when using an MAO inhibitor and that the patient consult with them prior to beginning any new medication, whether prescription or not.

Nonpharmacological Treatments. As mentioned above, many patients who are treated pharmacologically alone will experience a return of their symptoms when tapered off their drug, even after a year or more. Because these drugs do not appear to be curative, considerable attention has been devoted to nonpharmacological modalities. Several of these have been shown to be effective in panic disorder. Most treatments involve exposure to the phobic object or situation, relaxation therapy, cognitive-behavioral therapy, or some combination of these. Barlow (1990) has published the results of a fifteen-week controlled clinical trial of a cognitive-behavioral therapy, with and without training in relaxation procedures, for patients with panic disorder. The cognitive treatment involved "systematic structured exposure to feared internal sensations." At six- and twenty-four-month follow-up evaluations, the cognitive treatment groups had significantly more panic-free patients (60 and 80 percent) than the relaxation groups (10 and 40 percent) or the combined groups (50 and 40 percent), suggesting that cognitive therapy is an effective treatment for panic disorder and that relaxation interferes with its effectiveness. Klosko, Barlow, and Tassinari (1990) reported a study comparing alprazolam to placebo and cognitive-behavioral therapy; both active treatment groups did significantly better than placebo and not significantly different from each other, although the cognitive-behavioral therapy group showed a broader pattern of positive response than the alprazolam group.

Graded exposure to the phobic object or situation is generally straightforward and can be accomplished under the supervision of the primary physician. This involves identifying the source of avoidant fears and gradually exposing oneself to them under controlled circumstances, usually with a supportive companion. For example, a patient may be afraid of crowds. Graded exposure might entail visiting a shopping mall early in the morning when there are few people around, then repeating this exposure at progressively more crowded times until it is possible to tolerate this setting at peak hours. Cognitive-behavioral therapies, on the other hand, are somewhat more involved and should be undertaken by a clinician with specialized training. Because cognitive-behavior therapy requires a trained clinician, it is a potentially expensive intervention. If future studies, particularly of long-term follow-up, corroborate that a cognitive-behavioral approach can lead to long-term improvement in patients with panic disorder, it will assume a preeminent place over other treatment options.

Agoraphobia

Panic disorder may occur with or without agoraphobia. However, agoraphobia is usually present by the time the panic symptoms are accurately diagnosed. Since the agoraphobia is a secondary phenomenon, the astute clinician can expect to see the occasional patient who has not yet developed phobic avoidance patterns. These nonphobic patients may respond to lower doses of antipanic drugs than patients with accompanying agoraphobia.

The clinician may occasionally see a patient with agoraphobia but without panic, the converse of the situation described above. This clinical phenomenon is generally uncommon, and these patients are less likely than those with alarming somatic manifestations of a panic attack to initially seek out medical treatment. If the primary care provider does encounter a simple agoraphobic patient, graded exposure to the phobic object or situation, as described above, is the therapy of choice and is quite effective (Marks, 1985; Teboul & Chouinard, 1991).

All of the drugs described in the section on panic disorder have been documented to be effective not only for the symptoms of panic, but for agoraphobia as well.

Social Phobia and Performance Anxiety

MAO inhibitors, particularly phenelzine, are effective treatment for social phobia by randomized controlled trials (Liebowitz, Fyer, Gorman, Campeas, & Levin, 1986; Liebowitz, Gorman, & Fyer, 1988). Cognitive and behavioral strategies have likewise been shown to be effective (Heimberg, 1989).

A number of other drugs have been reported effective in clinical case reports or open clinical trials: the MAO inhibitor tranylcypromine (Versiani, Mundim, & Nardi, 1988), the beta-blocker atenolol (Gorman, Liebowitz, & Fyer, 1985), the alpha-blocker clonidine (Goldstein, 1987), the tricyclic imipramine (Benca, Matuzas, & Al-Sadir, 1986), and several benzodiazepines, particularly alprazolam (Reich & Yates, 1988) and clonazepam (Reiter, Pollack, Rosenbaum, & Cohen, 1990). Clonazepam at 1–3 mg a day looks particularly promising, and the literature may soon contain reports of controlled clinical trials of this and similar drugs for social phobia.

Performance anxiety, or stage fright, can be considered a special case of social phobia and is especially common among amateur and professional musicians. Beta-blockers are widely prescribed and even more widely used for this condition but have yet to be shown unequivocally effective (Nies, 1986). These drugs also reduce heart rate and tremor (Brantigan, Brantigan, & Joseph, 1979; James, Griffith, & Pearson, 1977; James & Savage, 1984; Neftel, Adler, & Kappeli, 1982), but they have little (James et al., 1977) or else no (Brantigan et al., 1979; James & Savage, 1984; Neftel et al., 1982) measurable effect on subjective anxiety. Benzodiazepines reduce subjective anxiety but impair performance, presumably via an adverse effect on psychomotor activity (James & Savage, 1984).

In a well-executed, controlled study comparing buspirone to placebo, both with and without a five-session cognitive-behavioral intervention, brief cognitive-behavioral therapy was effective in reducing anxiety and improving performance, but buspirone was no more effective than placebo in producing either of these outcomes (Clark & Agras, 1991). Therefore, the treatment of choice at this time would be considered brief cognitive-behavior therapy, but ongoing research activity in this area may soon demonstrate the efficacy of other therapies.

Simple Phobia

Graded exposure therapy is generally considered the treatment of choice for this extremely common but circumscribed condition (Marks, 1985). The patient's degree of fear and general physical condition as well as the degree of interference with everyday life are useful indicators to determine the speed and duration needed for exposure to the feared object or situation. The clinician does not necessarily have to be physically present during the exposure. Significant improvement generally occurs in four to twenty sessions and often lasts up to four years.

Obsessive-Compulsive Disorder

Traditionally, this disorder has been regarded as one of the more intractable neuroses. However, significant breakthroughs have recently occurred in the management of obsessive-compulsive disorder. Since the primary physician will only occasionally be called on to treat someone with this disorder, the treatment modalities will be briefly outlined.

Many authorities would now consider the treatment of choice

to be a particular form of behavior therapy involving graded exposure to the stimuli that provoke the obsessional fears coupled with prevention of the ritualistic response (March, Johnston, & Greist, 1989; O'Sullivan, Noshirvani, Marks, Monteiro, & Lelliott, 1991). Benefits of this modality tend to be at least as pronounced as those attained with pharmacotherapy, with 90 percent of patients achieving at least moderate improvement (Foa, Steketee, & Ozarrow, 1985). Moreover, the benefits tend to be longer lasting (O'Sullivan et al., 1991). However, only about 75 percent of patients are willing to endure the discomfort of this procedure, which should last for several hours a day for at least six weeks. The procedure is straightforward and not time consuming for the physician and has been found to be effective even when self-administered (Marks, Lelliott, & Basoglu, 1988). In fact, an effective self-help manual is available for this purpose (Greist, Jefferson, & Marks, 1986).

A number of drugs have been shown to be effective for this disorder. Greist recommends pharmacotherapy if behavioral therapy fails, is not available, is refused, or if the patient is obsessional without ritualistic behavior or is severely depressed (Greist, 1990). While most antidepressants have been ineffective against obsessive-compulsive disorder, at least three drugs in this class—clomipramine, fluvoxamine, and fluoxetine—have shown some efficacy. Clomipramine is the best studied and perhaps the most effective of these drugs (Rapoport, 1988), having been shown efficacious in repeated controlled clinical trials (DeVeaugh-Geiss, Katz, & Landau, 1989; Perse, 1988). About 75 percent of patients will show significant improvement, which may not manifest for four to six weeks, at dosages of about 200 mg a day. Fluvoxamine has been shown effective in at least one controlled clinical trial at a dose of about 300 mg a day (Goodman, Price, & Rasmussen, 1989), whereas fluoxetine has been shown to be effective in at least several open clinical trials (Jenicke, Baer, & Buttolph, 1991; Jenicke, Buttolph, & Baer, 1989). These results await replication in controlled clinical trials.

At least one controlled clinical trial (Pato et al., 1991) has shown buspirone at a mean daily dose of about 60 mg to be as effective as clomipramine in the acute treatment of obsessive-compulsive disorder. This trial, which used a crossover design and showed some degree of a carryover effect, will also need to be replicated.

Treatment with any of the drugs described above should be maintained for at least eight weeks, preferably ten, before judging the effectiveness. Despite the sometimes dramatic improvement in symptomatology brought about by these drugs, about 25 percent of patients will not respond. In this case, another drug can be added to augment the effect of the first medication. Both lithium (600–900 mg a day) (Rasmussen, 1984) and buspirone (60 mg a day) (Jenicke et al., 1991) have been shown in open trials to be effective when used in this supplemental manner.

As a last resort, refractory patients can be referred for psychosurgery, which is surprisingly safe (1–10 percent complication rate, usually seizures controlled with phenytoin) and effective (greater than 50 percent success rate for patients who have failed all other modalities) (Jenicke et al., 1991). Four neurosurgical procedures are being performed for obsessive-compulsive disorder, but the most common at this time is computerized tomography-guided stereotactic radiofrequency thermal anterior cingulotomy. This procedure generally results in a small, discrete ablation that causes no measurable neurological or neuropsychiatric deficits. The procedure often must be repeated for maximum benefit.

Post-Traumatic Stress Disorder

The first step in the management of post-traumatic stress disorder (PTSD) is careful attention to diagnostic issues. PTSD commonly occurs together with other psychiatric diagnoses, particularly generalized anxiety disorder and depression (Shore, Vollmer, & Tatum, 1989). In addition, the trauma that precipitates PTSD may itself have caused brain injury, particularly postconcussive syndrome. PTSD may in fact be more than one entity and certainly consists of a heterogeneous aggregation of symptoms that respond differentially and at times unpredictably to treatment. Nevertheless, some medications have been shown to be helpful for limited symptoms in some patients. This small but rapidly expanding literature should be watched for further developments.

Whenever phobic-avoidant symptoms are part of the clinical

picture of PTSD, graded exposure therapy (as described in the section on panic disorder) is somewhat helpful (Marks, 1985). This modality generally plays an adjunctive role and is used in concert with pharmacotherapy, which tends to be more effective against the "positive" symptoms of autonomic arousal such as irritability, hypervigilance, insomnia, nightmares, and outbursts of anger.

Several tricyclics have been studied in controlled trials, including amitriptyline (which showed a modest improvement in depression scores, although most subjects still met diagnostic criteria for PTSD) (Davidson, Kudler, & Smith, 1990), desipramine (no improvement in symptoms of PTSD after four weeks) (Reist, Kauffmann, & Haier, 1989), and imipramine (improvement in nightmares, flashbacks, and intrusive memories at 240 mg a day) (Kosten, Frank, Dan, McDougle, & Giller, 1991).

Phenelzine has been directly compared to placebo and to imipramine in at least one controlled trial (Kosten et al., 1991) and shown to be superior to both, at a dose of about 70 mg a day. However, neither of the active drugs affected the pattern of avoidant behavior.

A number of other drugs have shown promise in open trials, and the literature should be monitored for corroborating reports. Among these promising agents are carbamazepine, valproate, lithium, alprazolam, propranolol, and clonidine. Silver, Sandberg, & Hales (1990) recommended initiating treatment with a tricyclic such as imipramine and adding or changing drugs according to the response and residual symptom patterns. Remember that a high proportion of patients suffering from PTSD have abused alcohol or other drugs, and benzodiazepines should be used cautiously.

Generalized Anxiety Disorder

A number of nonpharmacological treatments have been reported to be useful in the treatment of generalized anxiety disorder (GAD), including supportive psychotherapy, exposure therapy, cognitive therapy, and deep relaxation (Marks, 1985). Controlled clinical trials will be necessary to conclusively document the efficacy of these interventions (Gorman, 1987).

Three classes of drugs are employed in the pharmacotherapy

of GAD: benzodiazepines, tricyclics, and azapirones. The benzodiazepines are undoubtedly the most widely used drugs for this disorder. At least in the short term, the efficacy of these agents is beyond question, confirmed by scores of clinical trials. A meta-analysis of some benzodiazapine trials suggests that about two-thirds of patients get an acceptable clinical response from these drugs (Quality Assurance Project, 1985).

GAD should probably be conceptualized as a chronic, intermittent disorder, although the natural history needs to be better elucidated. This conceptualization raises questions about the long-term efficacy of the benzodiazepines, the potential for abuse, the development of tolerance, and the optimal duration of treatment. The issue of abuse has been fairly well delineated, as discussed in the section on panic disorder: the benzodiazepines are rarely abused except by people who abuse other drugs, but unfortunately this includes a fair number of patients with GAD. A careful drug and alcohol use history should always be taken. The other questions are less well worked out and need further research. What is particularly needed are long-term placebo-controlled trials with diagnostically distinct patient groups to examine potential for abuse, development of tolerance, and optimal duration of treatment. Rickels and colleagues found no evidence for an attenuation of the effectiveness of diazepam after twenty-two weeks (Rickels, Case, Winokur, & Swenson, 1984), whereas other trials have shown reduced efficacy after less than eight weeks (Kahn et al., 1981). On the basis of the admittedly incomplete but currently available evidence, several authorities (Gorman, 1987; Lader, 1988) recommend treatment with a benzodiazepine for as long as the anxiety persists, with frequent attempts at tapering the patient off the drug.

One benzodiazepine is probably as effective as another, but for long-term use, a drug with a long half-life—such as diazepam (5–20 mg a day) or clonazepam (0.5–2.0 mg a day)—is usually recommended. Some authors recommend using shorter-acting benzodiazepines in the elderly to prevent the buildup of long-acting metabolites, but careful attention to the clinical status of the patient will eliminate the need for this restriction.

At least one multicenter study unequivocally supports the superiority of imipramine (150–200 mg a day) over both chlordiazepoxide (60–80 mg a day) and placebo in anxious outpatients, even when controlling for baseline levels of depression and when eliminating the subset of patients with panic disorder. This support is based on the results from a well-designed study of 223 volunteers with clinical anxiety recruited from the community (Kahn, McNair, & Lipman, 1986). Doxepin has also been extensively studied for the treatment of GAD, and a number of reviews of these doxepin treatment studies have been published (see Gorman, 1987). Gorman calls for more and better studies but interprets the available evidence as suggestive of an anxiolytic effect with many antidepressants comparable to the effect of benzodiazepines. However, the antidepressants have a slower onset of action, a higher side effect profile, and a higher patient dropout rate. Doxepin is not clearly superior to other antidepressants.

Buspirone is also approved for treatment of anxiety. It is as effective as diazepam for this indication (Goa & Ward, 1986), with advantages including the absence of sedation, minimal cognitive and psychomotor impairment, and low abuse potential. The disadvantages of this agent are slow onset of action (two to four weeks) and poor acceptance by patients previously treated with benzodiazepines. The usual dose is 10–60 mg a day, in two or three divided doses. Abrupt withdrawal causes no reaction.

A number of other drugs have been used for generalized anxiety. Lader (1988) summarizes these agents as follows: antihistamines are sedating but ineffective as anxiolytics; barbiturates and meprobamate both have unfavorable benefit-risk ratios; antipsychotics may be useful for patients previously dependent on other drugs and patients with psychotic or schizoaffective features; and beta-blockers may be effective for somatic manifestations of anxiety, such as tachycardia or gastrointestinal upset, but do not cause improvement in the cognitive manifestations of anxiety.

Conclusion

In conclusion, the primary practitioner will frequently encounter patients with clinically significant anxiety syndromes; most of these disorders are amenable to successful treatment. The management of anxiety disorders is an interesting and lively field at the moment, and the clinician should monitor the literature for new developments that will make the management of these disorders safer and even more effective. The interested investigator will find the field ripe for research. What follows is a sampling of topics in need of investigation.

1. *Subthreshold disorders.* The most important subthreshold disorder is acute situational anxiety. This is a condition frequently managed by primary care clinicians, but the entity has no established diagnostic criteria. We need basic clinical and epidemiologic descriptions of this condition as it appears in the various primary care settings: How common is this disorder when defined rigorously? What are the typical and atypical presenting manifestations? What are the most common predisposing events or risk factors? What is the natural history of acute situational anxiety? Does it ordinarily resolve spontaneously without treatment? What proportion of patients ultimately get reassigned to another diagnostic category? Are there interventions that lessen the severity or duration of the condition? Who should undertake these interventions?

2. *Mixed anxiety-depression.* This heterogeneous diagnostic category is enjoying considerable investigative activity right now, but relatively little appears to be occurring in the primary care setting. This is ironic, since it has been shown in at least one primary care setting to be more common than any other RDC mental diagnosis (Barrett et al., 1988). Primary care investigators could help us by clarifying the forms and range of severity this condition takes in the primary medical setting. Also, controlled clinical trials in this setting of the various treatment regimens being advocated would be helpful.

3. *Somatized anxiety.* One frequently hears that certain DSM-III-R conditions occur in the primary medical setting in a somatized form. This needs to be documented. The anxiety disorders all have somatic manifestations; are these somatic manifestations really more pronounced in the medical setting? Are there anxiety diagnoses in which the *only* manifestations are somatic? To some extent, these questions have been addressed for panic disorder, but they have not been addressed for the others. Investigators interested in the phenomenology of anxiety in the primary care setting could learn much of value. Even more valuable would be clinical

trials for the treatment of these somatized variants, if they in fact exist.

4. *Anxiety-medical comorbidity studies.* There is a fascinating literature on the relationship between medical illness and mental disorders, most of which deals with depression and major medical illnesses, or depression and physical symptomatology. Much less is known about the relationship between anxiety disorders and ambulatory medical illnesses. Are high levels of anxiety (or the presence of an anxiety disorder) associated with more symptomatic ambulatory medical illnesses? Or with higher levels of dysfunction for a medical illness of a given severity? Or with longer recovery from medical illnesses? If so, are there treatments aimed at the anxiety that can lower the morbidity associated with a given medical illness? Conversely, are there medical illnesses that are particularly associated with anxiety diagnoses? What is the natural history of anxiety disorders when complicated with physical illness? There is no end to the questions one might ask about this anxiety-medical illness interface.

5. *Post-traumatic stress disorder.* This disorder may be one of the great underdiagnosed disorders in primary care. Certainly the requisite traumatic event is extremely common in the primary care setting: we know that about one-fourth of women family practice patients report severe physical violence from male partners (Rath, Jarratt, & Leonardson, 1989), 17 percent of women family practice patients report having experienced incest as children, and 30 percent of women family practice patients report having been raped (Walker, Torlkeson, Katon, & Koss, 1993). These patients report far more somatic complaints and have a much higher rate of most mental diagnoses than their nonvictimized cohorts. What is the relationship between this trauma and subsequent symptomatology? The DSM-III-R criteria for PTSD do not emphasize somatic manifestations, but the primary care clinician may be the person most likely to see somatized variants of this disorder. Careful epidemiologic work would be most welcome here.

This is the briefest outline of a research agenda for primary care, which should also include replicating most of the epidemiologic studies and clinical trials undertaken in the psychiatric setting. The curious investigator will not have any lack of interesting or important questions to answer about anxiety in the primary care setting.

References

Aden, G. C. (1987). Alprazolam's role in the treatment of anxious depression. In G. Racagni & E. Smeraldi (Eds.), *Anxious depression: Assessment and treatment* (pp. 189–208). New York: Raven Press.

Andreasen, N. C., & Wasek, P. (1980). Adjustment disorders in adolescents and adults. *Archives of General Psychiatry, 37,* 1166–1170.

Ballenger, J. C. (1991). Long-term pharmacologic treatment of panic disorder. *Journal of Clinical Psychiatry, 52*(Suppl.), 18–25.

Ballenger, J. C., Burrows, G. D., & Dupont, R. L., Jr. (1988). Alprazolam in panic disorder and agoraphobia: Results from a multicenter trial: 1. Efficacy in short-term treatment. *Archives of General Psychiatry, 45,* 413–422.

Barlow, D. H. (1990). Long-term outcome for patients with panic disorder treated with cognitive-behavioral therapy. *Journal of Clinical Psychiatry, 51*(12(Suppl. A)), 17–23.

Barrett, J. E., Barrett, J. A., & Oxman, T. E. (1988). The prevalence of psychiatric disorders in a primary care practice. *Archives of General Psychiatry, 45,* 1100–1106.

Benca, R., Matuzas, W., & Al-Sadir, J. (1986). Social phobia, MVP, and response to imipramine. *Journal of Clinical Psychopharmacology, 6,* 50–51.

Brantigan, C., Brantigan, T., & Joseph, N. (1979). The effect of beta blockade on stage fright: A controlled study. *Rocky Mountain Medical Journal, 76,* 227–233.

Bryant, S. G., & Brown, C. S. (1988). Major depressive disorders. In L. Y. Young & M. A. Koda-Kimble (Eds.), *Applied therapeutics: The clinical use of drugs* (pp. 1231–1254). Vancouver, British Columbia: Applied Therapeutics, Inc.

Charney, D. S., & Woods, S. W. (1989). Benzodiazepine treatment of panic disorder: A comparison of alprazolam and lorazepam. *Journal of Clinical Psychiatry, 50,* 418–423.

Charney, D. S., Woods, S. W., Goodman, W. K., Krystal, J. H.,

Naey, L. M., & Heninger, G. R. (1987). The efficacy of lorazepam in panic disorders. In *New Research Program and Abstracts, 140th Annual Meeting of the American Psychiatric Association* (Abstract No. NR165.119).

Clark, D. B., & Agras, W. S. (1991). The assessment and treatment of performance anxiety in musicians. *American Journal of Psychiatry, 148,* 598–605.

Coplan, J. D., & Gorman, J. M. (1990). Treatment of anxiety disorder in patients with mood disorders. *Journal of Clinical Psychiatry, 51*(Suppl.), 9–13.

Davidson, J., Kudler, H., & Smith, R. (1990). Treatment of posttraumatic stress disorder with amitriptyline and placebo. *Archives of General Psychiatry, 47,* 259–266.

Deltito, J. A., Argyle, N., & Klerman, G. L. (1991). Patients with panic disorder unaccompanied by depression improve with alprazolam and imipramine treatment. *Journal of Clinical Psychiatry, 52,* 121–127.

Derogatis, L. R., Morrow, G. R., & Fetting, J. (1983). The prevalence of psychiatric disorders among cancer patients. *Journal of the American Medical Association, 249,* 751–757.

DeVeaugh-Geiss, J., Katz, R. J., & Landau, P. (1989). Preliminary results from a multicenter trial of clomipramine in obsessive-compulsive disorder. *Psychopharmacol Bulletin, 25,* 36–40.

Diamond, E. L., & Grauer, K. (1987). The spectrum of anxiety disorders in family practice. *American Family Physician, 36,* 167–173.

Dubovsky, S. L. (1990). Understanding and treating depression in anxious patients. *Journal of Clinical Psychiatry, 51*(Suppl. 10), 3–8.

Dunner, D. L., Ishiki, D., Avery, D. H., Wilson, L. G., & Hyde, T. S. (1986). Effect of alprazolam and diazepam on anxiety and panic attacks in panic disorder: A controlled study. *Journal of Clinical Psychiatry, 47,* 458–460.

Engel, G. L. (1988). How much longer must medicine's science be bound by a seventeenth century world view? In K. L. White (Ed.), *The task of medicine: Dialog at Wickenberg* (pp. 113–136). Menlo Park, CA: Henry J. Kaiser Family Foundation.

Fawcett, J. (1988). Predictors of early suicide: Identification and appropriate intervention. *Journal of Clinical Psychiatry, 49* (Suppl. 10), 7-8.

Fawcett, J. (1990). Targeting treatment in patients with mixed symptoms of anxiety and depression. *Journal of Clinical Psychiatry, 51*(Suppl. 1), 40-43.

Foa, E. B., Steketee, G. S., & Ozarrow, B. J. (1985). Behavior therapy with obsessive compulsives: From theory to treatment. In M. Mavissakalian, S. M. Turner, & L. Michelson (Eds.), *Obsessive-compulsive disorder: Psychological and pharmacological treatment* (pp. 49-129). New York: Plenum Press.

Fyer, A. J., Liebowitz, M. R., & Gorman, J. M. (1987). Discontinuation of alprazolam treatment in panic patients. *American Journal of Psychiatry, 144,* 303-308.

Goa, K. L., & Ward, A. (1986). Buspirone: A preliminary review of its pharmacological properties and therapeutic efficacy as an anxiolytic. *Drugs, 32,* 114-129.

Goldstein, S. (1987). Treatment of social phobia with clonidine. *Biological Psychiatry, 22,* 36.

Goodman, W. K., Price, L. H., & Rasmussen, S. A. (1989). Efficacy of fluvoxamine in obsessive-compulsive disorder: A double-blind comparison with placebo. *Archives of General Psychiatry, 46,* 36-44.

Gorman, J. M. (1987). Generalized anxiety disorders. In D. F. Klein (Eds.), *Anxiety.* Basel, Switzerland: Karger.

Gorman, J. M., Liebowitz, M., & Fyer, A. (1985). Treatment of social phobia with atenolol. *Journal of Clinical Psychopharmacology, 5,* 298-301.

Gorman, J. M., Liebowitz, M. R., & Fyer, A. J. (1987). An open trial of fluoxetine in the treatment of panic attacks. *Journal of Clinical Psychopharmacology, 7,* 329-332.

Greist, J. H. (1990). Treating the anxiety: Therapeutic options in obsessive compulsive disorder. *Journal of Clinical Psychiatry, 51*(Suppl. 11), 29-34.

Greist, J. H., Jefferson, J. W., & Marks, I. M. (1986). *Anxiety and its treatment: Help is available.* Washington, DC: American Psychiatric Press.

Griffiths, R. R., & Roache, J. D. (1985). Abuse liability of benzodiazepines: A review of human studies evaluating subjective and/

or reinforcing effects. In D. E. Smith & D. R. Wesson (Eds.), *The benzodiazepines: Current standards for medical practice.* Lancaster, England: MTP Press.

Heimberg, R. (1989). Cognitive and behavioral treatments for social phobia: A critical analysis. *Clinical Psychology Review, 9,* 107–128.

James, I., Griffith, D., & Pearson, R. (1977). Effect of oxprenolol on stage fright in musicians. *Lancet, 2,* 952–954.

James, I., & Savage, I. (1984). Beneficial effect of nadolol on anxiety-induced disturbances of performance in musicians: A comparison with diazepam and placebo. *American Heart Journal, 4,* 1150–1155.

Jenicke, M. A., Baer, L., Ballantine, T., Martuza, R. L., Tynes, S., Giriunas, I., Buttolph, L., & Cassem, N. H. (1991). Cingulotomy for refractory obsessive-compulsive disorder: A long-term followup of 33 patients. *Archives of General Psychiatry, 48,* 548–555.

Jenicke, M. A., Baer, L., & Buttolph, L. (1991). Buspirone augmentation of fluoxitine in patients with obsessive compulsive disorder. *Journal of Clinical Psychiatry, 52,* 13–14.

Jenicke, M. A., Buttolph, L., & Baer, L. (1989). Fluoxitine in obsessive-compulsive disorder: A positive open trial. *American Journal of Psychiatry, 146,* 909–911.

Kahn, R. J., McNair, D. M., Covi, L., Downing, R. W., Fisher, S., Lipman, R. S., Rickels, K., & Smith, V. (1981). Effects of psychotropic agents on high anxiety subjects. *Psychopharmacology Bulletin, 17,* 97–100.

Kahn, R. J., McNair, D. M., & Lipman, R. S. (1986). Impiramine and chlordiazepoxide in depressive and anxiety disorders. *Archives of General Psychiatry, 43,* 79–86.

Klerman, G. L. (1990). Depression and panic anxiety: The effect of depressive co-morbidity on response to drug treatment of patients with panic disorder and agoraphobia. *Journal of Psychiatric Research, 24*(Suppl. 2), 27–41.

Klosko, J. S., Barlow, D. H., & Tassinari, R. (1990). A comparison of alprazolam and behavior therapy in treatment of panic disorder. *Journal of Consulting and Clinical Psychology, 58,* 77–84.

Kosten, T. R., Frank, J. B., Dan, E., McDougle, C. J., & Giller, E.

L. (1991). Pharmacotherapy for posttraumatic stress disorder using phenelzine or imipramine. *Journal of Nervous and Mental Disorders, 179,* 366–370.

Lader, M. (1988). Long-term treatment of anxiety: Benefits and drawbacks. In D. E. Casey & A. V. Christensen (Eds.), *Psychopharmacology: Current trends* (pp. 169–179). Berlin: Springer-Verlag.

Landry, M. J., Smith, D. E., McDuff, D. R., & Baughman, O. L. (1991). Anxiety and substance use disorders: The treatment of high-risk patients. *Journal of the American Board of Family Practice, 4,* 447–456.

Liebowitz, M. R., Fyer, A. J., & Gorman, J. M. (1988). Tricyclic therapy of the DSM-III anxiety disorders: A review with implications for further research. *Journal of Psychiatric Research, 22*(Suppl. 1), 7–31.

Liebowitz, M. R., Fyer, A. J., Gorman, J. M., Campeas, R., & Levin, A. (1986). Phenelzine in social phobia. *Journal of Clinical Psychopharmacology, 6,* 93–98.

Liebowitz, M. R., Gorman, J. M., & Fyer, J. J. (1988). Pharmacotherapy of social phobia: An interim report of a placebo-controlled comparison of phenelzine and atenolol. *Journal of Clinical Psychiatry, 49,* 252–257.

Liebowitz, M. R., Quitkin, F. M., & Stewart, J. W. (1984). Phenelzine versus imipramine in atypical depression. *Archives of General Psychiatry, 41,* 669–677.

Lydiard, R. B., & Ballenger, J. C. (1987). Antidepressants in panic disorder and agoraphobia. *Journal of Affective Disorders, 13,* 153–168.

McGlynn, T. J., & Metcalf, H. L. (Ed.). (1989). *Diagnosis and treatment of anxiety disorders: A physician's handbook.* Washington, DC: American Psychiatric Press.

Man, G. C., Hsu, K., & Sproule, B. J. (1986). Effect of alprazolam on exercise and dyspnea in patients with chronic obstructive pulmonary disease. *Chest, 90*(6), 832–836.

March, J. S., Johnston, H., & Greist, J. H. (1989). Obsessive-compulsive disorder. *American Family Physician, 39,* 175–182.

Marks, I. M. (1985). Behavioral psychotherapy for anxiety disorders. *Psychiatric Clinics of North America, 8,* 25–35.

Marks, I. M., Lelliott, P., & Basoglu, M. (1988). Clomipramine, self-exposure and therapist-aided exposure for obsessive-compulsive rituals. *British Journal of Psychiatry, 152,* 522–534.

Mellman, T. A., & Uhde, T. W. (1989). Sleep panic attacks: New clinical findings and theoretical implications. *American Journal of Psychiatry, 146,* 1204–1207.

Midgren, B., Hansson, L., Skeidsvoll, H., & Elmquist, D. (1989). The effects of nitrazepam and flunitrazepam on oxygen desaturation during sleep in patients with stable hypoxemic nonhypercapnic COPD. *Chest, 95*(4), 765–768.

Nagy, L. M., Krystal, J. H., & Woods, S. W. (1989). Clinical and medication outcome after short-term alprazolam and behavioral group treatment in panic disorder: 2.5 year naturalistic followup study. *Archives of General Psychiatry, 46,* 993–999.

Neftel, K., Adler, R., & Kappeli, L. (1982). Stage fright in musicians: A model illustrating the effect of beta blockers. *Psychosomatic Medicine, 44,* 461–469.

Nies, A. S. (1986). Clinical pharmacology of beta-adrenergic blockers. *Medical problems of performing artists, 1,* 25–29.

Noyes, R., Jr., Anderson, D. J., Clancy, J., Crowe, R. R., Slymen, D. J., Ghoneim, M. M., & Hinrichs, J. V. (1984). Diazepam and propanolol in panic disorder and agoraphobia. *Archives of General Psychiatry, 41,* 287–292.

Noyes, R., Jr., Garvey, M. J., Cook, B. L., & Samuelson, L. (1989). Problems with tricyclic antidepressant use in patients with panic disorder or agoraphobia: Results of a naturalistic follow-up study. *Journal of Clinical Psychiatry, 50,* 163–169.

Noyes, R., & Perry, P. (1990). Maintenance treatment with antidepressants in panic disorder. *Journal of Clinical Psychiatry, 51*(12(Suppl. A)), 24–30.

O'Sullivan, G. O., Noshirvani, H., Marks, I., Monteiro, W., & Lelliott, P. (1991). Six-year follow-up after exposure and clomipraminetherapy for obsessive compulsive disorder. *Journal of Clinical Psychiatry, 52,* 150–155.

Pato, M. T., Pigott, T. A., Hill, J. L., Grover, G. N., Bernstein, S., & Murphy, D. L. (1991). Controlled comparison of buspirone and clomipramine in obsessive-compulsive disorder. *American Journal of Psychiatry, 148,* 127–129.

Pecknold, J. D., Swinson, R. P., Kuch, K., & Lewis, C. P. (1988). Alprazolam in panic disorder and agoraphobia: Results from a multicenter trial: 3. Discontinuation effects. *Archives of General Psychiatry, 45,* 429–436.

Perse, T. (1988). Obsessive-compulsive disorder: A treatment review. *Journal of Clinical Psychiatry, 49,* 48–55.

Petruzzello, S. J., Landers, D. M., & Hatfield, B. D. (1991). A meta-analysis on the anxiety-reducing effects of acute and chronic exercise: Outcomes and mechanisms. *Sports Medicine, 11,* 143–182.

Pollack, M. H., Tesar, G. E., & Rosenbaum, J. F. (1986). Clonazepam in the treatment of panic disorder and agoraphobia: A one-year followup. *Journal of Clinical Psychopharmacology, 6,* 302–304.

Quality Assurance Project. (1985). Treatment outlines for the management of anxiety states. *Australia and New Zealand Journal of Psychiatry, 19,* 138–151.

Rapoport, J. L. (1988). The neurobiology of obsessive-compulsive disorder. *Journal of the American Medical Association, 260,* 2888–2890.

Rasmussen, S. A. (1984). Lithium and tryptophan augmentation in clomipramine-resistant obsessive-compulsive disorder. *American Journal of Psychiatry, 141,* 1283–1285.

Rath, G. D., Jarratt, L. G., & Leonardson, G. (1989). Rates of domestic violence against adult women by men partners. *Journal of the American Board of Family Practice, 2,* 227–233.

Reich, J., & Yates, W. (1988). A pilot study of treatment of social phobia with alprazolam. *American Journal of Psychiatry, 145,* 590–594.

Reist, C., Kauffmann, C. D., & Haier, R. J. (1989). A controlled trial of desipramine in 18 men with posttraumatic stress disorder. *American Journal of Psychiatry, 146,* 513–516.

Reiter, S. R., Pollack, M. H., Rosenbaum, J. F., & Cohen, L. S. (1990). Clonazepam for the treatment of social phobia. *Journal of Clinical Psychiatry, 51,* 470–472.

Rickels, K., Case, W. G., Winokur, A., & Swenson, C. (1984). Long-term benzodiazepine therapy: Benefits and risks. *Psychopharmacology Bulletin, 4,* 608–615.

Robinson, D. S., Alms, D. R., & Shrotriya, R. C. (1989). Serotonergic anxiolytics and treatment of depression. *Psychopathology, 22*(Suppl. 1), 27–36.

Schatzberg, A. F. (1990). Anxiety and adjustment disorder: A treatment approach. *Journal of Clinical Psychiatry, 51,* 20–24.

Schatzberg, A. F., & Ballenger, J. C. (1991). Decisions for the clinician in the treatment of panic disorder: When to treat, which treatment to use, and how long to treat. *Journal of Clinical Psychiatry, 52*(Suppl.), 26–32.

Sheehan, D. V. (1987). Benzodiazepines in panic disorder and agoraphobia. *Journal of Affective Disorders, 13,* 169–181.

Shore, J. H., Vollmer, W. M., & Tatum, E. L. (1989). Community patterns of posttraumatic stress disorders. *Journal of Nervous and Mental Disorders, 177,* 681–685.

Silver, J. M., Sandberg, D. P., & Hales, R. E. (1990). New approaches in the pharmacotherapy of posttraumatic stress disorder. *Journal of Clinical Psychiatry, 5*(Suppl. 10), 33–38.

Spier, S. A., Tesar, G. E., Rosenbaum, J. F., & Woods, S. W. (1986). Treatment of panic disorder and agoraphobia with clonazepam. *Journal of Clinical Psychiatry, 47,* 238–242.

Teboul, E., & Chouinard, G. (1991). A guide to benzodiazepine selection: 2. Clinical aspects. *Canadian Journal of Psychiatry, 36,* 62–73.

Tesar, G. E., Rosenbaum, J. F., Pollack, M. H., Otto, M. W., Sachs, G. S., Herman, J. B., Cohen, L. S., & Spier, S. A. (1991). Double-blind, placebo-controlled comparison of clonazepam and alprazolam for panic disorder. *Journal of Clinical Psychiatry, 52,* 69–76.

Versiani, M., Mundim, F., & Nardi, A. (1988). Tranylcypromine in social phobia. *Journal of Clinical Psychopharmacology, 8,* 279–283.

Walker, E. A., Torlkeson, N., Katon, W. J., & Koss, M. P. (1993). The prevalence rate of sexual trauma in a primary care clinic. *Journal of the American Board of Family Practice, 6,* 465–471.

Wedzicha, J. A., Wallis, P. J., Ingram, D. A., & Empey, D. W. (1988). Effect of diazepam on sleep in patients with chronic airflow obstruction. *Thorax, 43*(9), 729–730.

Weiss, D. S., & Billings, J. H. (1988). Behavioral medicine techniques. In H. H. Goldmann (Ed.), *Review of general psychiatry* (pp. 574–579). East Norwalk, CT: Appleton & Lange.

Woods, J. H., Katz, J. L., & Winger, G. (1988). Use and abuse of benzodiazepines: Issues relevant to prescribing. *Journal of the American Medical Association, 260,* 3476–3480.

Kelly Kelleher
Vaughn I. Rickert

14

Management of Pediatric Mental Disorders in Primary Care

Mental disorders in childhood and adolescence result in a tremendous cost to society through increased suicide, drug abuse, disability days, school dropout, and chronic impairment. Society is further impacted by the effects of the emotional trauma to individual youth and their families (Kazdin, 1989; U.S. Congress, 1986). Studies of the prevalence of mental disorders in childhood and adolescence in community-based samples suggest that 12 to 22 percent of youth are afflicted with diagnosable mental disorders (Costello, 1989a). Approximately 3 to 5 percent of the pediatric population have severe and chronic conditions (National Institute of Mental Health, 1990).

Concerns about the mental health care of children and adolescents have been raised by professionals throughout this century (U.S. Congress, 1986). In spite of the high visibility and elaborate recommendations of numerous commissions and task forces, disturbed youth remain one of the most underserved populations in the United States (National Institute of Mental Health, 1990). Investigators studying the response of the mental health specialty sector to common disorders of youth note that mental health specialists serve less than 2 percent of children and adolescents in the United States in any year (Burns, Taube, & Taube, 1990). These youth are often inappropriately served because of inadequate coordination between service sectors, insufficient providers, and an overreliance on restrictive forms of care such as psychiatric hospitalization and residential treatment centers. Thus, as many as 80 percent of children and adolescents with emotional and behavioral disorders fail to be seen in the mental health sector, and some of those in care are not receiving appropriate treatment (Costello, 1989b).

In the United States, the lack of adequate psychiatric treatment services for children and adolescents with mental disorders, coupled with concerns about labeling and stigma in childhood, have strained other service sectors that care for youth with behavioral and emotional disorders. The service sectors bearing the additional burden are schools, child welfare services, correctional facilities, and nonpsychiatric health care providers. Although little is known about mental health services for children and adolescents in the educational, welfare, or correctional systems (National Institute of Mental Health, 1990), a growing body of research sheds some light on the management of mental disorders among children and youth by pediatricians and family and general practitioners as primary health care providers. This research will be carefully reviewed by third-party payers and others as they consider the effectiveness of mental health care for children and adolescents in primary care settings. To date, there are no completed studies of the outcomes of primary care management of child and adolescent behavioral and emotional disorders. Nevertheless, some information on current primary care provider practices is available.

Children or adolescents with psychosocial problems constitute a large part of the practice of providers in primary care settings. At least 12 percent of children seen in one study of office-based practice met criteria for DSM-III-R diagnoses (Costello, Edelbrock, et al., 1988). In other primary care settings, as many as one-quarter of children evaluated are reported to have significant psychological problems requiring some type of intervention (Starfield et al., 1980). An additional 10 to 15 percent may have maternal mental health problems (Bailey, Graham, & Boniface, 1978). Pediatricians report that youth with behavioral, emotional, and developmental problems take up as much as 40 percent of office staff time (Garralda & Bailey, 1986; Bailey et al., 1978) and that these children and adolescents with psychiatric conditions are more likely than adults to be treated only in the general health care sector (Regier et al., 1982). Thus, these conditions represent a significant portion of visits to primary care settings by children and adolescents.

A number of barriers to the delivery of effective mental health care exist in primary care settings. Effective care requires efficacious treatments, access to care, accurate diagnoses, appropriate treatment provision, and organizational and financial systems that promote suitable care. First, considerable debate about the efficacy of treatments for many of the emotional and behavioral problems of childhood continues even among mental health specialists. No standards of ideal care have been developed (Mechanic, 1990). Second, in a small series of studies during the past decade (Hankin, Goodman, & Starfield, 1986; Costello, Edelbrock, et al., 1988), pediatricians have recognized only 20 to 35 percent of children with diagnosable mental disorders as measured by psychiatric screening instruments or structured interviews. More recent research has clarified some of this disparity by using provider-friendly classification systems to document recognition at higher rates than previously reported (Horwitz, Leaf, Leventhal, Forsyth, & Speechley, 1992). Further analyses have also revealed that providers recognized some cases with symptomatic complaints and social problems not detected by psychiatric interviews (Garralda & Bailey, 1986). Pediatricians may be particularly sensitive to certain types of social disruptions in the family and childhood behavioral symptoms, but less so to anxiety and depressive symptoms. While detection is a concern, time and reimbursement for providers caring for pediatric patients with psychosocial problems also continue to be problematic. Primary care providers are frequently not reimbursed, or reimbursed at substantially reduced rates for the treatment and management of mental disorders. Finally, patients with insurance may not have mental health benefits or may be covered with larger copayments for mental health care, further increasing the difficulty in receiving treatment for psychosocial problems in primary care (Mechanic, 1990).

Despite these and other barriers, pediatricians, family practitioners, and general practitioners should continue to play a key role in the care of children and adolescents with psychosocial disorders because of their longitudinal relationships with families, their place as the point of access to the health care system, the limited number of mental health providers for children, and the sheer volume of patients they see (Wallen & Pincus, 1988; Haggerty, 1983). In the United States, these three groups of physicians see approximately 75 percent of the 135 million child visits to office-based practices each year, while psychiatrists account for less than 1 percent (Kelleher, Hohmann, & Larson, 1989). Therefore, investigators and policy-makers interested in mental health services for children and adolescents should understand the care delivered by these primary care physicians to youth with emotional and behavioral problems.

The few studies that examine the management of childhood mental disorders in general health care settings focus on one or two specific components of the treatment provided. Traditionally, investigators have examined counseling or psychotherapy, psychotropic drug-prescribing practices, and referral to mental health settings. Additionally, some have considered the use of both on- and off-site consultation-liaison services with psychiatrists or psychologists.

Counseling

Primary care physicians report that they provide treatment for the majority of emotional and behavioral problems that children and adolescents experience (Costello, 1989b). Counseling is the most frequently cited type of treatment offered by primary care physicians; counseling is provided to over 80 percent of pediatric patients identified with psychosocial problems. In addition, counseling or supportive therapy may be used in conjunction with other forms of treatment such as medication or suggesting environmental changes (Chamberlin, 1982; Goldberg, Roghmann, McInerny, & Burke, 1983). Graham (1982) suggests that counseling may be an important intervention, especially for commonly seen pediatric problems such as nocturnal awakenings, enuresis, and phobias. Further, short-term psychotherapy and physician assurance may shorten the course of emotional disorders (Graham, 1982). However, counseling in primary care is vaguely defined in professional literature and appears to include the provision of anticipatory guidance, supportive counseling, information giving, behavior modification techniques, and psychotherapy to children, adolescents, and their families (Haggerty, 1982; Goldberg et al., 1983). These interventions may occur during well-child visits, during acute-illness visits, or when the chronically ill child returns for a follow-up appointment. Few studies have differentiated between the various forms of counseling interventions, and none have examined their effectiveness when delivered in a primary care setting.

The development of well-child visits designed to provide anticipatory guidance (educational information designed to prevent problem behaviors) has gathered much attention and theoretical support (Reisinger & Bires, 1980). In addition to providing medical screening, the prevention of psychosocial morbidities is an unstated goal of anticipatory guidance (Chamberlin, 1982; Haggerty, 1982). However, anticipatory guidance is often time limited and decreases as children age (Reisinger & Bires, 1980). Although some evidence exists that these interventions may decrease the prevalence of parent-child interactional problems in early childhood, the effectiveness of primary care prevention for mental disorders is largely unexamined.

Prevention and early intervention have also been promulgated for psychosocial problems of adolescence (Reisinger & Bires, 1980; Millstein, 1989). An adolescent wellness schedule has been proposed to minimize the impact of the often-destructive behaviors and consequences that this population experiences (Blum, 1987). However, a standard psychosocial screening procedure suggested for adolescents may take thirty to forty-five minutes or more of physician time (Marks & Fisher, 1987). A recently completed national survey found that over 60 percent of adolescent visits to a physician lasted less than ten minutes (D'Angelo & Delozier, 1986). Further, a large majority of older adolescents surveyed reported that they never received any information from their regular primary care provider about depression, suicide, or stress, even though they desired counseling on these topics (Joffe, Radium, & Gall, 1988). Time constraints of busy practitioners, lack of financial reimbursement, and professional discomfort in treating this population have all been cited as significant obstacles that need to be overcome in order to develop an appropriate wellness schedule for adolescents (Rickert, Jay, & Gottlieb, 1990). Finally, easily administered interventions for this population have not been developed in either the primary care or allied health care literature.

The impact of supportive counseling for psychosocial concerns of parents is even less well understood, although these communications may represent from 10 to 21 percent of all interactions between pediatricians and their patients and families (Wasserman, Barriatua, Carter, & Lippincott, 1984). Supportive counseling has been defined as reassurance, empathy, and encouragement, with reassurance being the most commonly occurring physician communicative behavior in pediatric settings. Only one study has examined these communications and used parent satisfaction as the only outcome measure (Wasserman et al., 1984). Reassurance had no impact on parental satisfaction with care provided, whereas encouragement and empathy increased parental satisfaction and improved perceptions of pediatricians.

Counseling by primary physicians for psychosocial problems provided to chronically ill children, adolescents, and their families is another underexamined area in the research literature, especially in light of the number of chronically ill children seen by primary care providers. Chronic illnesses or related conditions are present in approximately 7.5 million children and adolescents (Haggerty, 1983). The chronically ill child represents about 10 to 14 percent of care given in the pediatric primary care setting (Gortmaker & Sappenfield, 1984). Further, studies have suggested that less than 20 percent receive any social or mental health services (Walker, Gortmaker, & Weitzman, 1991; Cadman, Boyle, & Offord, 1986). The effects of chronic illness on children's emotional and psychological status remain unclear (Garrison & McQuiston, 1989). However, estimates in chronically ill populations suggest a two- to fourfold increase in the risk of psychiatric problems during the childhood and adolescent period (Garrison & McQuiston, 1989). Families of these children and adolescents, on the whole, seem to function well, but increased psychological distress and maladjustment have been reported (Garrison & McQuiston, 1989). The primary care physician is a likely gatekeeper and initial contact for these patients and their families, especially when environmental stressors increase.

Psychotropic Drug Prescriptions

The use of psychotropic drugs, especially stimulants, for children has received increased critical attention in both the scientific and lay press during the last few years (Kelleher et al., 1989). This attention is likely a result of the lack of consensus on the appropriate treatment for childhood mental disorders and of the prevalence of reported cases of inappropriate use of stimulants. Although children and adolescents are less likely than any other age group to receive psychotropic drugs during outpatient visits, it is important to understand current practice patterns, because these drugs are often expensive, have frequent interactions with other medications, may have the potential for addiction, and may affect the long-term growth and cognition of children (Koch, 1983).

Psychotropic drug prescriptions are a relatively rare event, occurring in only 1.5 percent of all pediatric visits when nonpsychiatric indications are excluded (Kelleher et al., 1989). Nonpsychiatric indications, such as the use of benzodiazapines for muscle spasm, account for approximately 5 to 15 percent of all psychotropic prescriptions for adults (Jencks, 1985). However, the cumulative effect may be significant, especially for stimulants in the treatment of attention deficit disorder. In Sweden, up to 12 percent of all children may have received a psychotropic drug by the age of six, with the most common indication for prescriptions being sleep disturbances or hyperactive syndromes (Rasmussen, 1988). In the United States, as many as 3 percent of children in school surveys are reported to be taking methylphenidate at any one time. This represents as many as 600,000 children nationally on stimulant medication. Overall, providers report that they prescribe psychotropic drugs for 15 to 50 percent of the children they diagnose with behavioral or emotional disorders (Costello, 1989b), although these numbers may be decreasing, at least for older children. High school seniors reported a decline in prescription tranquilizer use from 18 to 12 percent between 1975 and 1986, whereas prescription amphetamines declined from 15 to 8 percent during the same period (Johnston, O'Malley, & Bachman, 1989). Studies of providers in one region document similar declines, with psychotropic prescriptions decreasing from 16 percent of those with recognized childhood emotional or behavioral disorders in 1979 to 11 percent in 1984 (Goldberg et al., 1983).

Prescribing practices are noticeably affected by a number of factors, including the age of the child or adolescent (Kelleher et al., 1989). Very young children receive few psychotropic drugs, while school-age children are frequently prescribed stimulants. Physicians write a decreasing number of prescriptions for stimulants for adolescents, but they receive a greater number of prescriptions for antidepressants and anxiolytics (Kelleher et al., 1989). However, most investigators counsel against the use of benzodiazepines for childhood and adolescent mental disorders (Dorsey et al., 1979).

Other factors are also associated with the prescription of psychotropic drugs in pediatric primary care: the presence of mental health symptoms as a reason for visits, a psychiatric diagnosis, male gender, and previous knowledge of the patient and symptoms by the provider (Kelleher et al., 1989). Furthermore, prescription practices may vary with type of practice setting (group versus solo), number of years in practice, and discipline (Ross & Duff, 1982). Pediatricians prescribe fewer drugs of all types and fewer psychotropics than family or general practitioners. Pediatricians are more likely to first intervene with psychosocial techniques for children and adolescents with emotional and behavioral problems. In a study of children referred to mental health settings from primary care (Kovacs, 1987), children and adolescents had experienced symptoms an average of thirty-two weeks for major depression and twenty-five weeks for adjustment disorder before referral. Most children received some psychosocial intervention by pediatricians before the referral, but few had received psychotropic drugs from their primary care providers for depression and adjustment disorders. Nevertheless, anxiolytics were the most commonly prescribed psychotropics for adolescents, especially by family and general practitioners in a national survey (Kelleher et al., 1989).

One of the most commonly prescribed classes of psychotropics includes the stimulants for attention or hyperactive disorders during the early school years. Stimulants comprise 25 to 40 percent of psychotropic drug prescriptions by pediatricians, and methylphenidate (Ritalin) is the preferred stimulant in 85 percent of treated cases (Safer & Krager, 1984). Boys are as much as seven times more likely to receive these medications than girls. For many children, the use of stimulants continues into adolescence (Johnston, O'Malley, & Bachman, 1989).

Unfortunately, many children who receive psychotropic drug prescriptions may not be receiving concurrent psychotherapy or the close follow-up care recommended when using these medications. In one study (Kelleher et al., 1989), only one-third of children receiving psychotropics were provided counseling or psychotherapy. Similarly, those receiving prescriptions were no more likely than children without these drugs to receive follow-up plans, even though most authors encourage close follow-up and concurrent psychosocial interventions in children receiving any psychotropics.

Referrals and Consultation-Liaison Services

Mental health referrals from primary care providers may represent a primary source of pediatric patients for specialty practices (Lewis, 1978; Jellinek, 1982). In fact, less than 10 percent of psychiatric patients present directly to psychiatry services (France, Weddington, & Houpt, 1978). Further, adult referrals from primary care physicians to specialists may generate an average of $3,000 in physician, laboratory, and hospital fees (Glenn, Lawler, & Hoerl, 1987).

Because of deficiencies in research, many facets of the complex relationship between physicians in general health care settings and mental health specialists remain unclear. Some of the confusion around the referral process for pediatric psychosocial problems is a result of the many service sectors—from education to child welfare—that provide mental health care for children and adolescents (National Institute of Mental Health, 1990). Nevertheless, some information on referral practices is available.

Studies on the frequency of referral for pediatric emotional or behavioral disorders usually count the percentage of children with recognized disorders receiving a recommendation to see a mental health specialist. These studies are predominantly conducted in managed care systems in the United States, although similar rates of referral seem to be present for general practitioners in the United Kingdom (Garralda & Bailey, 1986, 1987). Approximately 30 to 60 percent of the children with recognized behavioral or emotional problems who are going to pediatricians are already seeing mental health specialists or are referred to them (Kamerow, 1985; Costello, 1989b; Goldberg, Roghmann, McInerny, & Burke, 1983; Costello, Edelbrock, et al., 1988). This amounts to between 1 and 3.5 percent of children and adolescents seen in a year by primary care providers. Furthermore, special assessment units established to carefully evaluate children with psychosocial problems in high-risk populations and assist in referral may increase to two-thirds the number referred to mental health specialists (Bergman, Corbin, & Haber, 1982).

A number of provider, system, and patient factors appear pivotal in the referral decision for disturbed children in general health care settings. An important provider factor is physician time for, and interest in, counseling for behavioral problems (Starfield, 1982; Haggerty, 1982). With the average visit in pediatric settings lasting approximately 11.5 minutes (Goldberg et al., 1983), many physicians are discouraged from managing time-intensive problems such as emotional and behavioral disorders. In fact, 51 percent of pediatricians in one survey (Bergman & Fritz, 1985) reported they were too busy with "sick" patients to spend adequate time with childhood psychosocial problems. Physician attitudes about the causes of psychiatric problems, the effectiveness of mental health specialty care, and the importance of the general practitioners in providing comprehensive care for their patient population may also be important in the decision to refer. However, at least one study in an adult population (Link, Levav, & Cohen, 1982) suggests that these attitudes may affect identification rates but may not have any measurable impact on referral. The only exception noted was the providers' beliefs about their own effectiveness in handling such problems. Some investigators have attempted to change the attitudes of primary caregivers through increased educational exposure to child psychiatry during pediatric residency training (Hickson & Mann, 1985). While positive attitudinal changes toward psychiatrists were documented, no change was found in the number or quality of consultation requests from these pediatricians. Finally, provider educational background and length of time in practice may be related to referral patterns. Older pediatricians report much higher rates of referrals to all specialists ("The Pattern of Pediatric Referrals," 1988). It is unclear whether referral from primary care providers results in better outcomes for children with psychosocial problems or whether more referrals should be occurring.

The organization and financing of health care appear to be playing an increasingly important role in the decision to refer from primary care settings. In particular, some settings and reimbursement mechanisms may significantly enhance or inhibit referrals for child or adolescent mental health specialty care. Referral patterns for youth with psychosocial concerns in general health care settings are increasingly influenced by on-site mental health specialists. In a 1985 assessment (Fritz & Bergman, 1985), one-third of pediatricians reported the availability of a psychologist or social worker for psychosocial problems in their offices. These pediatricians were predominantly from group-practice settings (Fritz & Bergman, 1985), and previous work suggests that this setup increases both recognition of mental disorders and referrals (Jacobsen et al., 1980). Conversely, pediatricians in health maintenance organizations (HMOs) report fewer referrals of all types than do pediatricians in group or solo fee-for-service (FFS) settings, while neighborhood health centers may have the highest referral rates of all (Kamerow, 1985; "The Pattern of Pediatric Referrals," 1988). Rural sites have lower referral rates (Browder, 1983), although it is unclear whether this is a result of different practice patterns, increased stigma associated with psychiatric disorders in rural settings, or the severe shortage of mental health providers in rural areas.

Patient and family factors also influence referral decisions. Referral from pediatricians occurs more often for children with severe problems (Roghmann, Zastowny, & Babigian, 1984; Costello, 1989b; Costello, Burns, et al., 1988), problems of a chronic nature (Kamerow, 1985; Mitchell, 1984), or conduct problems (Kamerow, 1985). In surveys on referrals for specific disorders, pediatricians report that they refer to mental health professionals most suicide gestures (72 percent) and between 10 and 25 percent of children diagnosed with school phobias, encopresis, enuresis, and attention deficit disorder ("The Pattern of Pediatric Referrals," 1988). Parent or family objection to formal mental health care certainly may limit referrals (Fritz & Bergman, 1985; Goldberg et al., 1983; Bergman & Fritz, 1985).

When primary care providers refer children and adolescents

with psychosocial problems for additional mental health services, a number of factors may influence their choices of referral providers. In particular, pediatricians report that they are influenced by family preferences and perceived stigma, insurance concerns, mental health provider availability, and previous experiences (Bergman & Fritz, 1985). Many of these influences discourage referrals to child psychiatrists. For example, in the United States, psychiatrists are less likely to participate in Medicaid (Schurman, Kramer, & Mitchell, 1985) than other medical specialists. Furthermore, surveys in the United Kingdom (Mitchell, 1984; Marks, Wolkind, & Napper, 1981) and the United States (Prazar & Charney, 1980; Fritz & Bergman, 1985) report that providers believe that psychiatrists are the least available, and have the largest waiting lists, of all the mental health professionals involved in the care of children and adolescents. In some areas such as the rural South in the United States, fewer than one child psychiatrist per million population may be available full time (American Medical Association, 1990).

Not surprisingly, psychiatrists are not the preferred referral provider for most pediatricians. Only 13 percent of offices in a U.S. survey reported any referrals to psychiatrists. Apparently, pediatricians prefer to refer most common psychosocial problems requiring further care to behaviorally oriented pediatricians (Fritz & Bergman, 1985). Psychiatrists were the preferred providers only for depression and eating disorders in another survey. Results similar to these have been published in Australia (Murphy, Hudson, & King, 1982) and the United Kingdom (Garralda & Bailey, 1987; Marks et al., 1981), where pediatricians are the preferred referral provider for most family and general practitioners. Psychologists are preferred for many school and learning problems.

A number of authors have addressed the origins of the apparent schism between pediatrics and child psychiatry (Jellinek, 1982; Lewis, 1978). Numerous explanations have been offered for the lack of communication between these disciplines in a relationship that appears to be more polarized than the relationship between pediatrics and psychologists specializing in the care of children seen in the general health care sector. The most commonly cited factor is a lack of shared experiences between psychiatrists and pediatricians (Schurman et al., 1985; Jellinek, 1982). Bergman and Fritz (1985) note that 52 percent of pediatricians report less than 15 contacts with psychiatrists during all of their training.

While the studies noted above have examined the use of either counseling, drug prescriptions, or referrals from primary care for children with emotional and behavioral disorders, less than a handful have reported on the co-occurrence of these management strategies. These include the Monroe County study, which summarized treatment plans for 18,000 pediatric visits in New York (Goldberg et al, 1983); Garralda, who describes the English experience (Garralda & Bailey, 1987); and another study reporting on data from the United States in the National Ambulatory Medical Care Survey (Kelleher et al., 1989). The problem with these summaries of management strategies is that they rely on visit-based data, whereas primary care providers choose treatment modalities in a sequential fashion, frequently relying on counseling for new or less severe problems, then progressing to psychotropic drug prescriptions and referral for persistent problems (Kovacs, 1987; Aintson & Philipsborn, 1982; Mitchell, 1984). In other words, providers treat "episodes" of mental disorder rather than symptoms from individual visits (Salkever, Skinner, Steinwachs, & Katz, 1982). Another problem with the current research literature on primary care management of childhood emotional and behavioral disorders is the exclusive focus on pediatrician practices. Family and general practitioners, nurse clinicians, and other providers of primary care services have been excluded from U.S. research in this area, even though family practitioners alone account for one-third of pediatric visits to office practices in the United States (Starfield et al., 1984). In the United Kingdom, general practitioners have been the focus of this research.

The available research reveals little about primary care practices for children and adolescents with behavioral and emotional disorders, and considerable gaps in understanding these practices exist. First, most of these studies are over a decade old and do not take into account the substantial changes that have occurred in medical practices, especially those associated with managed care, utilization review, and insurance benefits. Second, no research on the outcomes of these various practices exists. Studies to compare different primary care management practices and to contrast these with specialist care practices using good measures of child and family outcomes are absent from the published literature.

Although symptom-level measures and functional outcomes have not been assessed, primary care investigators have begun to examine some other outcomes of relevance. In particular, parent satisfaction and use of health care services by children and adolescents have been used to assess the impact of some interventions (Mitchell, 1984). Finney et al. (1990) used a simple, brief prompting strategy prior to a scheduled health visit to enhance parent reporting of symptoms to providers. Parents were prompted to ask questions that were of interest to them and that also coincided with the recommended age-relevant anticipatory guidance content for visits developed by the American Academy of Pediatrics. The investigators found that parents who had been randomly assigned to this condition initiated significantly more interactions with providers, and more behavioral topics were discussed. Interestingly, both groups were equally satisfied with the health care services they had received.

Reductions in the use of health care after treatment for mental health problems, or the "offset" phenomenon, is another gauge of the impact of mental health services for children and adolescents in primary care settings (Jones & Vischi, 1979). Only a few studies have examined reductions in care after initiation of mental health services for youth with mental disorders in primary care settings. Although some caveats have been raised (Costello, Burns, et al., 1988), these studies find a small but consistent reduction in use of general health care services after referral to mental health specialists. In particular, use of nonpsychiatric specialty care appears to decrease (Kelleher & Starfield, 1990). No changes in primary care services have been described. Unfortunately, none of the published studies was designed as a randomized trial, and none considered the effect of counseling or drug prescriptions by primary care providers. A more recent study evaluated the impact of short-term psychological treatment on children's use of medical services (Finney, Riley, & Cataldo, 1991). Following a visit to an HMO, children with identified behavioral concerns were referred to mental health specialists where individualized treatment guided by problem-specific protocols were employed. Data collected found that children treated by a psychologist were significantly less likely to have subsequent acute visits to this health organization than a matched comparison group. Further, no overall increase in HMO utilization was found.

Although better studies on the structure and process of mental health treatment of children and adolescents in primary care settings will be necessary to improve care, a number of factors will probably impede studies of treatment outcome and development of guidelines for providers. First, the development of mental disorder classification systems appropriate to primary care settings for children and adolescents is being considered only now (Frances, Pincus, Widiger, Davis, & First, 1990). This task will require years of research and evaluation. Second, efficacious treatments for child and adolescent mental disorders need to be developed. The child and adolescent research initiatives sponsored by the National Institute of Mental Health (1990) in the United States and other similar efforts would facilitate this treatment research, but this also will require time.

Current structural features of care and the reimbursement system actively discriminate against pediatric patients with mental disorders. Because primary care physicians frequently do not receive reimbursement for the diagnosis and management of mental disorders, regardless of the availability and appropriateness of community mental health services, many children are likely not to be treated for their emotional problems. All of these barriers are being addressed at some level, but some years may be required before changes affect primary care practices.

In the meantime, an adequate number of child psychiatrists and psychologists are unlikely to be available to meet the anticipated needs for mental health services in the United States, especially for minority and rural children and adolescents (Haggerty, 1982; Jellinek, 1982). Nor is it likely that primary care physicians will ever have adequate time, interest, or training to deal with the many and varied mental disorders they encounter in day-to-day practice (Mitchell, 1984; Mechanic, 1990). Instead, closer working relationships between specialists and primary care providers and the use of family and other specialist "extenders" for children and adolescents with mental disorders is the logical solution for inadequate and inappropriate mental health services (Mitchell, 1984;

Mechanic, 1990). This approach was suggested almost fifteen years ago and remains relevant today. Some efforts to improve relationships between child mental health specialists and primary care physicians are underway through federally funded efforts to conduct weekly meetings of child psychiatrists and pediatricians and to encourage other cooperative initiatives between psychiatrists, pediatricians, and psychologists. The goal of the meetings is to develop better relationships, classification systems for pediatric mental disorders, and joint multisite research projects (M. Fishman, personal communication, July 1992).

Conclusion

While there are many barriers to effective mental health services for children and adolescents in primary care settings, family practitioners and pediatricians will continue to play an important role in the care of youth with emotional and behavioral problems. A large part of that care involves brief "counseling" provided to most children and adolescents with identified problems. Unfortunately, the term *counseling* is poorly defined, and no studies of effectiveness have been conducted. Primary care providers are also the largest prescribers of psychotropic drugs for children and adolescents. Stimulants are the most commonly administered agents during the early school years, and minor tranquilizers are increasingly being prescribed during adolescence. Physician and patient factors influence prescription writing for these drugs. Referral to, or concurrent use of, specialty mental health services probably occurs for approximately one-half of children with recognized disorders, although referral may constitute a behavior that occurs later in an episode of illness. All of these management strategies are affected by patient and family characteristics, provider factors, the availability of alternative sources of mental health care, and financial constraints. Unfortunately, the empirical basis for these conclusions rests on a few studies conducted in a small number of practices.

The task for investigators wishing to understand mental health services for children in primary care are formidable. Not only is primary care research fraught with uncertainties and confounding factors (Schwartz, 1990), but the rapidly changing system of health care in the United States adds considerable complexity to research design. Finally, the developmental nature of psychosocial problems during childhood and adolescence discourages many investigators. As a result, few investigators have tested the waters of primary care mental health services research.

Nevertheless, child mental health advocates acknowledge that most children with mental disorders will not receive specialty mental health service in our current health care delivery system. Therefore, it is imperative to put forth an ambitious research and training agenda to improve the knowledge base on services delivered in the primary care setting and to design effective interventions to address identified shortfalls in the quality and quantity of primary care mental health services for children and adolescents.

Because of the substantial nature of the methodological issues confronting investigators in primary care settings specifically and mental health services generally, methodological studies will necessarily precede content studies in the field. In particular, research exploring sampling issues, the developmental nature of child and adolescent psychopathology, the co-occurrence of psychiatric and nonpsychiatric disorders, and the measurement of outcomes of relevance to the health care system and families will be critical to the success of future studies on the effectiveness of interventions in primary care settings.

Although some of the sampling issues have been mentioned previously, two particular concerns bear repeating. First, few investigators have considered the impact of group and partner practices or practice structures on their sample. A growing body of evidence suggests that primary care providers are influenced by the practices of their colleagues and the presence of other specialties in the practice. Therefore, future studies should consider the possibility of cluster sampling when examining provider behavior or controlling for this contamination in other ways. In the same vein, the majority of primary care mental health studies to date have occurred in managed care settings because of the availability of management information systems and captive populations. While informative, these studies may not be representative of the majority of the population or of providers in rural, inner-city, or minority areas. Alternative types of practices and populations should be included wherever possible in mental health services research to improve the generalizability of study findings.

Two other issues that require careful attention in studies of mental health services for children and adolescents are the developmental nature of childhood psychopathology and the co-occurrence of psychiatric and nonpsychiatric disorders. The rapid maturation of children and adolescents coincides with changing symptom complexes for child and adolescent mental disorders. Research on depression, substance abuse, and other mental disorders suggests that the presentation of these conditions changes with the age of the child or adolescent. This is particularly important for longitudinal studies, which are the core of understanding the outcomes of primary care mental health services. In the same vein, the measurement of psychopathology in childhood and adolescence for primary care settings is further confounded by the frequent co-occurrence of acute and chronic medical conditions. Many scales currently used by investigators to access childhood mental disorders include somatic symptoms that may be a result of mental disorder or associated medical conditions. Without adequate consideration, children with chronic medical conditions may be diagnosed with psychiatric disorders inappropriately.

The last methodological issue that bears special attention is the range of outcomes and the ability to measure these outcomes for studies of interventions and services in primary care. First, it has become increasingly clear that reduction of symptoms and avoidance of harmful side effects, while important, are not sufficient criteria for treatment effectiveness studies. Other outcomes that need consideration are the overall health status of children and their families, the cultural and social acceptability of services or treatments, and the satisfaction of patients and their families with the care received. Outcomes of importance to society and health care systems will include the cost of treatment, changes in the use of related services, and the long-term functioning of individuals as productive members of society.

Some progress on these issues will determine, in part, the rate at which investigators explore the theoretical and practical aspects of mental health services in primary care settings for children and adolescents. To date, much of the work has been focused on identification and screening issues. This work has been limited in that classification systems rarely used in primary care systems have been employed and outcomes have almost never been considered. New studies are the first to include broadly based mental disorder classifications designed for primary care and randomized designs with an assessment of clinical outcomes.

Research on management by primary care providers has also been limited to studies of process, with little attention paid to the clinical outcomes of mental health services in the primary care sector. Outcomes assessment will clearly be central, as will careful matching of patients with treatment strategies. Increasingly, managed care systems and other third-party payers will require primary care physicians to justify services prescribed or recommended. Providers will need to stratify patients by the severity and chronicity of the identified problems and then choose the management strategy linked with that selection. For example, many children and adolescents with mild to moderate behavioral problems would benefit from behavior modification strategies that could be recommended by pediatricians or family physicians using tested protocols. For more intensive cases, consultation-liaison models of working with mental health professionals should be employed. In some high-risk populations, conjoint management by health and mental health professionals is probably indicated. To date, studies on management have treated all mental disorders as unitary phenomena instead of taking a staged approach, which recognizes the different degrees of severity and types of emotional and behavioral disorders that present in primary care settings.

Probably the least understood aspects of primary care mental health services for children and adolescents relate to the impact of the system and financing factors on the quality and effectiveness of care. Studies of system or financing factors generally require large samples from diverse settings to attain adequate sample size and variation to definitively answer questions about the organization of mental health services. These samples and settings have not been available to date. Newly developed or organized primary care research networks offer the potential to conduct the first large-scale trials in primary care settings of organizational and financial factors on a prospective basis. While some forms of these networks have been in existence for a number of years, it is only during the past five years that the two national networks of primary care providers for children have come into their own. The Ambulatory Sentinel Practice Network is a group of over 70 practices in the United States and Canada with more than 350 family practitioners and internists who care for children and adolescents. The Pediatric Research in Office Settings network is a group of almost 500 pediatricians in office-based practices nationwide. Together, these two networks have a pediatric patient base approaching one and a half to two million children and adolescents.

Regardless of where these studies are conducted, the need for this research is increasingly apparent, since the majority of children and adolescents are enrolled in plans with some component of managed care. Strategies used by managed care systems to control costs clearly affect referral rates, prescriptions, and even recognition of mental disorders, but the extent of their influence and which particular strategies change provider behavior is unclear. Research in this area will require careful attention to the changing regulatory structures and legislation, which may increasingly mandate particular benefits. Finally, the careful design of system, provider, and patient intervention studies will provide the important link to improve mental health services in the primary care settings for children and adolescents. System interventions that affect the strategies used by managed care systems to increase or decrease certain types of provider management will be important, as will provider interventions. Comprehensive reviews of the literature on interventions to affect changes in provider behavior suggest that personal communications regarding practice behaviors by respected members of the practicing community and ongoing review of provider practices are the most effective ways of changing primary care management for some conditions. Similarly, patient activation strategies to improve doctor-patient communication may enhance diagnosis and treatment.

All of this research should be used to inform the rapidly growing number of residencies and medical school rotations dealing with developmental and behavioral pediatrics at every stage of training. Only a small amount of mental health services research has filtered into the medical school training programs for primary care providers. Similarly, the training programs for mental health specialists have focused inadequate attention on the primary care setting and its link with specialty care. The result is the mental health specialist with little understanding of the primary care setting or patient. Attempts to increase interaction between the primary care setting and mental health specialists will improve communication and the continuity of care for children and adolescents with mental disorders.

References

Aintson, P. H., & Philipsborn, H. F. (1982). Pediatrician-parent communication in a continuity of care setting. *Clinical Pediatrics, 21*(5), 302-307.

American Medical Association. (1990). *AMA Physicians' Master File, County Hospital File.* Department of Commerce. Washington, DC: Government Printing Office.

Bailey, V., Graham, P., & Boniface, D. (1978). How much child psychiatry does a general practitioner do? *Journal of the Royal College of General Practitioners, 28,* 621-626.

Bergman, A. S., & Fritz, G. K. (1985). Pediatricians and mental health professionals: Patterns of collaboration and utilization. *American Journal of Diseases of Children, 139,* 155-159.

Bergman, D. A., Corbin, S., & Haber, J. (1982). Analysis of a program for mental health referrals from a pediatric clinic. *Development and Behavioral Pediatrics, 3*(4), 232-235.

Blum, R. (1987). Contemporary threats to adolescent health in the United States. *Journal of the American Medical Association, 257,* 3390-3395.

Browder, J. A. (1983). Pediatric diagnosis and management of children with developmental disabilities. *Developmental and Behavioral Pediatrics, 4*(2), 99-102.

Burns, B. J., Taube, C. A., & Taube, J. E. (1990). *Background paper for U.S. Congress OTA Adolescent Health Project.* Washington, DC: U.S. Congress.

Cadman, D., Boyle, M. H., & Offord, D. R. (1986). Chronic illnesses, medical conditions, and limitations in Ontario children. *Canadian Medical Association Journal, 9,* 117-121.

Chamberlin, R. W. (1982). Prevention of behavioral problems in young children. *Pediatric Clinics of North America, 29*(2), 239-247.

Costello, E. J. (1989a). Developments in child psychiatric epidemiology. *Journal of the American Academy of Child and Adolescent Psychiatry, 28*(6), 836-841.

Costello, E. J. (1989b). Primary care pediatrics and child psychopathology: A review of diagnostic, treatment, and referral practices. *Pediatrics, 78,* 1044-1051.

Costello, E. J., Burns, B. J., Costello, A. J., Edelbrock, C., Dulcan, M., & Brent, D. (1988). Service utilization and psychiatric diagnosis in pediatric primary care: The role of the gatekeeper. *Pediatrics, 82,* 435-441.

Costello, E. J., Edelbrock, C., Costello, A. J., Dulcan, M. K., Burns, B. J., & Brent, D. (1988). Psychopathology in pediatric primary care: The new hidden morbidity. *Pediatrics, 82,* 415-424.

D'Angelo, L. J., & Delozier, J. (1986). Who provides care for adolescents: A reappraisal of NAMCS. *Journal of Adolescent Health Care, 7,* 290-292.

Dorsey, R., Ayd, F. J., Cole, J., Klein, D., Simpson, G., Tupin, J., & Di Mascio, A. (1979). Psychopharmacological screening criteria development project. *Journal of the American Medical Association, 241,* 1021-1031.

Finney, J. W., Brophy, C. J., Friman, P. C., Golden, A. S. (1990). Promoting parent-provider interaction during young children's health-supervision visits. *Journal of Applied Behavior Analysis, 23*(2), 207-213.

Finney, J. W., Riley, A. W., & Cataldo, M. F. (1991). Psychology in primary health care: Effects of brief targeted therapy on children's medical care utilization. *Journal of Pediatric Psychology, 16,* 447-461.

Fishbane, M., & Starfield, B. (1981). Child health care in the United States: A comparison of pediatricians and general practitioners. *New England Journal of Medicine, 305,* 552-556.

France, R. D., Weddington, W. W., & Houpt, J. L. (1978). Referral of patients from primary care physicians to a community mental health center. *Journal of Nervous and Mental Disease, 166*(8), 594-598.

Frances, A., Pincus, H. A., Widiger, T. A., Davis, W. W., & First, M. B. (1990). DSM-IV: Work in progress. *American Journal of Psychiatry, 147*(11), 1439–1448.

Fritz, G. K., & Bergman, A. S. (1985). Child psychiatrists seen through pediatricians' eyes: Results of a national survey. *Journal of the American Academy of Child Psychiatry, 24,* 81–86.

Garralda, E. M., & Bailey, D. (1986). Psychological deviance in children attending general practice. *Psychological Medicine, 16,* 423–429.

Garralda, E. M., & Bailey, D. (1987). Psychosomatic aspects of childrens consultations in primary care. *European Archives of Psychiatry and Neurological Sciences, 237,* 319–322.

Garrison, W. T., & McQuiston, S. (1989). *Chronic illness during childhood and adolescence: Psychological aspects.* Newbury Park, CA: Sage.

Glenn, J. K., Lawler, F. H., & Hoerl, M. S. (1987). Physician referrals in a competitive environment: An estimate of the economic impact of a referral. *Journal of the American Medical Association, 258*(14), 1920–1924.

Goldberg, I. D., Roghmann, K. J., McInerny, T. K., & Burke, J. D. (1983). Mental health problems among children seen in pediatric practice. *Pediatrics, 73,* 278–293.

Gortmaker, S. L., & Sappenfield, W. (1984). Chronic childhood disorders: Prevalence and impact. *Pediatric Clinics of North America, 31,* 3–18.

Graham, P. (1982). Child psychiatry in relation to primary health care. *Social Psychiatry, 17*(2), 109–116.

Haggerty, R. (1982). Behavioral pediatrics: Can it be taught? Can it be practiced? *Pediatric Clinics of North America, 29*(2), 391–398.

Haggerty, R. (1983). Foreword to symposium on chronic disease in children. *Pediatric Clinics of North America, 31,* 1–2.

Hankin, J. R., Goodman, A. C., & Starfield, B. H. (1986). *Management of psychosocial problems by pediatricians: Final progress report for Grant MH 38810.* Unpublished report.

Hickson, L., & Mann, E. M. (1985). The relationship between attitudinal and behavioral change in pediatric residents in a psychiatric liaison teaching program: A pilot study. *International Journal of Psychiatry in Medicine, 15*(1), 61–73.

Horwitz, S. M., Leaf, P. J., Leventhal, J. M., Forsyth, B., & Speechley, K. N. (1992). Identification and management of psychosocial and developmental problems in community-based, primary care pediatric practices. *Pediatrics, 89,* 480–485.

Jacobsen, A. M., Goldberg, I. D., Burns, B. J., Hoeper, E. W., Hankin, J. R., & Hewitt, K. (1980). Diagnosed mental disorder in children and use of health services in four organized health care settings. *American Journal of Psychiatry, 137,* 559–565.

Jellinek, M. S. (1982). The present status of child psychiatry in pediatrics. *New England Journal of Medicine, 306,* 1227–1229.

Jencks, S. F. (1985). Recognition of mental distress and diagnosis of mental disorder in primary care. *Journal of the American Medical Association, 253,* 1903–1907.

Joffe, A., Radium, S., & Gall, M. (1988). Health counseling for adolescents: What they want, what they get, and who gives it. *Pediatrics, 82,* 481–485.

Johnston, L. D., O'Malley, P. M., & Bachman, J. G. (1989). *Drug use, drinking, and smoking: National survey results from high school, college, and young adult populations, 1978–1988.* Ann Arbor: University of Michigan, Institute for Social Research.

Jones, M., & Vischi, T. (1979). Impact of alcohol, drug abuse, and mental health treatment on medical care utilization. *Medical Care, 17,* 1–18.

Kamerow, D. (1985). *Mental health problems among children seen in pediatric practice: Referral practices.* Unpublished manuscript.

Kazdin, A. E. (1989). Developmental psychopathology: Current research, issues, and directions. *American Psychologist, 44*(2), 180–187.

Kelleher, K. J., Hohmann, A. A., & Larson, D. B. (1989). Prescription of psychotropics to children in office-based practice. *American Journal of Diseases of Children, 143,* 855–859.

Kelleher, K. J., & Starfield, B. (1990). Health care use by children receiving mental health services. *Pediatrics, 85*(1), 114–118.

Koch, H. (1983). Utilization of psychotropic drugs in office-based ambulatory care, NAMCS, 1980 and 1981. *Advance data from vital and health statistics, No. 90* (DHHS Publication No. (PHS) 83-1250). Hyattsville, MD: National Center for Health Statistics.

Kovacs, M. (1987). Depression in childhood. In S. M. Channabasavanna & S. A. Shah (Eds.), *Affective disorders: Recent research and related developments* (pp. 195–203). Bangalore, India: National Institute of Mental Health and Neurosciences.

Lewis, M. (1978). Child psychiatric consultation in pediatrics. *Pediatrics, 62*(3), 359–364.

Link, B., Levav, I., & Cohen, A. (1982). The primary medical care practitioner's attitudes toward psychiatry: An Israeli study. *Social Science and Medicine, 16,* 1413–1420.

Marks, A., & Fisher, M. (1987). Health assessment and screening during adolescence. *Pediatrics, 803*(Suppl.), 131–158.

Marks, F. M., Wolkind, S. N., & Napper, R. (1981). Primary care workers' perception of disturbed children and the agencies they use to help these children. *Child: Care, Health, and Development, 7,* 217–228.

Mechanic, D. (1990). Treating mental illness: Generalist versus specialist. *Health Affairs,* Winter, 61–75.

Millstein, S. G. (1989). Adolescent health: Challenges for behavioral scientists. *American Psychologist, 44,* 837–842.

Mitchell, A. K. (1984). Psychiatrists in primary health care settings. *British Journal of Psychiatry, 147,* 371–379.

Murphy, G. C., Hudson, A. M., & King, N. J. (1982). Perceptions of child psychologists held by parents of Australian school children. *Psychological Reports, 51,* 47–51.

The pattern of pediatric referrals. (1988). *Contemporary Pediatrics, 5*(12), 20–30.

Prazar, G., & Charney, E. (1980). Behavioral pediatrics in office practice. *Pediatric Annals, 9,* 220–228.

Rasmussen, F. (1988). *Self-care, medical care, and prescription drugs in early childhood.* Uppsala, Sweden: Uppsala University.

Regier, D. A., Goldberg, I. D., Burns, B. J., Hankin, J., Hoeper, E. W., & Nycz, G. R. (1982). Specialist/generalist division of responsibility for patients with mental disorders. *Archives of General Psychiatry, 39,* 219–223.

Reisinger, K. S., & Bires, J. A. (1980). Anticipatory guidance in pediatric practice. *Pediatrics, 66,* 889–892.

Rickert, V. I., Jay, M. S., & Gottlieb, A. A. (1990). Adolsescent wellness: Facilitating compliance on social morbidities. *Medical Clinics of North America, 74,* 1135–1148.

Roghmann, K. J., Zastowny, T. R., & Babigian, H. M. (1984). Mental health problems of children: Analysis of a cumulative psychiatric case register. *Pediatrics, 73*(6), 781–790.

Ross, C. E., & Duff, R. S. (1982). Medical care, living conditions, and children's well-being. *Social Forces, 61*(2), 457–474.

Safer, D. J., & Krager, J. M. (1984). Trends in medication therapy for hyperactivity. *Advances in Learning and Behavior Disability, 3,* 125–149.

Salkever, D. S., Skinner, E. A., Steinwachs, D. M., & Katz, H. (1982). Episode-based efficiency comparisons for physicians and nurse practitioners. *Medical Care, 20*(2), 143–153.

Schurman, R. A., Kramer, P. D., & Mitchell, J. B. (1985). The hidden mental health network. *Archives of General Psychiatry, 42,* 89–94.

Schwartz, J. S. (1990). Changing provider behavior. In *Primary care research: An agenda for the 90s—AHCPR conference proceedings* (pp. 45–54). Washington, DC: U.S. Department of Health and Human Services.

Starfield, B. (1982). Behavioral pediatrics and primary health care. *Pediatric Clinics of North America, 29*(2), 377–391.

Starfield, B., Gabriel, I., Livingston, G., Benson, P., Hankin, J., Horn, S., & Steinwachs, D. (1984). Morbidity in childhood: A longitudinal view. *New England Journal of Medicine, 310,* 824–829.

Starfield, B., Gross, E., Wood, M., Pantell, R., Allen, C., Gordon, I. B., Moffatt, P., Drachman, R., & Kratz, H. (1980). Psychosocial and psychosomatic diagnoses in primary care of children. *Pediatrics, 66,* 159–167.

U.S. Congress. (1986). *Children's Mental Health: Problems and Services.* Washington, DC: U.S. Government Printing Office.

U.S. Department of Health and Human Services, (1990). *National Plan for Research on Child and Adolescent Mental Disorders.* Rockville, MD: Author.

Walker, D., Gortmaker, S., & Weitzman, M. (1991). *Chronic illness and psychosocial problems among children in Genesee County.* Boston: Harvard School of Public Health.

Wallen, J., & Pincus, H. A. (1988). Care of children with psychiatric disorders at community hospitals. *Hospital and Community Psychiatry, 39,* 167–172.

Wasserman, R. C., Barriatua, R. D., Carter, W. B., & Lippincott, P. (1984). Pediatric clinicians' support for parents makes a difference: An outcome-based analysis of clinician-parent interaction. *Pediatrics, 74*(6), 1047.

15

Junius J. Gonzales
Grayson Norquist

Mental Health Consultation-Liaison Interventions in Primary Care

Despite the substantial number of people with mental disorders receiving services from primary care practitioners (Regier, Goldberg, & Taube, 1978; Kessler et al., 1987), research has demonstrated that these providers often underrecognize and misdiagnose mental disorders (Jones, Badger, Ficken, Leeper, & Anderson, 1987; Ormel et al., 1990; Perez-Stable, Miranda, Muñoz, & Ying, 1990). Even if the condition is recognized, people with mental disorders may not be treated appropriately (Hohmann, Larson, Thompson, & Beardsley, 1991; Wells, Goldberg, Brook, & Leake, 1988) or as intensively as warranted (Katon, Von Korff, Lin, Bush, & Ormel, 1992; Magruder-Habib et al., 1989). Furthermore, few of those with mental disorders receiving service from primary care physicians are referred to mental health specialists (Fauman, 1983; Jones et al., 1987). Even when primary care providers do make referrals, many patients do not actually obtain mental health care (Olfson, 1991), regardless of insurance status or availability of mental health services (Ware, Manning, Duan, Wells, & Newhouse, 1984).

Note: The authors would like to thank Emily Fair for her help.

Mental health consultation-liaison (C-L) interventions hold promise for improving the care of mental disorders in primary care. Fortunately, these interventions are more integral a part of standard clinical practice than the research literature would indicate (Schulberg, 1991; Schulberg & Burns, 1988). This chapter provides a brief history of C-L psychiatry and its role in ambulatory primary care settings, as well as a brief overview of the conceptual models of C-L interventions. The chapter also reviews the research on mental health C-L interventions in outpatient primary care. The conclusion offers recommendations for a research agenda in this area.

For the purpose of this chapter, the following definitions of *consultation-liaison* and *primary care* will be used. "Mental health consultation and liaison" (C-L) refers to any clinical or educational intervention provided for general medical personnel by mental health specialists, usually clinicians. Clearly the term *consultation-liaison* applies to a wide range of consultants providing services to a clinical group of consultees. The consultants include physicians (psychiatrists), nurses, psychologists, and social workers, and the consultees include professionals in medical, social service, legal, and educational settings. This chapter will primarily evaluate consultation by psychiatrists to physicians.

The setting for consultation most appropriate to this book is primary care. According to Hibbard and Nutting (1991, p. 2), primary care is "distinguished by being 'front-line' or 'firstcontact' care, person-centered (rather than disease or organ system-centered), and comprehensive in scope, rather than being limited to illness episodes or by the organ system or disease process involved. . . . Primary care practitioners deal with ambulatory patients at the initial interface of the individual with the health care system." This chapter will evaluate psychiatric consultation to primary care physicians.

Consultation-Liaison Psychiatry: History and Links to Primary Care

Historically, mental health consultation became prominent in the 1920s with an initial focus on comprehensive child health. Early interventions were community based—with an emphasis on prevention—and were delivered in child guidance clinics. Diverse professional groups and individuals likely to have direct contact with mental health issues were targeted, including physicians, nurses, educators, the clergy, social welfare workers, and those in the legal and judicial systems. Over time, each mental health discipline that provided mental health services has developed its own traditions and orientation and has made unique contributions to the area of consultation.

The term *liaison,* although now attached to consultation, originated as a separate conceptual area of expertise in the field of psychiatry. Liaison is the process of linking or joining two separate disciplines with the common goal of increasing awareness of mental health issues. This term, most often used in psychiatry and nursing, is now more widely accepted, as the primary care literature shows. While the terms *consultation* and *liaison* may be used separately, in this chapter they will be used together to fit our definition above. Those readers more interested in mental health consultation should read Caplan's classic text *The Theory and Practice of Mental Health Consultation* (1970).

More than any other area of psychiatry, C-L psychiatry has had the most direct and active connection to the rest of medicine, but some believe the connection can still be improved (Fink, 1985; Wise, 1985). C-L psychiatry developed within the conceptual rubric of psychosomatic medicine in the 1930s (Kaplan, 1989; Oken, 1989) and expanded with the active use of the biopsychosocial paradigm (Engel, 1977) for patient care. However, as early as 1929, George Henry—a psychiatrist at Cornell Medical College—described the clinical practice of psychiatric consultation (Henry, 1929), and the Rockefeller Foundation granted funds in 1934 for the introduction of psychiatry departments in general hospitals.

The actual phrase *liaison psychiatry* was used in Billings's 1939 article "Liaison Psychiatry and Intern Instruction." From the early post–World War II period through the 1960s, C-L psychiatry remained at a standstill due to a dissociation of psychiatry from general medicine. An exceptional growth in formal training for C-L psychiatry in the 1970s and early 1980s revitalized psychiatry's connection to medicine by training primary care physicians in psychosocial issues, one of several C-L psychiatry endeavors that received federal fiscal support (Eaton, Goldberg, Rosinski, & Allerton, 1977). This growth was further supported by the emergence of other C-L mental health professionals such as nurses, social workers, and psychologists, and by the National Institute of Mental Health (NIMH)-supported fellowships for C-L psychiatry (Saravay, Steinberg, Solomon, & Hong, 1984).

The community mental health center and the neighborhood health center movements in the 1960s and 1970s and the President's Commission on Mental Health (1978) prioritized better linkage of primary care and mental health services. In fact, in the late 1970s, the NIMH nearly doubled its funds (from about $6 to $10.2 million) for mental health training in primary care (Pincus, Strain, Houpt, & Gise, 1983).

The hyphenated name *consultation-liaison* was derived from two movements that were closely allied. Oken (1983, pp. 1168–1169), distinguished the two functions of consultation and liaison work in terms of "scope and focus" and stressed that "the concern of the liaison psychiatrist is with the operation of psychological and social factors in *every* illness. . . . The consultant, in contrast, is called in to deal with overt aberrant behavior and to identify and treat *psychiatric* disorders, including the clarification as to whether physical symptoms 'arise from' a psychiatric condition." In theory, the distinguishing feature of liaison work is that it does not involve direct clinical patient care but instead involves working collaboratively with medical and surgical staff in providing clinical education. Today, the separation of the two processes has been obliterated, and most C-L psychiatrists function in both capacities.

Pasnau (1982) provided a comprehensive description of the tasks of a C-L psychiatrist. This practitioner is "concerned with the study, diagnosis, treatment and prevention of psychiatric morbidity in the physically ill, of psychological factors affecting physical conditions, and of somatopsychic and psychosomatic interactions."

Today, the overwhelming majority of C-L psychiatric work takes place in the inpatient sector of general hospitals. Hales (1985, p. 214) predicted that C-L psychiatry in the general hospital could be influential in "fostering closer primary care–psychiatry cooperation and more comprehensive treatment of patients." He not only believed that C-L psychiatry could make a contribution to linking with primary care through direct training of primary care providers in mental health issues, but that by virtue of some C-L work itself, this relationship could be enhanced. Other potential indirect benefits for primary care providers included the increased recognition of psychiatric morbidity in inpatients, the potential impact of C-L intervention on length of stay, and the possible impact on health care utilization.

Mayou (1991, p. 261) supported this contention and noted that the general hospital is often an entry point for patients to use mental health services, especially in Britain—"in some countries, C-L psychiatrists are developing extensive liaison links with general practitioners." Primary care physicians often admit to general hospitals and follow their patients during inpatient stays.

The more natural link to primary care would seem to be made in the outpatient sector. One review (Epstein & Gonzales, 1992) found only eleven published reports of outpatient C-L psychiatry clinics between 1948 and 1991. These reports revealed a wide range of programs staffed primarily by medical personnel—psychiatrists, other physicians (medicine, family practice), psychiatry trainees (fellows and residents), and medical students. The review also summarized six unique educational advantages of outpatient C-L psychiatry over traditional inpatient C-L psychiatry:

1. Continuity of care
2. Ambulatory psychiatric diagnoses in the medically ill
3. Ambulatory medical problems
4. Liaison and collaborative care
5. Acquiring and honing therapeutic skills
6. Research

The first and fourth advantages have direct implications for strengthening the linkage between psychiatry and primary care. Not only can trainees benefit from following inpatients into the outpatient sector, but primary care providers may be more likely to request consultations if they are aware this mode of continuous psychiatric care exists. Active liaison and collaboration in the integrated care of a patient is another potential advantage of outpatient C-L psychiatry. This can be especially useful for primary care providers who care for the medically ill with comorbid psychiatric conditions. These advantages prepare the psychiatric trainee for the "real-world" patients, their problems, and management.

Von Korff, Katon, Lin, and Wagner (1987) surveyed primary care providers and found further support for coordinating general medical and mental health services. In their study, 74.3 percent of general medical providers felt there was a "lack of coordination between mental health service and primary care." Furthermore, physician self-ratings for management of mental health problems were low. Given general physician attitudes, the opportunities for outpatient C-L psychiatry to join with primary care, whether it be in service delivery or training, seem limitless.

Conceptual Models of Consultation-Liaison Interventions in Primary Care

While no one theoretical model dominates the C-L field, derivations of psychological or psychiatric theory, together with contributions from the social sciences, have influenced the practice of consultation-liaison. Mannino, Trickett, Shore, Kidder, and Levin (1986) describe several conceptual models, including the "traditional" or psychodynamic approach, the cognitive-behavioral approach, and the organizational development approach.

In addition, Schwab (1986) describes the importance of general systems theory in the evolution of C-L psychiatry. General systems theory was incorporated into the field because this model emphasizes multilevel assessments in the clinical evaluation of patients, including organizational factors—both intersystem and intrasystem—that might influence treatment response.

In reviewing the history of mental health liaison, Pincus (1980, 1987) proposed six models that linked general medical and mental health systems of care and described relationships between the primary care provider and the mental health professional. He based these six models on three key elements of linkage:

1. Contractual, which "consist of the nature and content of formal or informal agreements between the two settings"
2. Functional, including "aspects of the relationship actually encountered by the patient"
3. Educational—that is, "aspects of the relationship that serve to establish and reinforce the primary care provider's knowledge and skills in mental health"

Pincus (1980, p. 316) based his models on a "generalized theory of . . . linkages without being limited to specific levels or settings" (a limiting aspect of previous models); instead, each is potentially applicable in a variety of settings. The linkage is modified by the level of administrative and clinical participation that each sector has. At one end of the spectrum, the agreement model is characterized by linkage established in a contractual way between two separate parties, in which each party renders separate services. The triage, service delivery team, consultation and service, and supervision and education models follow, whereas the last model, an integrated health care team, is described by Pincus (1980, p. 315) as "a fluid synthesis of the three elements of the relationship"—a team that routinely includes a mental health professional as a regular colleague.

Strathdee (1987) conducted research on a liaison-attachment model of consult-liaison treatment. Mental health professionals were part of the general health care team. She found perceived advantages of such a liaison scheme. In addition, psychiatrists reported that this model could improve clinical care and help to diminish the stigma associated with seeing a psychiatrist. In this study, 98 percent of general practitioners reported that the process was facilitated, 82 percent had regular clinical discussions with psychiatrists, and 79 to 86 percent felt that their knowledge of psychiatric illness and treatments had increased. Interestingly, the general practitioners felt that health services delivery had been significantly improved. In fact, 97 percent believed that hospital admissions had been prevented, and 93 to 98 percent felt that mental health services delivery had been improved in all three survey domains.

Research on Mental Health Consultation-Liaison in Primary Care

As the above descriptions of conceptual bases and clinical practicalities indicate, mental health C-L efforts may improve recognition, diagnosis, and management of persons with mental disorders seen in primary care settings. Several papers have discussed C-L in primary care (Kamerow & Burns, 1987; Schulberg, 1987; Von Korff & Myers, 1987), and one even stated that "psychiatric consultation-liaison in primary care is a promising approach to the solution of several important public health problems" (Schulberg & Burns, 1988, p. 80). However, the research on C-L interventions in primary care is inconclusive: the number of studies is limited, the study populations are diverse, the interventions are varied, and the multiple outcomes measured are derived from various domains. The lack of conceptually driven interventions is a major problem. Consequently, the research reporting positive findings has limited generalizability. These and related issues will be further discussed in the final section.

This section will review the C-L research literature with particular emphasis on recent studies of primary care settings that were not detailed in two recent reviews (Kamerow & Burns, 1987; Balestrieri, Williams, & Wilkinson, 1988). Table 15.1 is a compilation of the mental health C-L clinical trials in the literature, including the two published reviews and our own literature reviews (including Medline and index searches).

The following is an attempt to summarize the clinical studies that evaluate the effect of mental health C-L intervention in a primary care setting. The intervention can be a time-limited direct clinical service (consultation or intervention), a liaison interaction, or a referral process. The providers studied included any mental health professional from any discipline as long as they were based in the primary care practice setting. Studies where the intervention occurred after a referral had been made, or where the intervention was in the specialty mental health sector, were not included. It should be noted that there have been C-L intervention studies of medical/surgical inpatients (Fulop, 1992; Levenson, Hamer, & Rossiter, 1992; Strain et al., 1991), but these were excluded since we focus here on outpatient primary care settings.

Table 15.1 provides a listing by author, year, provider type, number of experimental subjects (*N*), outcome variables (specific measures are not denoted), and results of overall effect for twenty-one studies. Positive effect (+) means the intervention had a beneficial effect on a clinical or service outcome. For example, a positive effect on primary care visits indicates that these were reduced by the C-L intervention, while a positive effect on mental health status indicates a clinical improvement.

Open or Uncontrolled Studies

Of the twenty-one studies noted in Table 15.1, eight were neither controlled nor randomized. Although five of the eight studies showed positive results, the absence of a control group makes conclusions about effectiveness impossible. As Kamerow and Burns (1987, p. 113) concluded, "Although all of these studies report encouraging results, they all suffer from a lack of control patients, nonstandardized evaluation procedures, and selection biases."

Controlled Studies

In this section, we review experimental studies that used a control group.

The diversity of C-L interventions in controlled studies can be best viewed by using a simple spectrum of specificity. At the end of less specificity is a general, open-ended, not time-limited intervention (apart from the study duration). For example, Cooper et al. in 1975 evaluated the effect of integrating a social worker into a primary care practice. The intervention provided a range of services, including direct recommendations to the primary care provider, referral to mental health services, and direct social support. Subjects were chosen by International Classification of Diseases (ICD) diagnoses or "chronic neurotic illness." Results showed trends that the experimental group received fewer psychotropic medications and improved mental health.

At the other end of the specificity spectrum is the application

Table 15.1. Studies on Mental Health Consultation-Liaison Interventions in Ambulatory Primary Care.

Study	*Mental Health C-L Provider*	*N*	*Length of Study (Months)*	*Outcomes*	*Results (+,– Effects)*
Cooper, Harwin, Depla, & Shepherd, 1975	Social worker	92	12	Mental health	+
				Social functioning	+
				Prescriptions[b]	+
				Primary care visits	+
				Specialty mental visits	+/–
Anderson & Hasler, 1979	Nurse	80	2	Mental health	+
				Primary care visits	+
Ives, 1979[a]	Psychologist	123	3–12	Mental health	+
Koch, 1979[a]	Psychologist	30	12	Mental health	+
				Prescriptions	+
				Primary care visits	+
Jannoun, McDoweel, & Catalan, 1981[a]	Psychologist	15	3	Mental health	+
				Medication use	+
Corney, 1984	Social worker	41	6	Mental health	+/–
				Social functioning	+/–
				Primary care visits	+/–
				Prescriptions	+/–
McKechnie, Philip, & Ramage, 1981[a]	Psychiatrist	72	24	Specialty mental health visits	+/–
				Mental health admissions	+
Thompson, Stoudemire, & Mitchell, 1982[a]	Psychiatrist	40	c	Assessment of mental health	+
Earll & Kincey, 1982	Psychologist	23	7	Mental health	+/–
				Social functioning	–
				Prescriptions	+/–
				Primary care visits	+/–
				Specialty mental health visits	+
Brodaty & Andrews, 1983	Psychologist	18	6	Mental health	+/–
				Social functioning	+/–
				Prescriptions	+/–

Robson, France, & Bland, 1984	Psychologist	229	12	Mental health	+/–
				Social functioning	+/–
				Prescriptions	+
				Primary care visits	+
Teasdale, Fennell, Hibbert, & Amies, 1984	Psychologist	17	4	Mental health	+
Tyrer, Seivewright, & Wollerton, 1984[a]	Psychiatric clinics	185	24	Specialty mental health visits	–
				Mental health admissions	+
Marks, 1985	Nurse	46	12	Mental health	+
				Social functioning	+
				Prescriptions	–
				Primary care visits	+/–
Ross & Scott, 1985	Social worker	30	3	Mental health	+
Blakey, 1986	Psychologist	25	36	Primary care visits	+
				Prescriptions	+
Smith, Monson, & Ray, 1986	Psychiatrist	38	9	Mental health	–
				Social functioning	–
				Primary care visits	+
Klerman et al., 1987	Nurse	64	3–12	Mental health	+
				Social functioning	+
				Specialty mental health visits	+/–
				Primary care visits	+/–
Katon, 1991; Katon et al., 1992; Katon & Gonzales, in press	Psychiatrist	119	12	Change in diagnosis/treatment	+
Scott & Freeman, 1992	Psychiatrist Psychologist Social worker	121	16	Mental health	+
				Patient satisfaction	+
				Costs	–

[a]Uncontrolled studies. [b]Psychotropic prescriptions. [c]Cross-sectional study.

of treatments derived from specialty mental health settings (for example, psychopharmacology and psychotherapy) into primary care settings. What makes them C-L interventions is their time-limited nature and practice in the primary setting. Most of the studies fall into this group. Two studies conducted in Great Britain (Brodaty & Andrews, 1983; Teasdale et al., 1984) compared the same interventions: group cognitive behavioral therapy versus special sessions with a family practitioner versus usual medical care. The later study used a specific patient population—people with major depression defined by research criteria—not just people with psychological distress on a screening instrument, and it had follow-up assessments with depression scales. Although the first study reported no improved outcome as a result of treatment, the second demonstrated some positive results—decreased depressive symptomatology at the end of the study—which were not sustained at three months.

Ross and Scott (1985, p. 239) followed up on these studies by evaluating "the effectiveness of individual and group cognitive therapy in the treatment of depressed patients in an inner city health centre." They found that depressive symptoms improved in both group and individual treatments compared to the control and that therapeutic gains were maintained at the twelve-month follow-up. An interesting part of their analysis was to include patients who failed to respond to the interventions or dropped out, since, "this was a more realistic representation of the situation encountered in general practice."

Klerman et al.'s 1987 study was unique in that it utilized nurse practitioners to provide a modified standard mental health intervention—interpersonal counseling (IPC) was based on interpersonal therapy, consisted of up to six thirty-minute sessions, and focused on current life stressors. Here psychological distress measured by a screening instrument, the General Health Questionnaire (GHQ), was used for entry and follow-up, even though experimental patients underwent a structured interview. Clinical improvement was observed in the experimental group, but there were no significant differences between the two groups in medical care utilization.

The last study using highly specialized mental health interventions was conducted by Scott and Freeman (1992). Patients were randomized to one of four groups: tricyclic antidepressant prescribed by a psychiatrist, cognitive-behavioral therapy with a psychologist, counseling/case work by a social worker, or usual care by the general practitioner. Results showed that at four weeks, patients in the medication group were most improved, but that at sixteen weeks, patients who received the social work intervention seemed most improved. Patients were more satisfied with the psychological treatments than with medications. Finally, the costs for all interventions were at least twice as much as for usual care.

In the middle of the intervention specificity spectrum are two other studies. The Smith et al. study (1986) is one of the few U.S. studies in this field. Featuring a randomized, controlled crossover design, the study of patients with somatization disorder involved a *single* psychiatric consultation, with patient management suggestions then sent to referring primary care providers. Health care costs for the experimental group were significantly less, although changes in health status or patient satisfaction measures were not found.

Focusing on psychologically distressed high utilizers of medical care, Katon and colleagues conducted a randomized trial of a liaison psychiatric intervention in a primary care setting (Katon et al., 1990). High utilizers (n = 767) were screened for distress and randomly assigned to either an experimental or a control group. The two-part intervention began with a structured interview by a psychiatrist, followed by a joint examination involving a shorter structured interview with the same psychiatrist and the patient's primary care physician. The two physicians jointly discussed treatment recommendations and then presented the plan to the patient. Major patient outcome variables in this study were psychiatric symptom change, use of services, associated illness behaviors, health care expenditures, and patient satisfaction with care. The effect of the C-L intervention on primary care providers was also measured. The most common psychiatric diagnoses among these patients were major depression (23.5 percent), generalized anxiety disorder (21.8 percent), somatization disorder (20.2 percent), and dysthymia (16.8 percent). Although the intervention did increase the number of patients receiving antidepressants, there was no significant effect on adequate dosing or duration. These data, as well as other research on higher prescribing of newer antidepressants, raise questions about the process of patient knowledge about depression and adherence to antidepressants. While the data do not appear to be encouraging, numerous factors may account for the absence of significant findings, as we will discuss in the summary of the research.

These findings stimulated interest in an extension project currently underway with the same research team that is designed to target both primary care providers and depressed patients, to improve provider recognition and management, and to encourage patient adherence and problem solving. Using a two part multilayered intervention design—a training intervention for physicians and an educational one for patients—the program seeks to evaluate the effects of these interventions on various provider and patient outcome variables.

Summarizing the Research

As illustrated by the preceding review of the literature (see Table 15.1), the research on mental health C-L interventions in outpatient primary care is diverse. The studies reviewed took place in both Great Britain and the United States, with a predominance in the former, and span a sixteen-year period. The mental health professionals involved in these interventions were from various disciplines—social work, psychology, nursing, and psychiatry—and research protocols ranged from two to thirty-six months. The interventions included consultation (such as Ross & Scott, 1985; Katon et al., 1990; Smith et al., 1986), time-limited focused therapy (Klerman et al., 1987), and an internist liaison program (Thompson et al., 1982). While some studies utilized standardized interventions, many offered clinical flexibility dependent on the patients' needs or complaints.

Some level of patient psychological distress was an inclusion criterion for entry into studies, but the range of this distress varied from nonspecific as measured by general screening instruments (for example, the GHQ), to more symptom specific by disorder screening instruments (for instance, the Beck Depression Inventory), to frank mental disorder by structured interviews (the Diagnostic Interview Schedule). Unfortunately, the unknown extent of symptom heterogeneity in the first two groups limits the generalizability of these findings. Furthermore, other patient characteristics such as psychiatric comorbidity and medical comorbidity were usually not addressed. Other possible confounding factors, including the extent of available social supports, were also not usually evaluated.

Most studies examined multidimensional outcomes, but some examined only change in clinical or mental health status. The use of nonclinical outcome measures, although important, brings the research another set of difficulties. For example, prescriptions written by the primary care provider may be assessed as a measure of how the provider responds to an educational intervention, but the measure does not account for patient adherence or nonadherence, either of which is determined by multiple factors not connected to the provider educational intervention.

Additionally, process variables, such as the physician-patient relationship, were not directly addressed in any of these reports. One study (Thompson et al., 1982) did compare physician sensitivity to patients' psychosocial concerns with patients' ratings of their psychosocial status, but other issues such as length of provider-patient relationship, physician attitudes/knowledge, and patient attitudes/knowledge were not assessed.

Finally, diverse clinical settings may be possible confounds, influencing the effect of interventions. For example, two of the U.S. studies (Katon et al., 1990; Klerman et al., 1987) were set in prepaid health plans. Structural variables in a health maintenance organization setting like length of visit or frequency of follow-up visits could affect patient outcomes such as medication adherence. In this context, Kamerow and Burns (1987) commented on the public health nature of British studies. Recent international primary care mental health studies have set an example by comparing, for example, disability and depression in various countries (Ormel et al., 1990).

Methodologic Issues in Mental Health Consultation-Liaison Primary Care Research

Several reports have summarized methodological issues in undertaking mental health C-L research in primary care settings (Kamerow & Burns, 1987; Schulberg, 1987; Von Korff & Myers, 1987; Wittchen & Essau, 1990), whereas others have addressed methodology in C-L psychiatry research (Dimsdale, 1991; Levenson, Colenda, Larson, & Bareta, 1990; Lyons, Hammer, Wise, & Strain, 1985; Mitchell & Thompson, 1985). This section will highlight the major methodologic issues for C-L research in primary care and will also suggest general research priorities.

The efficacy and effectiveness of reported mental health C-L intervention research cannot be determined, given the heterogeneity of research designs, study populations, and specific interventions. Some authors have recommended applying gold standard designs such as the randomized clinical trial to C-L interventions (Von Korff, Katon, Lin, & Wagner, 1987), while others have suggested that randomized trials are most appropriate when groups of patients with specific, diagnosed psychiatric disorders are being treated (Schulberg, 1991). We believe that the lack of a conceptual basis for C-L interventions poses difficulty for a randomized clinical trial and also argue for increased specificity and intensity of the experimental condition.

Along with the issues of specificity and intensity of an intervention, primary care researchers who have experienced the practical and theoretical difficulties of applying the gold standard of experimental design—the randomized clinical trial (RCT)—in naturalistic practice settings call for other methodologies (U.S. Department of Health and Human Services, 1991; Norton, Stewart, Tudiver, Bass, & Dunn, 1991) to gather data. The dynamic tension between the design concerns and clinical interventions in an RCT is evident where the treatment is standardized (for example, manual) and where this standardized format may impede the natural physician-patient interaction. This issue is incisively addressed in Schulberg et al.'s paper titled "Investigating Primary Care Treatments for Depression Through Culturally Synchronous Clinical Trials" (1991).

The design chosen depends on the questions of the investigation, but basic descriptive questions regarding primary care patients with mental health problems have not been answered. The epidemiology of people with mental disorders in primary care has not been well established. Subthreshold conditions such as minor depression and mixed anxiety-depression are not well described (Broadhead, Blazer, George, & Tse, 1990) but have been shown to impair functioning and well-being over time (Wells, Burnam, Rogers, Hays, & Camp, 1991). Popkin, Colon, Callies, and MacKenzie (1991) described a similar proposal for more epidemiologic research in C-L psychiatry dealing with comorbid physically and mentally ill populations, since the impact of medical illness can be a factor in influencing outcome. The heterogeneity of the primary care population's health needs is both challenging and appealing to investigators.

Schulberg (1987) delineated three clusters of patient groups that would benefit from further study:

1. Undiagnosed, poorly differentiated problems that may or may not achieve a clinical diagnosis since they often are subthreshold or transitory in nature
2. Highly specific comorbidity in which organic pathology is accompanied by psychiatric disturbance—for example, cancer and depression
3. Well-diagnosed chronic conditions in which secondary psychosocial management issues play a significant, if not dominating, role

Special populations posing more methodological challenges but needing further study include urban minority persons, especially in poorly studied urban areas (Miranda, Schreckengost, & Gonzales, 1991), people in rural areas where mental health resources are scarce, and people with co-occurring substance use and/or medical problems with mental disorders. Finally, studies on mental health C-L interventions in pediatric primary care are infrequent and much needed.

Most cited studies did not consider specific provider characteristics that may substantially influence outcome results. For example, in Brodaty and Andrews's study (1983), one study group had sessions with a family practitioner, but various approaches in primary care physician style, attitudes, length of relationship, knowledge, and response to consultations were not considered. Depending on the focus of the C-L intervention, the study group can be patients, providers, or both. For example, Katon's study (1991) did randomize physicians to control for spillover of knowledge. However, their CLPE intervention was aimed at the primary care provider, not just at the patient. Primary care provider characteristics play a role in physician-patient process issues but may also be prominent in the physician-consultant process. Both interactive processes can have little or significant influence on patient outcomes.

Some have more explicitly advocated use of health services research paradigms to inform C-L research (Katon & Gonzales, in press). The issues addressed thus far—patient and provider characteristics, structural variables, and outcomes—all fall naturally into these paradigms. The relationships between these components are complex and often indirect. Since C-L interventions are diverse and varied processes, clarity about process components can be guided by using these models. Finally, authors have proposed useful conceptual domains for outcome measurement in mental health services research (Hargreaves & Shumway, 1989), but considering the primary care setting, other clinical measures such as general health status measures would seem to be a necessity for most studies (Lohr, 1992).

For instance, social and occupational functioning measures are crucial for primary care C-L research. As an example, disability days have been studied and may serve to indicate extent of dysfunction rather than meeting diagnostic criteria for a disorder, again given the primary care setting (Broadhead et al., 1990). Other outcomes refer to those concerned with the well-being and quality of life of patients, their families, and caregivers. Such measures should include quality of life, patient and caregiver satisfaction, and family burden.

This section has cursorily covered some major issues facing primary care mental health C-L research. Clearly, the complexities of the research extend beyond experimental design problems and call for vigorous scrutiny of the structure, process, and outcome issues in various components of a C-L intervention (Katon & Gonzales, in press).

Conclusion

This chapter has provided a brief overview of mental health C-L interventions in primary care—from history to models to research to methodology. There is no doubt about Schulberg's (1987, p. 132) conclusion and recommendation: "Mental health consultation in primary care is a diverse, complex technology requiring rigorous scientific study and validation if we are to know when, where, and how to utilize it. . . . A flexible rather than restrictive approach is needed, therefore, with the hope that investigators will create appropriate scientific designs for unraveling consultation's persisting mysteries." Our research recommendations are in line with those of others and fall under some methodological issues addressed above. Many issues facing primary care mental health research in general need consideration in doing C-L research. The research data thus far are inconclusive regarding the effectiveness of C-L interventions in primary care. Primary care C-L research so far lacks hypothesis-driven investigation, standard operationalization of variables, and, most important, theoretical or conceptual frameworks.

Nevertheless, priorities specific to mental health C-L research should include:

1. Research on mental health C-L interventions where specialty mental health resources are scarce—such as in rural settings—or for special populations (for example, minority groups, children)
2. Continued research on the impact of C-L interventions on short- and long-term recognition and management of mental disorders
3. Studies on the barriers to C-L interventions in primary care (for instance, setting, structural, attitudinal, knowledge deficiency, reimbursement), whether they be at the provider, institutional, or patient level
4. Research on the types, quality, and effectiveness of mental health C-L interventions
5. Studies on innovative mental health C-L models in primary care
6. Research on the nature and effectiveness of C-L interventions that link primary care, mental health care, and other potential systems of care (for example, schools, social services)

A majority of people who suffer from mental disorders are seen in the general health care sector, especially primary care. Effective and efficient C-L interventions hold tremendous promise but need to be carefully and creatively researched. The primary care community is an active voice calling for more research in mental health (Katerndahl, 1991; Poynton & Higgins, 1991; Like, 1991). Finally, two of the mental health objectives in the Department of Health and Human Services's strategic planning document, *Healthy People 2000* (1991, p. 219), are related to primary care; mental health C-L work can make a direct contribution to these objectives:

> Increase to at least 50 percent the proportion of primary care providers who routinely review with patients their patients' cognitive, emotional, and behavioral functioning and the resources available to deal with any problems that are identified.
>
> Increase to at least 75 percent the proportion of providers of primary care for children who include assessment of cognitive, emotional, and parent-child functioning, with appropriate counseling, referral, and follow-up, in their clinical practices.

References

Anderson, A., & Hasler, J. C. (1979). Counselling in general practice. *Journal of the Royal College of General Practitioners, 29,* 352–356.

Balestrieri, M., Williams, P., & Wilkinson, G. (1988). Specialist mental health treatment in general practice: A meta-analysis. *Psychological Medicine, 18,* 711–717.

Billings, E. G. (1939). Liaison psychiatry and intern instruction. *Journal of the Association of American Medical Colleges, 14,* 375–385.

Blakey, R. (1986). Psychological treatment in general practice: Its effect on patients and their families. *Journal of the Royal College of General Practitioners, 36,* 209–211.

Broadhead, W. E., Blazer, D., George, L., & Tse, C. K. (1990). Depression, disability days, and days lost from work in a prospective epidemiologic survey. *Journal of the American Medical Association, 264,* 2524–2528.

Brodaty, H., & Andrews, G. (1983). Brief psychotherapy in family practice: A controlled prospective intervention trial. *British Journal of Psychiatry, 143,* 11–19.

Caplan, G. (1970). *The theory and practice of mental health consultation.* London: Tavistock.

Cooper, B., Harwin, B. G., Depla, C., & Shepherd, M. (1975). Mental health care in the community: An evaluative study. *Psychological Medicine, 5,* 372–380.

Corney, R. H. (1984). The mental and physical health of clients referred to social workers in a local authority department and a general practice attachment scheme. *Psychological Medicine, 14,* 137–144.

Dimsdale, J. E. (1991). Challenges, problems, and opportunities in consultation-liaison psychiatry research. *Psychiatric Medicine, 9,* 641–648.

Earll, L., & Kincey, J. (1982). Clinical psychology in general practice: A controlled clinical evaluation. *Journal of the Royal College of General Practitioners, 32,* 32–37.

Eaton, J. S., Goldberg, R., Rosinski, E., & Allerton, W. S. (1977). The educational challenge of consultation liaison psychiatry. *American Journal of Psychiatry, 134,* 20–23.

Engel, G. (1977). The need for a new medical model: A challenge for biomedicine. *Science, 196,* 129–136.

Epstein, S. A., & Gonzales, J. J. (1992). *Outpatient consultation-liaison psychiatry: A valuable addition to the training of advanced psychiatry residents.* Unpublished manuscript.

Fauman, M. A. (1983). Psychiatric components of medical and surgical practice: 2. Referral and treatment of psychiatric disorders. *American Journal of Psychiatry, 140,* 760–763.

Fink, P. J. (1985). Psychiatry and primary care: Can a working relationship develop? *General Hospital Psychiatry, 7,* 205–209.

Fulop, G. (1992). *Geriatric co-morbidity: Hospital course and cost* (NIMH Grant R29 MH43378). Unpublished manuscript.

Hales, R. E. (1985). The benefits of a psychiatric consultation-liaison service in a general hospital. *General Hospital Psychiatry, 7,* 214–218.

Hargreaves, W. A., & Shumway, M. (1989). Effectiveness of mental health services for the severely mentally ill. In C. A. Taube, D. Mechanic, & A. A. Hohmann (Eds.), *The future of mental health services research* (DHHS Publication No. 89-1600). Washington, DC: U.S. Government Printing Office.

Healthy People 2000. (1991). (DHHS Publication No. (PHS) 91-50212). Washington, DC: U.S. Government Printing Office.

Henry, G. W. (1929). Some aspects of psychiatry in general hospital practice. *American Journal of Psychiatry, 9,* 481–499.

Hibbard, H., & Nutting, P. A. (1991). Research in primary care: A national priority. In *AHCPR Conference Proceedings, Primary Care Research: Theory and Methods* (AHCPR Publication No. 91-0011). Washington, DC: U.S. Government Printing Office.

Hohmann, A. A., Larson, D. B., Thompson, J. W., & Beardsley, R. S. (1991). Psychotropoic medication prescription in U.S. ambulatory care. *DICP: The Annals of Pharmacotherapy, 25,* 85–89.

Ives, G. (1979). Psychological treatment in general practice. *Journal of the Royal College of General Practitioners, 29,* 343–351.

Jannoun, L., McDoweel, I., & Catalan, J. (1981). Behavioural treatment of anxiety in general practice. *Practitioner, 225,* 58–62.

Jones, L. R., Badger, L. W., Ficken, R. P., Leeper, J. D., & Anderson, R. L. (1987). Inside the hidden mental health network: Examining mental health care delivery of primary care physicians. *General Hospital Psychiatry, 9,* 287–293.

Kamerow, D. B., & Burns, B. J. (1987). The effectiveness of mental health consultation and referral in ambulatory primary care: A research lacuna. *General Hospital Psychiatry, 9,* 111–117.

Kaplan, H. I. (1989). History of psychosomatic medicine. In H. I. Kaplan & B. J. Sadock (Eds.), *Comprehensive textbook of psychiatry* (Vol. 4). Baltimore, MD: Williams & Wilkins.

Katerndahl, D. A. (1991). Panic disorder in primary care settings: Research agenda for the '90s. *Family Practice Research Journal, 11,* 3–7.

Katon, W. (1991). The development of a randomized trial of consultation-liaison psychiatry in distressed high utilizers of primary care. *Psychiatric Medicine, 9,* 577–591.

Katon, W., & Gonzales, J. (in press). A review of randomized trials of psychiatric consultation liaison studies in primary care. *Psychosomatics.*

Katon, W., Von Korff, M., Lin, E., Bush, T., & Ormel, J. (1992). Adequacy and duration of antidepressant treatment in primary care. *Medical Care, 30,* 67–76.

Katon, W., Von Korff, M., Lin, E., Lipscomb, P., Russo, J., Wagner, E., & Polk, E. (1990). Distressed high utilizers of medical care: DSM-III-R diagnoses and treatment needs. *General Hospital Psychiatry, 12,* 355–362.

Kessler, L. G., Burns, B. J., Shapiro, S., Tischler, G. L., George, L. K., Hough, R. L., Bodison, D., & Miller, R. H. (1987). Psychiatric diagnoses of medical service users: Evidence from the Epidemiologic Catchment Area Program. *American Journal of Public Health, 77,* 18–24.

Klerman, G. L., Budman, S., Berwick, D., Weissman, M. M., Damico-White, J., Demby, A., & Feldstein, M. (1987). Efficacy of a brief psychosocial intervention for symptoms of stress and distress among patients in primary care. *Medical Care, 25,* 1078–1088.

Koch, H. C. (1979). Evaluation of behavior therapy intervention in general practice. *Journal of the Royal College of General Practitioners, 29,* 337–340.

Levenson, J. L., Colenda, C., Larson, D. B., & Bareta, J. C. (1990). Methodology in consultation-liaison research: A classification of biases. *Psychosomatics, 31,* 367–376.

Levenson, J. L., Hamer, R. M., & Rossiter, L. F. (1992). A randomized controlled study of psychiatric consultation guided by screening in general medical inpatients. *American Journal of Psychiatry, 149,* 631–637.

Like, R. C. (1991, September). *Primary health care for adults with chronic mental illness: Clinical findings from a model service demonstration project.* Poster presentation at the fifth annual NIMH International Research Conference on the Classification, Recognition, and Treatment of Mental Disorders in General Medical Settings, Bethesda, MD.

Lohr, K. N. (1992). Overview of the third annual Conference on Advances in Health Status Assessment. *Medical Care, 30*(Suppl. 5), 1–14.

Lyons, J. S., Hammer, J. S., Wise, T. N., & Strain, J. J. (1985). Consultation-liaison psychiatry and cost-effectiveness research: A review of methods. *General Hospital Psychiatry, 7,* 302–308.

McKechnie, A., Philip, A. E., & Ramage, J. G. (1981). Psychiatric services in primary care: Specialized or not? *Journal of the Royal College of General Practitioners, 31,* 611–614.

Magruder-Habib, K. M., Zung, W. W. K., Feussner, J. R., Alling, W. C., Saunders, W. B., & Stevens, H. A. (1989). Management of general medical patients with symptoms of depression. *General Hospital Psychiatry, 11,* 201–207.

Mannino, F. V., Trickett, E. J., Shore, M. F., Kidder, M. G., & Levin, G. (Eds.). (1986). *Handbook of mental health consultation* (DHHS Publication No. 86-1446). Washington, DC: U.S. Government Printing Office.

Marks, I. (1985). Controlled trial of psychiatric nurse therapists in primary care. *British Medical Journal, 290,* 1181–1184.

Mayou, R. (1991). What should British consultation-liaison psychiatry be doing? *General Hospital Psychiatry, 13,* 261–266.

Miranda, J., Schreckengost, J., & Gonzales, G. (1991, September). *Treatment of depression in disadvantaged primary care patients.* Paper presented at the fourth annual NIMH International Research Conference on the Classification, Recognition, and Treatment of Mental Disorders in General Medical Settings, Bethesda, MD.

Mitchell, W. D., & Thompson, T. L. (1985). Research problems for consultation-liaison psychiatry in the DRG era. *General Hospital Psychiatry, 7,* 349–352.

Norton, P. G., Stewart, M., Tudiver, F., Bass, M. J., & Dunn, E. V. (Eds.). (1991). *Primary care research: Traditional and innovative approaches.* Newbury Park, CA: Sage.

Oken, D. (1983). Liaison psychiatry. *Advances in Psychosomatic Medicine, 11,* 23–51.

Oken, D. (1989). Current theoretical concepts in psychosomatic medicine. In H. I. Kaplan & B. J. Sadock (Eds.), *Comprehensive textbook of psychiatry* (Vol. 4). Baltimore, MD: Williams & Wilkins.

Olfson, M. (1991). Primary care patients who refuse specialized mental health services. *Archives of Internal Medicine, 151,* 129-132.

Ormel, J., van den Brink, W., Koeter, M. W. J., Giel, R., van der Meer, K., van de Willige, G., & Wilmink, F. W. (1990). Recognition, management, and outcome of psychological disorders in primary care: A naturalistic follow-up study. *Psychological Medicine, 20,* 909-923.

Pasnau, R. O. (1982). *Consultation-liaison psychiatry.* Kalamazoo, MI: Upjohn Company.

Perez-Stable, E. J., Miranda, J., Muñoz, R. F., & Ying, Y. (1990). Depression in medical outpatients: Underrecognition and misdiagnosis. *Archives of Internal Medicine, 150,* 1083-1088.

Pincus, H. A. (1980). Linking general health and mental health systems of care: Conceptual models of implementation. *American Journal of Psychiatry, 3,* 315-320.

Pincus, H. A. (1987). Patient-ordered models for linking primary care and mental health care. *General Hospital Psychiatry, 9,* 95-101.

Pincus, H. A., Strain, J. J., Houpt, J. L., & Gise, L. H. (1983). Models of mental health training in primary care. *Journal of the American Medical Association, 249,* 3065-3068.

Popkin, M. K., Colon, E. A., Callies, A. L., & MacKenzie, T. B. (1991). The shift from outcome studies to epidemiological studies of specific medical illnesses in consultation-liaison psychiatry. *Psychiatric Medicine, 9,* 607-621.

Poynton, A., & Higgins, P. (1991). Role of general practitioners in care of long-term mentally ill patients. *British Journal of Psychiatry, 159,* 703-706.

President's Commission on Mental Health. Report to the President. (1978). Washington, DC: U.S. Government Printing Office.

Regier, D. A., Goldberg, I. D., & Taube, C. A. (1978). The de facto mental health services system. *Archives of General Psychiatry, 35,* 685-693.

Robson, M. H., France, R., & Bland, M. (1984). Clinical psychologist in primary care: Controlled clinical and economic evaluation. *British Medical Journal, 288,* 1805-1808.

Ross, M., & Scott, M. (1985). An evaluation of the effectiveness of individual and group cognitive therapy in the treatment of depressed patients. *Journal of the Royal College of General Practitioners, 35,* 239–242.

Saravay, S. M., Steinberg, H., Solomon, S. P., & Hong, G. K. (1984). A confirmation of NIMH training objectives for consultation-liaison residents. *American Journal of Psychiatry, 141,* 1437–1440.

Schulberg, H. C. (1987). Ambulatory mental health liaison research: A review and preview. *General Hospital Psychiatry, 9,* 126–134.

Schulberg, H. C. (1991). Mental disorders in the primary care setting: Research priorities for the 1990s. *General Hospital Psychiatry, 13,* 156–164.

Schulberg, H. C., & Burns, B. J. (1988). Mental disorders in primary care: Epidemiologic, diagnostic, and treatment research directions. *General Hospital Psychiatry, 10,* 79–87.

Schulberg, H. C., et al. (1991). Investigating primary care treatments for depression through culturally synchronous clinical trials. (manuscript under review)

Schwab, J. J. (1986). The psychiatrist's roles and functions in the 1980s. In F. V. Mannino, E. J. Trickett, M. F. Shore, M. G. Kidder, & G. Levin (Eds.), *Handbook of Mental Health Consultation* (DHHS Publication No. 86-1446). Washington, DC: U.S. Government Printing Office.

Scott, A. I., & Freeman, C. P. (1992). Edinburgh primary care depression study: Treatment outcome, patient satisfaction, and cost after 16 weeks. *British Medical Journal, 304,* 883–887.

Smith, G. R., Monson, R. A., & Ray, D. C. (1986). Psychiatric consultation in somatization disorder: A randomized controlled study. *New England Journal of Medicine, 314,* 1407–1413.

Strain, J. J. Lyons, J. S., Hammer, J. S., Fahs, M., Lebovits, A., Paddison, P. L., Snyder, S., Strauss, E., Burton, R., Nuber, G., Abernathy, T., Sacks, H., Nordlie, J., & Sacks, C. (1991). Cost offset from a psychiatric consultation-liaison intervention with elderly hip fracture patients. *American Journal of Psychiatry, 148,* 1044–1049.

Strathdee, G. (1987). Primary care-psychiatry interaction: A British perspective. *General Hospital Psychiatry, 9,* 102–110.

Teasdale, J. D., Fennell, M. J. V., Hibbert, G. A., & Amies, P. L.

(1984). Cognitive therapy for major depressive disorder in primary care. *British Journal of Psychiatry, 144,* 400–466.

Thompson, T. L., Stoudemire, A., & Mitchell, W. D. (1982). Effects of a psychiatric liaison program on internists' ability to assess psychosocial problems. *International Journal of Psychiatry in Medicine, 12,* 153–160.

Tyrer, P., Seivewright, N., & Wollerton, S. (1984). General practice psychiatry clinics: Impact on psychiatric services. *British Journal of Psychiatry, 145,* 15–19.

U.S. Department of Health and Human Services. (1991). *AHCPR Conference Proceedings, Primary Care Research: Theory and Methods* (AHCPR Publication No. 91-0011).

Von Korff, M., Katon, W., Lin, E. H. B., & Wagner, E. H. (1987). Evaluation of psychiatric consultation-liaison in primary care settings. *General Hospital Psychiatry, 9,* 102–110.

Von Korff, M., & Myers, L. (1987). The primary care physician and psychiatric services. *General Hospital Psychiatry, 9,* 235–240.

Ware, J. E., Manning, W. G., Duan, N., Wells, K. B., & Newhouse, J. P. (1984). Health status and the use of outpatient mental health services. *American Psychologist, 39,* 1090–1100.

Wells, K. B., Burnam, M. A., Rogers, W., Hays, R., & Camp, P. (1992). The course of depression in adult outpatients: Results from the medical outcomes study. *Archives of General Psychiatry, 49,* 788–794.

Wells, K. B., Goldberg, G., Brook, R., & Leake, B. (1988). Management of patients on psychotropic drugs in primary care clinics. *Medical Care, 26,* 645–656.

Wise, T. N. (1985). Commentary: Psychiatry and primary care. *General Hospital Psychiatry, 7,* 202–204.

Wittchen, H., & Essau, C. A. (1990). Methodological challenges in the assessment of mental disorders in primary care. In C. N. Stefanis, A. D. Rabavilas, & C. R. Soldatos (Eds.), *Psychiatry: A world perspective.* London: Elsevier Science.

Part Five

Service Use and Economic Consequences of Mental Disorders in Primary Care

16

Philip J. Leaf

Psychiatric Disorders and the Use of Health Services

We have long known that many individuals seeking general medical services suffer from significant emotional distress (Goldberg, 1972; Hankin & Oktay, 1979; Sartorius et al., 1990; Shepherd, Cooper, Brown, & Kalton, 1966) and that a substantial proportion of the health services related to mental illness and distress are provided through the general medical sector rather than through the mental health specialty sector (Horgan, 1985; Regier et al., 1982; Regier, Goldberg, & Taube, 1978). Although this partly reflects the frequent occurrence of psychiatric disorders in the general population and well-defined patterns of helpseeking, concern with the impact of psychiatric disorders on the use of health services is growing because the prevalence of these disorders is increasing and the age of onset decreasing (Cross-National Collaborative Group, 1992; Klerman & Weissman, 1989).

Primary care providers may not be capable of offering adequate services to their patients with psychiatric disorders. These providers fail to detect most psychiatric disorders in their patients (Barrett, Barrett, Oxman, & Gerber, 1988; Coulehan, Schulberg, & Block,

1989), so that it is impossible to provide appropriate treatment. Inadequate treatment may increase the overall use of health care and result in unnecessary morbidity and mortality. Thus, the impact of psychiatric disorders on the use of health care is an important consideration in increasing the effectiveness of health care, developing health care policy, and creating a rational basis for the financing of health services.

The actual impact of psychiatric disorders on the use of general health services is difficult to determine. Considerable attention has been paid to developing more reliable and valid criteria for identifying psychiatric disorders, but disagreement concerning the relevance of these criteria for the types of problems presented in primary care settings remains. Psychiatric disorders frequently cooccur with other illnesses (Kessler, Tessler, & Nycz, 1983), but adequate measures of these other disorders are rarely included in studies focusing on the psychopathology. Most researchers employ either categorical measures of psychiatric disorder or measures of distress, but both specific symptoms and the level of distress to an individual and his or her family are important factors in the use of health care services.

In this chapter, we review recent research focusing on the impact of psychiatric disorders on the use of health services. We summarize the current perspective on the impact of psychiatric disorders on the use of health services. We then examine limitations in this research and identify issues yet to be resolved.

Prevalence of Psychiatric Disorders

Much of the data concerning the prevalence of psychiatric disorders in the United States and the use of services for the treatment of mental and emotional disorders comes from the Epidemiologic Catchment Area (ECA) project conducted in the early 1980s (Eaton & Kessler, 1985). This study is based on large surveys of community residents and persons living in institutions in or near New Haven, Connecticut; Baltimore, Maryland; Durham, North Carolina; St. Louis, Missouri; and Los Angeles. Data from these surveys indicate that between 20 and 28 percent of all adult Americans—or as many as forty-five million people—experience a psychiatric disorder during a twelve-month period (Regier, Narrow, Rae, Manderscheid, Locke, & Goodwin, 1993; Robins & Regier, 1991).

If individuals having only addictive disorders are excluded, Regier et al. (1993) estimate the one-year prevalence rate to be twenty-two per one hundred adults, equivalent to approximately thirty-five million persons. In addition, data from the ECA project indicate that between 32 and 44 percent of all American adults experience a psychiatric disorder at some point in their lives (Regier et al., 1993; Robins & Regier, 1991). Recent epidemiologic studies have also found high rates of psychiatric disorders in children and adolescents (McGee, Feehan, Williams, & Anderson, 1992; Offord et al., 1987).

Using data from the ECA study, Regier et al. (1993) combine reports from the initial and follow-up interviews to examine both the prevalence of psychiatric disorders and the use of mental health services. They estimate that 6.4 percent of the adult population, or ten million people, received mental health services in the general medical sector during 1980, compared to 5.6 percent of the adult population or about nine million people receiving outpatient services from the mental health specialty or addictive treatment sector. In addition, many individuals with psychiatric disorders are treated by nonphysicians in both the mental health specialty sector and the human services sector, with services provided by social service agencies and schools. For 1980, Regier et al. (1993) estimated that approximately 3 percent of the adult population or 4.8 million people received mental health services in the human services sector.

Despite the enormous expansion of mental health services during the past two decades, most individuals with psychiatric and substance abuse disorders do not receive treatment for these disorders (Leaf et al., 1985; Shapiro et al., 1984). Regier et al. (1993) estimate that only 28.5 percent of individuals with a mental/addictive disorder receive any mental/addictive service during the year they manifest the disorder. This situation is not unique to the United States. In a study of 1,498 adults living in Christchurch, New Zealand, Hornblow, Bushnell, Wells, Joyce, and Oakley-Brown (1990) found that only 29 percent of the subjects identified as having a disorder through a community survey had a mental health-related contact during the six-month period being investigated.

Persons having a psychiatric disorder are as likely to be served in the general medical sector as in the specialty mental/addictive sector, with approximately 13 percent of all those with a disorder served in each sector (Regier et al., 1993). The likelihood of being treated in the general medical sector varies by disorder. Only 9.8 percent of those with an alcohol use disorder are being treated for a mental health or substance problem in the general medical sector (Regier et al., 1993). People with somatization are more likely to be treated in the general medical sector than in the mental health specialty sector. Persons with other disorders, such as schizophrenia, are more likely to receive mental health services in the mental health specialty sector than in the general medical sector.

However, it is important to remember that many individuals talking to health professionals about mental or emotional problems do not meet criteria for any specific psychiatric disorder. This is especially true of patients reporting contacts with the general medical sector. The failure of a user of health services to meet standard diagnostic criteria for a psychiatric disorder reflects at least three factors. First, structured psychiatric interviews do not assess all psychiatric disorders, and the reliability of the assessments made varies from disorder to disorder. Second, treatment for mental disorders can be effective. This means that symptoms are reduced while patients are in treatment. Patients assessed during later stages of an episode of illness may no longer meet all diagnostic criteria. Third, patients may talk to doctors about problems to be reassured that they do not have a disorder. Not everyone who seeks clinical services will be determined to be in need of treatment.

Regier et al. (1993) estimate that 15 percent of adults use the de facto mental/addictive disorders service system during a year, irrespective of whether they actually met criteria for a psychiatric disorder. The de facto mental health system consists of all persons—both professionals and nonprofessionals—who provide treatment or mental health-related services (Regier, Goldberg, & Taube, 1978). In the United States, 40 percent of those reporting the use of some services rely on the specialty mental/addictive sector and 43 percent rely on the general medical sector. Only 25 percent rely solely on the specialty mental health service sector and 32 percent rely solely on the general medical sector for services. Thus, the general medical sector is an important source of services for individuals with mental health-related problems.

Besides examining the likelihood that an individual will use general medical services for a mental health problem, it is also important to examine the quantity of mental health-related services being provided in the general medical sector. Using data from the ECA project, Narrow, Regier, Rae, Manderscheid, and Locke (1993) estimate that in a one-year period, 22.8 million adults used ambulatory services for mental or addictive disorder treatment, with 54 percent meeting Diagnostic Interview Schedule (DIS) / DSM-III diagnostic criteria for a mental disorder during the year and another 37.4 percent having had a history of a psychiatric disorder or "significant psychiatric symptoms." Although the study found that many individuals talked to doctors in the general medical sector about their emotional or mental health problems, these individuals tended to have fewer mental health services-related contacts than persons using the mental health specialty sector. Narrow et al. (1993) estimate that 11.1 percent of all mental health-related visits are to the general medical sector, compared to 40.5 percent of the total visits to the mental and addictive disorder specialty settings and 27 percent of the contacts to support networks of friends, relatives, or self-help groups. This suggests the need for future studies to examine separately the propensity to use the health sector for mental health services and the quantity of mental health services utilized.

There is no national system for monitoring the use of ambulatory mental health services (Leaf, 1985). To assess the utility of the reports of service utilization generated by the ECA project, Manderscheid, Rae, Narrow, Locke, and Regier (1993) have compared the reports of service use from the ECA project with estimates generated by the following sources: the National Institute of Mental Health (NIMH) National Reporting Program; the National Drug and Alcoholism Treatment Utilization Survey (NDATUS), conducted jointly by the National Institute of Alcohol Abuse and Alcoholism and the National Institute of Drug Abuse; the National Medical Care Utilization and Expenditure Survey; and the National Ambulatory Medical Care Surveys, conducted by the National Center for Health Statistics (Manderscheid, Witkin, Rosenstein, & Bass,

1986). Although data for mental health specialty services generated from the ECA were similar to estimates from the NIMH National Reporting system, greater inconsistencies existed for the estimates of mental health services provided in the general medical sector. Here the estimates from the ECA project tended to be higher than those generated from other studies.

Self-reported mental health visits may overestimate actual service provision because clinicians may not provide any treatment during these contacts even if the patient reports that mental health or emotions were discussed during the visit. The study by Manderscheid et al. (1993) tends to support this hypothesis. On the other hand, the analyses conducted by Manderscheid et al. confirm the important role played by the general medical sector in the treatment of persons with psychiatric disorders.

Impact of Mental Health Status on Use of Health Services

Although many studies have found that people seen by physicians frequently have mental or emotional problems, fewer studies have addressed the role of mental disorders and psychological distress in the use of health services. Research on the relationship between mental health status and use of health services is important, because this research has implications for reducing the morbidity that accompanies psychiatric disorders and because unnecessary or poorly targeted mental health-related services add to the overall cost of health care. Most earlier research on the relationship between mental health status and service use focused on the relationship between distress and use of health services. For example, Tessler, Mechanic, and Dimond (1976) found in a study of 327 persons enrolled in a prepaid group practice plan that psychological distress, as measured by five questions ascertaining subjective assessments of stress, was related to both total visits and visits initiated by patients with symptoms. The variance associated with distress after controlling for sociodemographic, attitudinal, and health status variables was between 2 and 4 percent, depending on the measure of service use employed in the analysis.

Other researchers—such as Levkoff, Cleary, and Wetle

(1987)—have found distress to be related to use of services, although the residual variance explained by the measures of distress is less than 4 percent. For example, in a recent study of 1,009 Medicare recipients, Berkanovic and Hurwicz (1989) found that psychological distress, measured by life events, life strains, and demoralization, showed little relationship to use of physicians. Factors such as the seriousness of the illness, as measured by the perceptions of the subject, and the number of restricted activity days were much more important in predicting visits to the doctor. Psychological distress explained only 3 percent of the variance in patient requested visits and accounted for only 1 percent of the variance when examined in conjunction with self-rated health and the number of chronic conditions.

Using data from the RAND Health Insurance Experiment, Manning and Wells (1992) examined the effects of mental health status on the use of general medical services. This study goes beyond earlier investigations because it examines the effects of mental health on both inpatient and outpatient general medical services and total expenditures for services in six different communities. On the other hand, several groups were excluded in this study: individuals sixty-two years of age or older at the time of enrollment, individuals with incomes greater than $25,000 in 1973 (equivalent to $61,000 in 1985), individuals in the military or their dependents, individuals eligible for Medicare disability, and veterans with service-connected disabilities. The data used in this study represented 16,319 person-years.

In this study, indicators of physical health, general health perceptions, and mental health status were available, with mental health status determined by indicators of both psychological distress and psychological well-being. In examining the effects of mental health status on the use of general medical services, Manning and Wells employed statistical analyses with a series of nested models. As had been found in earlier studies (Hoeper et al., 1980; Leaf, Bruce, Tischler, Weissman, & Myers, 1988; Mechanic, Cleary, & Greenley, 1982; Tessler, Mechanic, & Dimond, 1976), Manning and Wells found that in the absence of adjustments for other health status, a summary measure of mental health and measures of psychological well-being and psychological distress demonstrate statistically significant associations with various measures of the use of general medical services. Of the measures examined in this study, psychological distress displayed the greatest effect on the annual probability of any medical care, the annual probability of any inpatient medical care, and total medical care expenditures. This held true even when the model controlled for physical health and psychological well-being.

When Manning and Wells (1992) added sociodemographic factors, health status, and insurance coverage as covariates, the composite measure of mental health status was not related to service use. Psychological well-being and psychological distress had statistically significant but opposite effects on medical use. People with higher levels of psychological well-being used more services when controlling for all factors, including psychological distress, but people with greater psychological distress used more services when controlling for all additional factors including psychological well-being. It is unclear whether this finding is due to the correlation between the two indicators of mental health or whether those who feel better about their lives use more services when experiencing distress.

Another important feature of the RAND study is its attention to issues related to inpatient services. Manning and Wells (1992) point out that inpatient services related to mental disorders generate greater costs than ambulatory services. Here, their findings consistently show that mental health status is related to use of general medical inpatient services, even when controlling for other factors related to the use of these services. They estimate that the occurrence of a new episode of a major psychiatric disorder would increase the likelihood of an inpatient medical episode by 10 percent. Most epidemiologic surveys of mental health services have not examined the use of inpatient general medical services by persons experiencing psychiatric disorders; the RAND study suggests that greater attention should be paid to this potential cost of mental illness.

These studies highlight the need to differentiate between factors related to different aspects of service utilization. Future research needs to pay greater attention to specific aspects of distress and disease and to control for other factors related to the use of health services, such as physical health and the existence of chronic health conditions. For example, in their analysis of data from the New Haven, Connecticut ECA project, Leaf et al. (1988) examined the effects of several indicators of mental health while controlling for a variety of predisposing and enabling factors. Subjective assessments of the subject's mental health, the existence of a recent or psychiatric disorder as assessed by the DIS (Robins, Helzer, Croughan, & Ratcliff, 1981), and reports of disability due to mental or emotional problems were correlated with the use of mental health services in both the mental health specialty and the general medical sector. When predisposing and enabling factors were examined in the same statistical models, each indicator of mental health had an independent effect on the use of the mental health specialty sector, but only indicators of recent psychiatric disorder and subjective assessment of mental health were related to reports of mental health services in the general medical sector.

It is clear from the earlier research that something about psychiatric disorders leads individuals and/or family members to seek advice from health professionals. Because individuals with different psychiatric disorders have different probabilities of seeking help from the general health care sector, it is equally clear that assessing psychiatric status alone is inadequate if we want to understand why persons seek help for their psychiatric disorders and where help will be sought. Leaf et al. (1988) examined several indicators of need for mental health services, psychiatric status, self-reported mental health, and disability due to mental health problems. They found that in the absence of some indicator of a need for mental health services, none of the enabling or predisposing factors had an effect on the use of general medical services for the treatment of mental or emotional problems.

Self-reports of disability attributed to mental health problems was the only indicator of service need that differentiated the use of general medical services from the use of the mental health specialty sector. Reports of physical dysfunction increased the likelihood that the mental health services would be provided in the general medical sector. This suggests that distress is one aspect of psychiatric disorders that leads to service use and that the nature of this distress may influence the type of person from whom help is sought. This research also suggests that greater attention needs to be paid to the specific measures used to assess disorder and distress and their relationships to use of health services. Indicators of disorder and distress may not be interchangeable, even if each has a significant impact on the use of general medical services for the treatment of mental or emotional disorders. If we want to understand why some people seek help from the primary medical care sector, we not only need to include measures of symptoms and services that will allow us to determine who is in need of mental health services; we also have to include measures that will allow us to differentiate who will seek services from the general medical sector and who will turn to mental health professionals.

In addition, it is important to recognize that treatment settings differ in the likelihood that patients seen by a primary care provider will have a psychiatric disorder. Bruce, Tischler, and Leaf (1992) examined the data from the five ECA sites to determine whether individuals differing in their usual source of medical services also differed in terms of the likelihood of having a psychiatric disorder. People whose usual source of medical care was a health plan were least likely to have any psychiatric disorder as measured by the DIS, with 16 percent of the subjects meeting criteria for one or more DIS/DSM-III psychiatric disorders. Persons using an emergency room as their usual source of medical care (28.1 percent) and those using outpatient clinics (24.9 percent) were the most likely to meet criteria for a DIS/DSM-III psychiatric disorder. Reports of not having a usual source of care varied from 5.8 percent in Baltimore to 25.4 percent in Los Angeles.

Use of the mental health specialty services also varied by usual source of care. For those whose usual source of care was a health plan, 5.7 percent reported using a service in the mental health specialty sector during the six months before being interviewed. People using private practitioners had the lowest rates of specialty mental health service use (3 percent). Future research will need to pay greater attention to the organization and financing of general medical services when investigating the impact of mental disorders on the use of these services.

Alternative Strategies

Although most research investigating the impact of mental disorders on the use of health services involves observational studies, data from clinical trials are also relevant for understanding factors related to the use of general medical services for the treatment of individuals with psychiatric disorders. Katon et al. (1992) conducted one of the few studies of the impact of psychiatric consultation interventions on patients who frequently use primary care providers. They examined patients of eighteen physicians in two primary care clinics. Patients receiving psychiatric consultations were more likely to be prescribed antidepressant medications and were more likely to be using these medications six months after the consultation. The study did not, however, find significant differences at six or twelve months in utilization of health care services, and thus no offset benefits could be documented. On the other hand, Smith, Monson, and Ray (1986) showed that the costs associated with providing health care to persons with somatization disorder could be significantly reduced by providing general practitioners with psychiatric consultation. Additional research is needed to determine how the organization and financing of primary care services affect the quantity of services used by individuals with psychiatric disorders and the nature of the services used.

Detection of Psychiatric Disorders in Primary Care Settings

Several studies have shown that few individuals with psychiatric disorders receive services from mental health specialists and that the majority receive no treatment for their disorders (Leaf et al., 1985; Shapiro, Skinner, Kramer, Steinwachs, & Regier, 1985). An important component of the lack of treatment is the failure of primary care providers and other general physicians to detect the existence of psychiatric disorders in their patients. Shapiro et al. (1987) attempted to improve detection by providing feedback to providers using the General Health Questionnaire (GHQ), a psychiatric screening instrument. Their randomized clinical trial of patients in a large group practice produced only minor increases in detection. Although detection was lower among older individuals, the feedback provided to clinicians resulted in significantly higher detection of older individuals with mental health problems (German et al., 1987). Smith et al. (1986) have shown that providing psychiatric consultation in the care of patients with somatization disorder reduces subsequent cost of treatment through a reduction in the use of hospitalization. Hankin, Goodman, and Starfield (1987) found little impact on physician practice when they provided pediatricians with the results from the Child Behavior Checklist. Too few randomized clinical trials have been conducted in general medical settings to investigate the impact of alternative treatment strategies on the subsequent use of health care services for patients with specific psychiatric disorders. Studies providing feedback to physicians have not necessarily structured the information so that the physicians could make best use of this information (see Chapter Ten).

Use of Health Services by Children with Psychiatric Disorders

In 1975, Haggerty, Roghmann, and Pless (1975) sought to focus the attention of health care providers on "the new morbidity," the psychiatric and psychosocial problems being encountered by pediatricians with increasing frequency. Since then, a number of studies have identified high rates of psychiatric, psychological, and social morbidity in children seen in pediatric practices (Costello, Edelbrock, Costello, Dulcan, & Brent, 1988; Garralda & Bailey, 1986; Giel et al., 1981; Goldberg, Regier, McInerny, Pless, & Roghmann, 1979; Goldberg, Roghmann, McInerny, & Burke, 1984; Horwitz, Leaf, Leventhal, Forsyth, & Speechley, 1992; Lavigne et al., 1992) and more frequent use of health services by children with these problems (Nader, Ray, & Brink, 1981; Starfield et al., 1985). Research on the use of health services by children with psychiatric disorders has, however, lagged behind the research focusing on the use of services by adults.

Increased Utilization of Primary Health Care Services

Most studies of the use of health services by children with psychiatric disorders start with children sampled from providers. Offord and his colleagues (1987) conducted one of the few population-based surveys examining the impact of a child's mental health on his or her use of general medical services. This study involved 1,869 children aged four to sixteen years living in Ontario, Canada. Three measures of mental health were used in the study. The first measure consisted of a global assessment of the child's behavioral/emotional problems. The second consisted of twenty-one items assessing externalizing symptoms and twenty-five items assessing internalizing symptoms (Boyle et al., 1987). The third measure consisted of using the internalizing and externalizing symptoms to approximate the criteria for four psychiatric disorders that occur frequently in children: conduct disorder, hyperactivity, emotional disorder, and somatization.

The study also included four measures of health status, including (1) a four-item scale adapted from the RAND Measure of Children's Health, (2) an assessment of chronic medical conditions, (3) the existence of chronic physical limitations during the past six months, and (4) the existence of asthma or hay fever. These last two conditions were assessed separately because of their frequency (18.5 percent) in the population (Woodward et al., 1988).

Of the children included in this study, 58 percent had used some medical services during the six months preceding the study interview. Children identified by parents as having more mental health problems than their peers were more likely to use some health service. These children were also more likely to be among the small group of children (18 percent) who used ambulatory medical services three or more times during the preceding six months, accounting for two-thirds of all the services used. Frequent utilizers were seen by their parents to have more internalizing and externalizing problems than children who did not use medical services or those who had only one or two visits in the six months before the interview. Of the children identified as having more emotional problems than their peers, 38 percent were frequent utilizers of health services, compared to only 17 percent of those children not having more emotional problems than their peers.

In another report of data from the same study, Offord et al. (1987) examined the relationship between the existence of four psychiatric disorders (conduct disorder, hyperactivity, emotional disorder, and somatization) and the use of ambulatory medical services. In contrast to the report of Woodward et al. (1988), children with one or more of these disorders were no more likely to have used medical services in the six months prior to the interview than those without one of the four disorders (58.8 versus 59.4 percent), although children with a disorder were 1.8 times as likely to have received a special education service at some point in their lives.

When Woodward et al. (1988) examined in a single statistical model all the factors potentially affecting the use of ambulatory medical services, the parent's assessment of child mental health was not related to the use of ambulatory medical care services, although the general physical health scale, age, urbanicity, existence of chronic medical conditions, and mother's education level all exerted independent effects on utilization. This finding is consistent with the studies of adults reviewed earlier. Similar to the studies of adults, child mental health status did have a significant effect on the volume of services used for children having at least one ambulatory medical care visit, even after accounting for the other factors related to the use of health services. Other factors found to affect the volume of services were the child's general physical health, the existence of chronic medical conditions, and the parent's mental health. This raises questions about the best way to measure symptoms and distress in studies of health service use by children. It is not likely that parents examine the indicators of specific psychiatric disorders when considering consultations with primary care providers. A parent's perception of a problem rather than the actual severity of a symptom or the underlying disorder may be the critical factor in the use of medical services by a child.

Parents' own mental and emotional problems probably contribute to the overuse of medical services by children. Tessler and Mechanic (1978), examining utilization of pediatric services in a prepaid group practice, found psychological distress in the mother to predict the amount of service utilization for the children, but only in white females. Gortmaker, Eckenrode, and Gore (1982) found a significant increase in the probability of health service utilization for children associated with the presence of a stressful event in the family. Their results were similar to those reported in an earlier study by Roghmann and Haggerty (1973). Horwitz, Morgenstern, and Berkman (1985b), in a review of the literature, concluded that psychosocial stressors among parents did predict utilization for children, but that the link was weak. Their own study (Horwitz et al., 1985a) of 513 families in a prepaid group practice in a university community failed to find such links. They point out that a number of methodological problems exist that may account for often inconsistent results in studies examining this issue. In particular, they note the difficulty of conceptualizing and measuring stress and psychological distress, as well as the difficulty in obtaining measures of health status independent of utilization (Horwitz et al., 1985b).

Provision of Services

Although pediatricians and other primary care providers play an important role in the detection and treatment of psychiatric disorders, a number of questions can be raised concerning the adequacy with which they perform this role. Research conducted in medical settings consistently finds that few children with psychiatric disorder have these disorders identified by primary care providers. Costello (1986), reviewing a number of studies that investigated identification of mental health problems by primary care physicians, concluded that the physicians identified only about one-half of all children with mental health problems and referred only one-half of these children for treatment. In their study of 789 children aged seven to eleven years attending pediatric primary care clinics in a health maintenance organization (HMO), Costello et al. (1988) found that 25 percent met criteria based on the Child Behavior Checklist (Achenbach & Edelbrock, 1983), 6 percent were diagnosed by a pediatrician, and 12 percent met criteria on a structured interview with a parent for a psychiatric disorder. Only 17 percent of the children who were identified by the parental interview as meeting criteria for behavioral or emotional problems were identified by the pediatricians. Giel et al. (1981) reported that in the four study areas of the World Health Organization collaborative study on strategies for extending mental health services, the frequency of mental disorder was 12 to 29 percent among children presenting to primary care facilities. When the primary health care provider's assessment was compared to psychiatric assessments, only 10 to 22 percent of the mental health problems were recorded.

However, in a more recent study investigating nineteen randomly chosen pediatric practices, Horwitz et al. (1992) found that physicians identified at least one psychosocial or developmental problem in 27 percent of a sample of 1,886 children aged four to eight years. This study used an assessment instrument that was specifically structured for ease of physician recording and that employed a taxonomy developed for primary care settings. The investigators suggest that this may account in part for the increased reporting of problem behaviors. About one-half of the children who were identified were reported to have been offered treatment, either within the practice or through an outside specialty referral.

A number of reasons have been suggested for the underidentification of children's mental health problems by their primary physicians. Costello and colleagues (Costello & Edelbrock, 1985; Costello, Edelbrock, Kalas, Kessler, & Klaric, 1982) believe that pediatricians are more likely to identify the more severe psychiatric disorders in children. The authors suggest that the less severe problems reported by the parents represent subpathological levels that could be transient or developmentally related rather than being an indication of true psychiatric disorder. On the other hand, the failure to note these milder levels of distress could have implications for the provision of preventive care and early intervention.

Horwitz et al. (1992) point out that identification of psychosocial problems is more likely when the child is well known to the pediatrician or during well-child visits when, presumably, more time and opportunity exist to discuss behavioral issues. Certain child and family characteristics, such as the child's gender, the type of psychiatric disorder the child has, the marital status of the mother, or the socioeconomic level of the family, also may influence the likelihood of physician identification (Goldberg et al., 1984; Horwitz et al., 1992; Starfield et al., 1980). In addition, pediatricians may be more likely to diagnose psychiatric disorders among older children and adolescents (Goldberg et al., 1984). Since the majority of children seen in pediatricians' practices tend to be younger children, the problems of large numbers of young children could be overlooked in these settings.

Physicians must, of course, rely to a great extent on parents' reports in determining whether a child has a psychosocial problem; a child is unlikely to present a range of symptoms adequate for diagnosis in the course of an office visit. The willingness or propensity of parents to raise such issues has received some attention. Hickson, Altemeier, and O'Connor (1983) found in a sample of children presenting for care in private pediatric practices that while the main concern of a majority (70 percent) of mothers was centered around nonmedical, psychosocial issues, only a small percentage of these mothers (28 percent) discussed these issues with the pediatrician. The degree of concern the mother had about these issues did not predict whether the mother would raise the issue with the pediatrician. Starfield et al. (1980) found in an HMO that routinely screened for psychosocial difficulties that about two-thirds of the children were reported to have such problems, but only 5 to 14 percent (depending on the child's age, gender, and race) of the parents asked for appointments to discuss the problems.

Even when children are identified in primary care settings, methods of treatment are far from standardized, and there remains the issue of the capability of primary care physicians to treat the variety and complexity of problems that childhood disorders may present. Jensen, Xenakis, Shervette, Bain, and Davis (1989) examined the charts of sixty-eight children at two clinics in military general hospitals who were diagnosed as having attention deficit disorder and who were prescribed psychostimulant medication. The audit of the medical record found that only about half (52 percent) of the children actually met criteria for attention deficit disorder. The investigators judged the overall quality of treatment to be less than adequate in about two-thirds of the cases. Kelleher, Hohmann, and Larson (1989) reviewed the prescription of psychotropic medications, concurrent psychotherapy, and frequency of follow-up arrangements for children seen in pediatric settings using data from the 1985 National Ambulatory Medical Care Survey. They concluded that many children for whom psychotropic medication was prescribed were not receiving optimal treatment: few were receiving any special follow-up or concurrent psychotherapeutic services. Costello and Pantino (1987) have suggested that pediatricians may develop skills in treating a few of the more frequently encountered disorders but that it may be more cost effective to refer most children with suspected psychiatric disorders to specialty care. They note that even in the specialty care sector, it is not usual to find providers who can offer a complete range of treatment for the myriad psychosocial disorders they encounter among children.

Conclusion

There is clear evidence that people seen by primary care providers are more likely to have a psychiatric disorder than others in the general population, and that individuals with psychiatric disorders consume more health care resources and more expensive health care resources than individuals without psychiatric disorders. The few studies with community samples that have controlled for the effects of physical health status while examining the effects of psychiatric status have found that those with high levels of psychiatric symptoms are no more likely than others to present to the general medical sector for treatment. These studies suggest that some or most of the increase in the likelihood to use some health services are accounted for by the co-occurrence of physical and psychiatric disorders.

On the other hand, studies that have examined psychiatric and health status have found that those with psychiatric disorders are more likely to be hospitalized and have longer lengths of stay even when controlling for the effects of physical health status. Once there is some initial contact with a health care provider, psychiatric disorders may increase the cost of health care. Some increase in contacts may be due to the increase in the number of tests used by physicians as they attempt to differentiate between physical and mental illness. This is most pertinent with disorders such as somatization, where the existence of large number of physical symptoms is inherent in the disorder.

Greater attention needs to be paid to differentiating the cost of medical services related to physical problems from costs related to detecting and treating the psychiatric disorders. These studies will involve the use of standardized psychiatric and medical assessments and better monitoring of the provision of services.

The identification and treatment of children with emotional and behavioral problems in primary care settings present special problems. For identification, physicians are dependent to a large extent on parental reports, and parents may be reluctant to initiate discussions of these issues on their own. Although extensive psychiatric examinations may be inappropriate for general pediatric practices, it is certainly feasible in such practices for the physician to screen for psychiatric disorders with brief parent-completed questionnaires. Likewise, parents need to be able to recognize the signs of emotional and behavioral problems and bring these to the attention of physicians. This is not likely to occur unless the parent believes that the physician can do something to help the problem.

Additional research is needed to determine the extent to which the failure to provide effective services to children seen in primary care settings is the result of the failure of the parent or physician to recognize the problem, an unwillingness by the parent to discuss the problem with physicians, the lack of familiarity of the physician with the patient, an unwillingness to comply with treatment recommendations, or the existence of other barriers. Unless more attention is focused on the examination of alternative indicators of need, factors related to the detection of problems, and factors that predispose or enable a person to access health care, future research is likely to generate the same inconsistencies observed in earlier studies.

References

Achenbach, T., & Edelbrock, C. (1983). *Manual for the Child Behavior Checklist.* Burlington: University of Vermont.

Barrett, J. E., Barrett, J. A., Oxman, J. E., & Gerber, P. D. (1988). The prevalence of psychiatric disorders in a primary care practice. *Archives of General Psychiatry, 45,* 1100–1106.

Berkanovic, E., & Hurwicz, M. L. (1989). Psychological distress and the decision to seek medical care among a Medicare population. *Medical Care, 27,* 1058–1075.

Boyle, M. H., Offord, D. R., Hoffman, H. F., Catlin, G. P., Byles, J. A., Cadman, D. T., Crawford, J. W., Links, P. S., Rae-Grant, N., & Szatmari, P. (1987). Ontario Child Health Survey: Methodology. *Archives of General Psychiatry, 44,* 826–831.

Costello, A., Edelbrock, C., Kalas, R., Kessler, M., & Klaric, S. (1982). *National Institute of Mental Health Diagnostic Interview Schedule for Children.* Bethesda, MD: National Institute of Health.

Costello, E. J. (1986). Primary care pediatrics and child psychopathology: A review of diagnostic, treatment, and referral practices. *Pediatrics, 78,* 1044–1051.

Costello, E. J., & Edelbrock, C. (1985). Detection of psychiatric disorders in pediatric primary care: A preliminary report. *Journal of the American Academy of Child Psychiatry, 24,* 771–774.

Costello, E. J., Edelbrock, C., Costello, A. J., Dulcan, M. K., & Brent, D. (1988). Psychopathology in pediatric primary care: The new hidden morbidity. *Pediatrics, 82,* 415–424.

Costello, E. J., & Pantino, T. (1987). The new morbidity: Who should treat it? *Developmental and Behavioral Pediatrics, 8,* 288–291.

Coulehan, J. L., Schulberg, H. C., & Block, M. R. (1989). The efficiency of depression questionnaires for case finding in primary medical care. *Journal of General Internal Medicine, 4,* 541–547.

Cross-National Collaborative Group. (1992). The changing rate of major depression: Cross-national comparisons. *Journal of the American Medical Association, 268,* 3098–3105.

Eaton, W. W., & Kessler, L. (Eds.). (1985). *Epidemiological field methods in psychiatry: The NIMH Epidemiologic Catchment Area program.* Orlando, FL: Academic Press.

Garralda, M. E., & Bailey, D. (1986). Psychological deviance in children attending general practice. *Psychological Medicine, 16,* 423–429.

German, P. S., Shapiro, S., Skinner, E. A., Von Korff, M., Klein, L. E., Turner, R. W., Teitelbaum, M. L., Burke, J., Jr., & Burns, B. J. (1987). Detection and management of mental health problems of older patients by primary care providers. *Journal of the American Medical Association, 257,* 489–493.

Giel, R., de Arango, M. V., Climent, C. E., Harding, T. W., Jorahim, H. H. A., Ladrido-Ignacio, L., Srinvasa-Murthy, R., Salazar, M. C., Wig, N. N., & Younix, Y. O. A. (1981). Childhood mental disorders in primary health care: Results of observations in four developing countries. *Pediatrics, 68,* 677–683.

Goldberg, D. P. (1972). *The detection of psychiatric illness by questionnaire.* Oxford, England: Oxford University Press.

Goldberg, I. D., Regier, D. A., McInerny, T. K., Pless, I. B., & Roghmann, K. J. (1979). The role of the pediatrician in the delivery of mental health services. *Pediatrics, 63,* 898–909.

Goldberg, I. D., Roghmann, K. J., McInerny, T. K., & Burke, J. D., Jr. (1984). Mental health problems among children seen in pediatric practice: Prevalence and management. *Pediatrics, 73,* 278–293.

Gortmaker, S. L., Eckenrode, J., & Gore, S. (1982). Stress and the utilization of health services: A time series and cross-sectional analysis. *Journal of Health and Social Behavior, 23,* 25–28.

Haggerty, R. J., Roghmann, K. J., & Pless, I. B. (Eds.). (1975). *Child health and the community.* New York: Wiley.

Hankin, J. R., Goodman, A., & Starfield, B. (1987, June). *The impact of sharing the results of psychosocial screening on the psychosocial management of the child.* Paper presented at the first annual NIMH Conference on Mental Health in General Medical Settings, Seattle, WA.

Hankin, J. R., & Oktay, J. S. (1979). *Mental disorder and primary medical care: An analytical review of the literature.* Washington, DC: National Institute of Mental Health.

Hickson, G. B., Altemeier, W. A., & O'Connor, S. (1983). Concerns of mothers seeking care in private pediatric offices: Opportunities for expanding services. *Pediatrics, 72,* 619–624.

Hoeper, E. W., Nycz, G. R., Regier, D. A., Goldberg, I. D., Jacobson, A., & Hankin, J. (1980). Diagnosis of mental disorder in adults and increased use of health services in four outpatient settings. *American Journal of Psychiatry, 137,* 207–214.

Horgan, C. M. (1985). Specialty and general ambulatory mental health services. *Archives of General Psychiatry, 43,* 565–572.

Hornblow, A. R., Bushnell, J. A., Wells, J. E., Joyce, P. R., & Oakley-Brown, M. A. (1990). *New Zealand Medical Journal, 12,* 415–417.

Horwitz, S. M., Leaf, P. J., Leventhal, J., Forsyth, B., & Speechley, K. N. (1992). Identification and management of psychosocial and developmental problems in community-based, primary care pediatric practices. *Pediatrics, 89,* 480–485.

Horwitz, S. M., Morgenstern, H., & Berkman, L. F. (1985a). The impact of social stressors and social networks on pediatric medical care use. *Medical Care, 23,* 946–959.

Horwitz, S. M., Morgenstern, H., & Berkman, L. F. (1985b). The use of pediatric medical care: A critical review. *Journal of Chronic Diseases, 38,* 935–945.

Jensen, P. S., Xenakis, S. N., Shervette, R. E., Bain, M. W., & Davis, H. (1989). Diagnosis and treatment of attention deficit disorder in two general hospital clinics. *Hospital and Community Psychiatry, 40,* 708–712.

Katon, W., Von Korff, M., Lin, E., Bush, T., Russo, J., Lipscomb, P., & Wagner, E. (1992). A randomized trial of psychiatric consultation with distressed high utilizers. *General Hospital Psychiatry, 14,* 83–85.

Kelleher, K. J., Hohmann, A. A., & Larson, D. B. (1989). Prescription of psychotropics to children in office-based practice. *American Journal of Diseases of Children, 143,* 855–859.

Kessler, L. G., Tessler, R. C., & Nycz, G. R. (1983). Co-occurrence of psychiatric and medical morbidity in primary care. *Journal of Family Practice, 16,* 319–324.

Klerman, G. L., & Weissman, M. M. (1989). Increasing rates of depression. *Journal of the American Medical Association, 261,* 2229–2235.

Lavigne, J. V., Binns, H., Christoffel, K. K., Hayford, J., Sinacore, J., Rosenbaum, D., Arend, R., McGuire, P., & Pediatric Practice Research Group. (1992, October). *Social/psychological characteristics and health care use among pre-schoolers in fee-for-service office settings.* Paper presented at the sixth annual NIMH International Research Conference on Primary Mental Health Research, Tyson's Corner, VA.

Leaf, P. J. (1985). Mental health service systems research: Adequacy of available organizational and systems data. *American Behavioral Scientist, 28,* 619–638.

Leaf, P. J., Bruce, M. L., Tischler, G. L., Weissman, M. M., & Myers, J. K. (1988). Factors affecting the utilization of specialty and general medical mental health services. *Medical Care, 26,* 9–26.

Leaf, P. J., Livingston, M. M., Tischler, G. L., Weissman, M. M., Holzer, C. E., & Myers, J. K. (1985). Contact with health professionals for the treatment of psychiatric and emotional problems. *Medical Care, 23,* 1322–1337.

Levkoff, S. E., Cleary, P. D., & Wetle, T. (1987). Differences in determinants of physician use between aged and middle-aged persons. *Medical Care, 25,* 1148–1160.

McGee, R., Feehan, M., Williams, S., & Anderson, J. (1992). DSM-III disorders from age 11 to age 15 years. *Journal of the American Academy of Child and Adolescent Psychiatry, 31,* 50–59.

Manderscheid, R. W., Rae, D. S., Narrow, W. E., Locke, B. Z., & Regier, D. A. (1993). Congruence of service utilization estimates from the ECA and other sources. *Archives of General Psychiatry, 50,* 108–114.

Manderscheid, R. W., Witkin, M. J., Rosenstein, M. J., & Bass, R. D. (1986). The national reporting program for mental health statistics: History and findings. *Public Health Reports, 101,* 532–539.

Manning, W. G., Jr., & Wells, K. B. (1992). The effects of psychological distress and psychological well-being on use of medical services. *Medical Care, 30,* 541–553.

Mechanic, D., Cleary, P. D., & Greenley, J. R. (1982). Distress syndromes, illness behavior, access to care, and medical utilization in a defined population. *Medical Care, 20,* 361–372.

Nader, P. R., Ray, L., & Brink, S. G. (1981). The new morbidity: Use of school and community health care resources for behavioral, educational, and social-family problems. *Pediatrics, 67,* 53–60.

Narrow, W. E., Regier, D. A., Rae, D. S., Manderscheid, R. W., & Locke, B. Z. (1993). Use of services by persons with mental and addictive disorders: Findings from the NIMH ECA program. *Archives of General Psychiatry, 50,* 95–107.

Offord, D. R., Boyle, M. H. Szatmari, P., Rae-Grant, N. I., Links, P. S., Cadman, D. T., Byles, J. A., Crawford, J. W., Blum, H. M., Byrne, C., Thomas, H., & Woodward, C. A. (1987). Ontario Child Health Study: 2. Six-month prevalence of disorder and rates of service utilization. *Archives of General Psychiatry, 44,* 832–836.

Regier, D. A., Goldberg, I. D., Burns, B. J., Hankin, J., Hoeper, E. W., & Nycz, G. R. (1982). Specialist/generalist division of responsibility for patients with mental disorders. *Archives of General Psychiatry, 39,* 219–224.

Regier, D. A., Goldberg, I. D., & Taube, C. A. (1978). The de facto

U.S. mental health services system: A public health perspective. *Archives of General Psychiatry, 41,* 934–941.

Regier, D. A., Narrow, W. E., Rae, D. S., Manderscheid, R. W., Locke, B. A., & Goodwin, F. K. (1993). The de facto U.S. mental and addictive disorders service system: ECA prospective one-year prevalence and service use rates. *Archives of General Psychiatry, 50,* 85–94.

Robins, L. N., Helzer, J. E., Croughan, J., & Ratcliff, K. (1981). National Institute of Mental Health Diagnostic Interview Schedule: Its history, characteristics, and validity. *Archives of General Psychiatry, 38,* 381–389.

Robins, L. N., & Regier, D. A. (Eds.). (1991). *Psychiatric disorders in America.* New York: Free Press.

Roghmann, K. J., & Haggerty, R. J. (1973). Daily stress, illness, and use of health services in young families. *Pediatrics Research, 7,* 520–526.

Sartorius, N., Goldberg, D., de Girolamo, G., Silva, J. A. C., Lecrubier, Y., & Wittchen, H.-U. (Eds.). (1990). *Psychological disorders in general medical settings.* Toronto: Hogrefe & Huber.

Shapiro, S., German, P. S., Skinner, E. A., Von Korff, M., Turner, R. W., Klein, L. E., Teitelbaum, M. L., Kramer, M., Burke, J. D., Jr., & Burns, B. J. (1987). An experiment to change detection and management of mental morbidity in primary care. *Medical Care, 25,* 327–339.

Shapiro, S., Skinner, E. A., Kessler, L. G., Von Korff, M., German, P. S., Tischler, G. L., Leaf, P. J., Benham, L., Cottler, O. L., & Regier, D. A. (1984). Utilization of health and mental health services: Three Epidemiologic Catchment Area sites. *Archives of General Psychiatry, 41,* 971–978.

Shapiro, S., Skinner, E. A., Kramer, M., Steinwachs, D. M., & Regier, D. A. (1985). Measuring need for mental health services in a general population. *Medical Care, 23,* 1033–1043.

Shepherd, M., Cooper, B., Brown, A. C., & Kalton, G. (1966). *Psychiatric illness in general practice.* Oxford, England: Oxford University Press.

Smith, G. R., Jr., Monson, R. A., & Ray, D. C. (1986). Psychiatric consultation in somatization disorder: A randomized controlled study. *New England Journal of Medicine, 14,* 1407–1413.

Starfield, B., Gross, E., Wood, M., Pantell, R., Allen, C., Gordon, I. B., Moffatt, P., Drachman, R., & Katz, H. (1980). Psychosocial and psychosomatic diagnoses in primary care of children. *Pediatrics, 66,* 159–167.

Starfield, B., Hankin, J., Steinwachs, D. M., Horn, S., Benson, P., Katz, H., & Gabriel, A. (1985). Utilization and morbidity: Random or tandem? *Pediatrics, 75,* 241–247.

Tessler, R., & Mechanic, D. (1978). Factors affecting children's use of physician services in a prepaid group practice. *Medical Care, 41,* 33–46.

Tessler, R., Mechanic, D., & Dimond, M. (1976). The effect of psychological distress on physician utilization: A prospective study. *Journal of Health and Social Behavior, 17,* 353–364.

Woodward, C. A., Boyle, M. H., Offord, D. R., Cadman, D. T., Links, P. S., Munroe-Blum, H., Byrne, C., & Thomas, H. (1988). Ontario Child Health Study: Patterns of ambulatory medical care utilization and their correlates. *Pediatrics, 82,* 425–434.

17

Curtis J. Henke
Michael S. Pallak

Economic Analysis of Treatment of Mental Disorders in Primary Care

The past decade has witnessed an explosion of interest in the cost of health care treatments and technologies, as a complement to the long-standing interest in the effectiveness of these interventions. In part, this new interest in cost results from the continued growth of aggregate health care expenditures. National health care spending increased 166 percent between 1980 and 1990, while the gross national product (GNP) grew only 100 percent. Consequently the share of the GNP going to health care rose from 9.2 to 12.2 percent during that decade (Levit, Lazenby, Cowan, & Letsch, 1991). Perhaps more important, many health care services that are being utilized are providing results that are worth substantially less than their cost. As a result, an increasing number of evaluations of medical treatments and technologies are examining the costs as well as the consequences. Indeed, the Australian government now requires economic analyses in support of applications for listing of new drugs on its Schedule of Pharmaceutical Benefits (Henry, 1992; Freund, Evans, Henry, & Dittus, 1992), and the U.S. Health Care Financing Administration has proposed using cost-effectiveness in funding decisions (Leaf, 1989). One cornerstone of effective cost containment is the provision of only those services worth their cost.

The question of whether the results are worth the costs needs to be asked when evaluating the treatment of mental disorders in primary care as well. Mental disorders are responsible for a great amount of morbidity (Rice, Kelman, Miller, & Dunmeyer, 1990; Miller & Kelman, 1992), and the treatment of such disorders in primary care may significantly reduce these losses. But their treatment can also result in a substantial cost. In this chapter, we will discuss how economic analyses combine information on the consequences and costs of the treatment of mental disorders to come to a conclusion about which treatments are and which are not worth the cost. We first present the general analytical constructs that have been used in economic analyses of medical care and highlight some of the research about mental health care in general that has utilized each method. Then we explore the application of these techniques specifically to the examination of the treatment of mental disorders in primary care. Finally, we suggest some directions for future research.

Economic Appraisals of Medical Treatments

The essence of an economic analysis—or an *economic appraisal*—of medical treatments is a comparison of their costs and outcomes (Warner & Luce, 1982; Drummond, Stoddart, & Torrance, 1987; Eisenberg, 1989; Detsky & Naglie, 1990). The goal is to determine which treatments provide the greatest value for the least use of resources. To maximize the good accomplished by their efforts, primary care providers should use their time and other resources to treat the patients for whom they can provide the most value per unit of cost. Accordingly, they should treat mental disorders whenever the benefits of this treatment are greater than the benefits to be gained from other uses of the same resources. Or, considering it from the other direction, they should treat patients with mental disorders whenever the cost per unit of outcome is lower than in other uses of the same resources. This is exactly the same rule that is used to evaluate any other medical treatment or technology. Using this principle, economic analyses provide a standard for judging which treatments are appropriate, given the constraints of society's finite resources (Neumann & Weinstein, 1991). While the principle is simple, a number of complexities are involved in its application. These complexities relate to the measurement of cost, the measurement of value, and ways of comparing the two.

In the most fundamental sense, treating mental disorders involves a cost to society because it requires resources that could also be used for other worthwhile purposes. For example, when a physician devotes twenty minutes to counseling a patient with depression, this time is not available to treat another patient with hypertension. The real cost of using twenty minutes to counsel the depressed patient is the loss of whatever would have been accomplished in the visit with the hypertensive patient. Economists call this the *opportunity cost.* More precisely, the opportunity cost of using resources for one thing is the value of what these resources could accomplish if they were instead employed in their most productive alternative use—that is, the value that must be given up to use the resources for the first activity. Even if the provider accomplishes more good in the twenty minutes devoted to the patient with depression than in any other possible use of that time, society still loses the value of the foregone activities. This is why it is so important to consider the cost as well as the effectiveness of the treatment of mental disorders: use of resources for these treatments precludes their use in other valuable activities. Even when there may not appear to be a cost to the individual patient, collectively as a society we lose the value of whatever else the resources could do for us.

Four different types of economic appraisals have been used to evaluate medical care treatments (Freund & Dittus, 1992), and all have been applied to mental health care. They differ from one another primarily in the way the outcomes of care are measured.

Cost-Minimization Analysis

The simplest of the four techniques is *cost-minimization analysis* (CMA), also known as *cost-identification analysis.* CMA considers differences in cost only, under the assumption that the outcomes of the treatment alternatives in question are identical. The goal of CMA is to find the least costly way of achieving the outcome. All economic analyses of treatment cost generally begin by measuring the expenditure necessary to purchase the resources required for the treatment. This is appropriate if, in fact, these expenditures are closely related to opportunity costs. But if the evaluation is made from the perspective of society as a whole, as is generally appropriate, all of the resources required for the treatment should be included, whether or not they are actually purchased. For example, the patients' time and any donated services have opportunity costs, and their value should be included in the calculation of treatment cost. The costs of these additional resources are generally estimated by measuring the quantity of each resource used, then pricing each with a suitable unit cost.

Another important consideration in measuring the cost of treatment of mental disorders by primary care providers occurs because the patient is often under treatment for other conditions as well. In this situation, the cost of treating the mental disorder is only the increment to cost needed to add the mental health care to the other care that would be given anyway. If the patient makes frequent visits for a physical health problem, the additional cost of treating the mental disorder may be small.

The best examples of CMAs concerned with mental health care are the medical cost offset studies, which have addressed the question of whether using mental health services (generally from specialty providers) reduces medical care expenditures among people with mental health problems (Follette & Cummings, 1967; Mumford, Schlesinger, Glass, Patrick, & Cuerdon, 1984; Borus et al., 1985; Holder & Blose, 1987; Fiedler & Wight, 1989). The focus of these studies is entirely on cost differences; possible differences in outcome are not considered. Most of these studies have concluded that a small reduction in physical health care expenditures can be achieved, and a few have found a more substantial saving (Pallak, Cummings, Dorken, & Henke, 1993). If mental health treatment improves outcomes without increasing cost, it is clearly desirable. A CMA could never find this result, because by design it ignores differences in outcome.

The remaining three types of economic analysis of treatments begin with the cost measures developed in CMA and then incorporate differences in the outcomes of the treatments as well.

The primary difference among them is the way they measure the treatment outcomes.

Cost-Effectiveness Analysis

The most direct of these techniques used to compare treatments on the basis of their differences in costs and outcomes is *cost-effectiveness analyses* (CEA). CEA uses natural measures of treatment outcome, such as years of life saved, months of abstinence from alcohol, number of days disabled by depression, or the score on an instrument that measures anxiety symptoms. These analyses are useful when such a single measure of outcome captures all the important differences among the treatments and when that outcome measure is available for all of the treatments in question. The goal of CEA is to determine which treatment produces the outcome at the lowest cost per unit of outcome. When the more effective treatments are also more costly (per unit of outcome), it is important to calculate the incremental effectiveness to be gained from incremental expenditures, both compared to the most cost-effective alternative.

A hypothetical example will illustrate these concepts. Suppose treatment A for depression reduces the score on a depression scale an average of twenty points compared with no treatment, at a cost of $500. Its cost-effectiveness ratio is $500/20 = $25 per point. Treatment B, which produces twenty-five points of improvement at a cost of $1,000, has a cost-effectiveness ratio of $1,000/25 = $40 per point. The additional five points of improvement obtained by treatment B compared to treatment A come at an additional cost of $500, so the incremental cost-effectiveness ratio of treatment B compared to treatment A is $500/5 = $100 per point. In the simple analysis, treatment A would be preferred to treatment B because it is less costly per unit of outcome. Using treatment B would be wasteful because it produced the incremental improvement in depression for $100 per point instead of the $25 per point available under treatment A. The use of treatment B rather than treatment A would be warranted only if there were no other opportunities to produce medical care benefits equivalent to the value of a one-point improvement in depression at a cost of less than $100.

The primary disadvantage of CEA is that it provides no way

of evaluating whether $25 or $100 per point improvement is worthwhile in an absolute sense. Nor does it reveal whether it is preferable to spend $500 for a twenty-point improvement in depression rather than spending the $500 for a thirty-point improvement in another patient's anxiety (measured on a different scale). Only treatments that use exactly the same outcome measure can be compared, and the only conclusion that can be drawn is which of the treatments that are compared is preferred to the others. CEA is also inappropriate when the single measure of effectiveness fails to capture important differences between the treatments. Sometimes an index can be created that incorporates different dimensions of outcome to overcome this limitation.

CEA has been used widely in the evaluation of medical care. In the evaluation of mental health treatments, it has overwhelmingly been the method of choice. Clozapine, imipramine, and lithium have all been shown to be cost effective in certain populations, and the same is true of psychotherapy (Frank, 1992). Assertive case management for the severely mentally ill has been shown to be cost effective (Bond, Miller, Krumwied, & Ward, 1988; Jerrell & Hu, 1989; Hu & Jerrell, 1991). Treatment for alcoholism has been studied extensively using CEA (Holder, Longabaugh, Miller, & Rubonis, 1991).

Cost-Utility Analysis

The limitations of CEA have led to the development of *cost-utility analysis* (CUA). Rather than measuring the treatment outcomes in natural units, CUA identifies the different outcomes that can result from a treatment and rates the satisfaction (utility) associated with each outcome (Torrance, 1976; Kaplan & Bush, 1982; Torrance, 1986). A general measure of treatment outcome is calculated by summing the utilities, weighted by their probabilities of occurrence. Usually, this measure is calibrated as the number of quality-adjusted life years (QALY) that result from each treatment. These QALYs are the measures that are compared to cost in a CUA, in a manner equivalent to the comparison of costs and outcomes in a CEA.

The utility ratings used in CUA are developed through exercises with people similar to those for whom the results are meant to apply (Drummond, Stoddart, & Torrance, 1987). One common method, the standard gamble, is based on the theory of rational decision making under uncertainty developed by Von Neumann and Morgenstern (1953). The *standard gamble* typically elicits a person's assessment of whether he or she prefers a specific suboptimal health state with certainty, or a gamble with a certain probability of a specific good outcome and one minus that probability of a specific bad outcome. By varying the probabilities until the person is indifferent between the certain state and the gamble, the investigator can calculate the relative utilities of each outcome. A second technique used to develop utility measures is the *rating scale,* in which a person subjectively places each health state on a line extending from the best to the worst outcomes. A third method, the *time trade-off,* asks the subject to compare living in a specific unhealthy state for time duration t_1 versus living in a healthy state for time $t_2 < t_1$.

While these techniques are still under development, they have already received extensive research and are now in wide use. The primary disadvantage of CUA is the difficulty of developing utility measures that are consistent and comparable across a range of populations and treatment alternatives.

The primary advantage of CUA over CEA is that the utility measures can be compared over a wide variety of treatments. Not only does this permit a comparison of the value of using $500 to treat depression with the value of using $500 to treat anxiety, but it also allows the comparison of the treatment of mental disorders with a range of physical health treatments. For example, treatments that produce improved quality of life without lengthening it can be compared with treatments that lengthen life with no improvement in quality. Moreover, CUA expresses the outcomes of health care in units that are directly relevant to patient satisfaction, which may be the most appropriate way to measure outcomes. It is now fashionable for reports of CUAs to present tables of the cost per QALY across a range of studies (called *league tables*), so that the results from the current analysis can be put in perspective (Russell, 1989; Drummond, 1992). For example, even though one cannot say that a treatment costing $30,000 per QALY is "worth it" in an absolute sense, one can demonstrate that it has a cost-utility ratio similar to treatment of mild hypertension in men aged forty ($23,175) and estrogen therapy among postmenopausal women who have not had a hysterectomy ($32,760), and a cost-utility ratio much lower than continuous ambulatory peritoneal dialysis ($57,100) and hemodialysis in the hospital ($65,500) (Labelle & Hurley, 1992). This would establish the treatment under study as being preferred to the many others in current use that are more expensive.

CUAs have just begun to be used to evaluate mental health treatments. Kamlet, Wade, Kupfer, and Frank (1992) present an interesting analytical framework for the use of CUA in comparing imipramine to interpersonal psychotherapy (IPT) as maintenance treatment for recurrent depression. They employ a simple Markovian state-transition model to capture the recurrent periods of depression and control through long-term maintenance by each of the treatments. Preliminary results suggest that IPT costs about $10,000 per QALY for a forty-year-old woman (compared to no maintenance therapy). The results for imipramine are quite sensitive to variations in the utility measurement.

Cost-Benefit Analysis

Cost-benefit analysis (CBA) is the only one of this group of economic appraisals that results in a conclusion about whether or not a treatment produces outcomes whose values are greater than the costs. It can do this because it measures benefits in dollar terms. This measure is comprehensive, including societal benefits that extend beyond the personal benefits included in CUA and the single dimension of outcome of a CEA. If the measure of costs accurately represents the opportunity cost of the resources used, and the measure of benefits is similarly based on the true value of the outcomes, the fact that the benefits are larger than the costs indicates that the treatment should be done.

The strength of CBA is the measurement of all outcomes in dollar terms, but this is also its weakness. Many of the outcomes relevant to the evaluation of medical treatments are difficult, if not impossible, to price in dollars. Even though some investigators have developed measures of the value of a year of life or of particular types of infirmity, these estimates vary widely from study to study

(Jones-Lee, 1976) and often seem questionable. In addition, quantifying the dollar value of the great variety of health outcomes that need to be compared would require more assumptions than those needed for CUA, with little apparent advantage. Therefore, even though CBA has been used extensively for evaluation of construction and development projects, it is not widely employed in the economic evaluation of medical care.

The most notable example of the use of CBA in mental health care is the work done by Weisbrod and colleagues in Dane County, Wisconsin, as part of the evaluation of case management in the community versus hospitalization for the mentally ill (Stein & Test, 1980; Weisbrod, Test, & Stein, 1980; Weisbrod, 1981). They used a comprehensive measure of costs including direct and indirect treatment costs, law enforcement costs, and lost earnings of family members due to caring for the patient. The only benefits that were quantified in monetary terms were the earnings of the patients, although a number of other benefits were measured in their natural units. The results showed that treatment costs greatly exceeded the dollar benefits in both the community and the hospital programs, although the discrepancy was slightly less in the experimental group. This study clearly illustrates the difficulty of using CBA for the evaluation of mental health treatment.

Evaluating the Treatment of Mental Disorders

CMA, CEA, CUA, and CBA are the four tools of economic appraisal of medical treatments. They are not tools for individual clinical decisions about the treatment of specific patients. Rather, they have been developed to guide the use of our scarce health care resources so that the value of medical services is maximized overall. They perform this function by identifying which treatment alternatives generally provide beneficial outcomes for the smallest use of resources. These tools are useful for evaluating the treatment of mental disorders in primary care only when they compare the alternatives that are relevant in this setting and evaluate the costs and benefits as they occur in this setting. It is well established that patients with mental disorders seen in primary care are different from those seen by specialty mental health providers, and the treatments also differ (Kessler, Cleary, & Burke, 1985; Orleans, George, Houpt, & Brodie, 1985; Schurman, Kramer, & Mitchell, 1985; Kamerow, Pincus, & Macdonald, 1986; Ormel, Koeter, van den Brink, & van de Willige, 1991). Hence the preferred alternatives in the specialty mental health sector may be different from the ones most appropriate for primary care.

Two general sets of choices relate to the treatment of mental disorders by primary care providers. The first is whether a given type of patient in a primary care setting should be treated in that setting, referred to a specialty mental health provider, or left untreated. If a beneficial outcome can be obtained at a cost (per unit of outcome) less than or equal to the cost of obtaining beneficial outcomes in other patients the providers might see, clearly treatment of mental disorders is warranted. But if the amount of benefit resulting from a given expenditure for these treatments is significantly lower than the benefits of treating other types of problems, the economic appraisal would conclude that the mental disorders should not be treated. Because this comparison involves patients of all types with different kinds of outcomes, CUA or CBA would be needed.

The choice between the primary care and specialty providers depends on which setting can provide beneficial outcomes at the lowest cost per unit; if one setting provides outcomes that are both larger and more expensive per unit, an incremental analysis is required. A CEA would be appropriate for this comparison, since the outcomes in the two settings could use the same measure. It is well established that treatment of mental disorders by specialty providers is more expensive than treatment by primary providers (Horgan, 1985; Frank & Kamlet, 1990), but a simple CMA is not appropriate for this assessment because the outcomes are not necessarily equivalent. Both the assessment of whether to treat and the assessment of whether a patient should be seen in the primary or specialty setting will in general depend on the diagnosis, severity, and other characteristics of the patient. Hence the research in this area must be differentiated by type of patient.

The second set of choices concerns the type of treatment to be used for patients who are treated in the primary care setting. Primary care providers use a wide array of diagnostic and therapeutic services for their patients with psychiatric diagnoses (Schurman, Kramer, & Mitchell, 1985). Alternative methods of treatment need to be evaluated with a CEA to determine which are most cost effective. Here, too, the answer will depend on the characteristics of the patients. It may seem that the question of how to treat should be addressed only after it has been decided that particular patients should be treated in primary care practices, as we have discussed it here. But the reverse is more correct; the assessments of the costs and consequences of treatment by primary versus specialty providers is based on an assessment of the best treatment alternatives available if they were to be treated in each setting. Hence the question of whether a patient should be treated in the primary care sector can only be answered after the preferred treatment in each setting has been found.

One interesting aspect of the use of the economic appraisal tools to examine treatment of mental disorders in primary care is that many patients will also be under treatment for a physical health problem. There are at least three ramifications of this. First, the cost of providing the mental health treatment may be lower than it would be otherwise, because the patient is being seen anyway; it is only the additional cost of treating the mental disorder that counts in the economic assessment. Second, there may be a synergy between the mental and physical treatments in some patients, so that the final outcome is better than the sum of what would have been obtained if each problem were treated alone. In this case, all of the improvement above that which would have been obtained with treatment of the physical problem alone should be credited to the mental health treatment. The combination of low incremental cost and high incremental benefit may make treatment of mental disorders in primary care practices much more cost effective than treatment in specialty practices, at least for patients who have physical problems as well as mental disorders. The third ramification of treating patients for both physical and mental problems is that the primary care provider is likely to have a broader objective for treatment than the specialty provider. This may make it difficult to find a single effectiveness measure that is appropriate for both settings.

This discussion of the appropriate referral and treatment choices has ignored payment for services. Ample evidence exists that levels of insurance and reimbursement influence patients' willingness to receive, and providers' willingness to supply, the quantity of mental health services warranted by these analyses (Manning, Wells, Duan, Newhouse, & Ware, 1984; Kamerow, Pincus, & Macdonald, 1986). The economic appraisals are designed to determine the care that is most appropriate from a societal perspective, weighing both costs and benefits. If the health care financing system contains incentives that lead to too much or too little use of services, this is an indication that the financing system is promoting economic inefficiency and may be in need of reform.

Conceptually, all of these decisions for primary care providers can, and should, be investigated using economic appraisal. While there have been efficacy and effectiveness studies investigating the treatment of mental disorders in primary care, the published literature apparently contains not even one cost-effectiveness, cost-utility, or cost-benefit study. A computer search could not locate a single paper. It is important to reiterate that the patients with mental disorders who are treated in primary care practices are different from the patients treated in specialty mental health practices and that the treatments differ as well. Therefore, the results reported in economic analyses of patients of psychiatrists, psychologists, or mental health clinics, or for patients from all practice settings together, may not apply to primary care practices.

Conclusion

Economic analyses of the treatment of mental disorders in primary care are critically needed at this time. The National Institute of Mental Health is encouraging economic appraisals of mental health care (Larson et al., 1987; Krupnick & Pincus, 1992), and some work related specifically to primary care is in progress. Research that addresses the following six priorities will be particularly useful.

1. Standardized outcome measures should be used as much as possible. The results from different CEAs are directly comparable only if they use the same measures of outcome, and any single study is far more useful if its results can be compared to studies of similar

treatments. Standardized outcomes will also aid in comparing the effects of the same treatments on different populations.

2. Standard techniques for measuring costs should also be used, and the costs should be measured as comprehensively as possible.

3. While CEA may be the technique of choice for comparing treatments with similar outcomes, the more common treatments should also be evaluated with CUA. This is the only way that the cost-effectiveness of treating mental disorders can be compared to the cost-effectiveness of physical health treatments. During the current period of increased concern about health care costs, it will be crucial to demonstrate that mental health care is as cost effective as other commonly used medical services. Further work on the utility assessment methods must include the development of reliable ways to measure utilities associated with outcomes of mental disorders.

4. Economic analyses must concentrate specifically on primary care. The differences between the primary and specialty sectors are too great to generalize results from one setting to the other with confidence.

5. Primary care and specialty care need to be compared for a variety of psychiatric diagnoses and physical comorbidities. Undoubtedly primary care will be more cost effective for some types of patients, and specialty care will be more cost effective for other patients.

6. To understand the special role that a primary care provider can play in the treatment of mental disorders, research is needed to elucidate the interactions of mental and physical treatments in the determination of costs and outcomes. If a positive synergy exists for outcomes, treatment of mental and physical problems by the same provider may be particularly beneficial.

Randomized trials will be neither feasible nor suitable for many of these questions. Investigators performing economic analyses should have the skills to use a variety of nonexperimental research designs. But these research methods need to be utilized carefully, to avoid biases due to self-selection of patients into the different treatment groups.

The treatment of mental disorders in primary care must be subjected to economic appraisal if these therapies are to find their suitable place in an efficient medical care system. Now more than ever, health care resources are scarce when compared to the population's need and desire for medical care services. We cannot permit ourselves the luxury of wasting resources on services that are not cost effective when tens of millions of Americans are receiving inadequate medical care.

References

Bond, G. R., Miller, L. D., Krumwied, R. D., & Ward, R. S. (1988). Assertive case management in three CMHCs: A controlled study. *Hospital and Community Psychiatry, 39,* 411–418.

Borus, J. F., Olendzki, M. C., Kessler, L., Burns, B. J., Brandt, U. C., Broverman, C. A., & Henderson, P. R. (1985). The 'offset effect' of mental health treatment on ambulatory medical care utilization and charges. *Archives of General Psychiatry, 42,* 573–580.

Detsky, A. S., & Naglie, I. G. (1990). A clinician's guide to cost-effectiveness analysis. *Annals of Internal Medicine, 113,* 147–154.

Drummond, M. F. (1992). Basing prescription drug payment on economic analyses: The case of Australia. *Health Affairs, 11*(4), 191–196.

Drummond, M. F., Stoddart, G. L., & Torrance, G. W. (1987). *Methods for the economic evaluation of health care programs.* Oxford, England: Oxford University Press.

Eisenberg, J. M. (1989). Clinical economics: A guide to the economic analysis of clinical practices. *Journal of the American Medical Association, 262,* 2879–2886.

Fiedler, J. L., & Wight, J. B. (1989). *The medical offset effect and public health policy.* New York: Praeger.

Follette, W. T., & Cummings, N. A. (1967). Psychiatric services and medical utilization in a prepaid health plan setting. *Medical Care, 5,* 25–35.

Frank, R. G. (1992, September). *Cost effectiveness of treatment for mental disorders: Implications for mental health care financing policy.* Paper presented at the sixth biennial Research Conference on the Economics of Mental Health, Bethesda, MD.

Frank, R. G., & Kamlet, M. S. (1990). Economic aspects of patterns of mental health care: Cost variation by setting. *General Hospital Psychiatry, 12,* 11–18.

Freund, D. A., & Dittus, R. S. (1992). Principles of pharmacoeconomic analysis of drug therapy. *ParmacoEconomics, 1,* 20–31.

Freund, D. A., Evans, D., Henry, D., & Dittus, R. (1992). Implications of the Australian guidelines for the United States. *Health Affairs, 11*(4), 202–206.

Henry, D. (1992). Economic analysis as an aid to subsidisation decisions. *PharmacoEconomics, 1,* 54–67.

Holder, H. D., & Blose, J. O. (1987). Mental health treatment and the reduction of health care costs. In R. M. Scheffler & L. F. Rossiter (Eds.), *Advances in health economics and health services research* (Vol. 8). Greenwich, CT: JAI Press.

Holder, H., Longabaugh, R., Miller, W. R., & Rubonis, A. V. (1991). The cost effectiveness of treatment for alcoholism: A first approximation. *Journal of Studies on Alcohol, 52,* 517–540.

Horgan, C. M. (1985). Specialty and general ambulatory mental health services. *Archives of General Psychiatry, 42,* 565–572.

Hu, T.-W., & Jerrell, J. (1991). Cost effectiveness of alternative approaches in treating severely mentally ill in California. *Schizophrenia Bulletin, 17,* 461–468.

Jerrell, J. M., & Hu, T.-W. (1989). Cost effectiveness of intensive clinical and case management compared with an existing system of care. *Inquiry, 26,* 224–234.

Jones-Lee, M. W. (1976). *The value of life: An economic analysis.* Chicago: University of Chicago Press.

Kamerow, D. B., Pincus, H. A., & Macdonald, D. I. (1986). Alcohol abuse, other drug abuse, and mental disorders in medical practice. *Journal of the American Medical Association, 255,* 2054–2057.

Kamlet, M. S., Wade, M., Kupfer, D. J., & Frank, E. (1992). Cost-utility analysis of maintenance treatment for recurrent depression: A theoretical framework and numerical illustration. In R. G. Frank & W. G. Manning, Jr. (Eds.). *Economics and mental health.* Baltimore, MD: Johns Hopkins University Press.

Kaplan, R. M., & Bush, J. W. (1982). Health-related quality of life measurement for evaluation research and policy analysis. *Health Psychology, 1,* 61–80.

Kessler, L. G., Cleary, P. D., & Burke, J. D. (1985). Psychiatric disorders in primary care. *Archives of General Psychiatry, 42,* 583–587.

Krupnick, J. L., & Pincus, H. A. (1992). The cost effectiveness of psychotherapy: A plan for research. *American Journal of Psychiatry, 149,* 1295–1304.

Labelle, R. J., & Hurley, J. E. (1992). Implications of basing health-care resource allocations on cost-utility analysis in the presence of externalities. *Journal of Health Economics, 11,* 259–277.

Larson, D. B., Kessler, L. C., Burns, B. B., Pincus, H. A., Houpt, J. L., Fiester, L., & Chaitkin, L. (1987). A research development workshop to stimulate outcome research in consultation-liaison psychiatry. *Hospital and Community Psychiatry, 38,* 1106–1109.

Leaf, A. (1989). Cost effectiveness as a criterion for Medicare coverage. *New England Journal of Medicine, 321,* 898–900.

Levit, K. R., Lazenby, H. C., Cowan, C. A., & Letsch, S. W. (1991). National health expenditures, 1990. *Health Care Financing Review, 13*(1), 29–54.

Manning, W. G., Jr., Wells, K. B., Duan, N., Newhouse, J. P., & Ware, J. E., Jr. (1984). Cost sharing and the use of ambulatory mental health services. *American Psychologist, 39,* 1077–1089.

Miller, L. S., & Kelman, S. (1992). Estimates of the loss of individual productivity from alcohol and drug abuse and from mental illness. In R. G. Frank, & W. G. Manning, Jr. (Eds.). *Economics and mental health.* Baltimore: Johns Hopkins University Press.

Mumford, E., Schlesinger, H. J., Glass, G. V., Patrick, C., & Cuerdon, T. (1984). A new look at evidence about reduced cost of medical utilization following mental health treatment. *American Journal of Psychiatry, 141,* 1145–1158.

Neumann, P. J., & Weinstein, M. C. (1991). The diffusion of new technology: Costs and benefits to health care. In A. C. Gelijns & E. A. Halm (Eds.). *The changing economics of medical technology.* Washington, DC: National Academy Press.

Orleans, C. T., George, L. K., Houpt, J. L., & Brodie, H. K. H. (1985). How primary care physicians treat psychiatric disorders: A national survey of family practitioners. *American Journal of Psychiatry, 142,* 52–57.

Ormel, J., Koeter, M. W., van den Brink, W., & van de Willige, G. (1991). Recognition, management, and course of anxiety and depression in general practice. *Archives of General Psychiatry, 48,* 700–706.

Pallak, M. S., Cummings, N. A., Dorken, H., & Henke, C. J. (1993). Managed mental health treatment, Medicaid, and medical cost offset. In S. H. Feldman & W. Goldman (Eds.), *Managed Mental Health Care.* New Directions in Mental Health Care. San Francisco: Jossey-Bass.

Rice, D. P., Kelman, S., Miller, L. S., & Dunmeyer, S. (1990). *The economic costs of alcohol and drug abuse and mental illness: 1985.* Reports submitted to the Office of Financing and Coverage Policy of the Alcohol, Drug Abuse, and Mental Health Administration, U.S. Department of Health and Human Services. San Francisco: University of California, Institute for Health and Aging.

Russell, L. B. (1989). Some of the tough decisions required by a national health plan. *Science, 246,* 892–896.

Schurman, R. A., Kramer, P. D., & Mitchell, J. B. (1985). The hidden mental health network. *Archives of General Psychiatry, 42,* 89–94.

Stein, L. I., & Test, M. A. (1980). An alternative to mental hospital treatment: 1. Conceptual model, treatment programs, and clinical evaluation. *Archives of General Psychiatry, 37,* 392–397.

Torrance, G. W. (1976). Toward a utility theory foundation for health status index models. *Health Services Research, 11,* 349–369.

Torrance, G. W. (1986). Measurement of health state utilities for economic appraisal: A review. *Journal of Health Economics, 5,* 1–30.

Von Neumann, J., & Morgenstern, O. (1953). *Theory of games and economic behavior.* New York: Wiley.

Warner, K. E., & Luce, B. R. (1982). *Cost-benefit and cost-effectiveness analysis in health care: Principles, practice, and potential.* Ann Arbor, MI: Health Administration Press.

Weisbrod, B. A. (1981). Benefit-cost analysis of a controlled experiment: Treating the mentally ill. *Journal of Human Resources, 16,* 523–548.

Weisbrod, B. A., Test, M. A., & Stein, L. I. (1980). An alternative to mental hospital treatment: 2. Economic benefit-cost analysis. *Archives of General Psychiatry, 37,* 400–405.

Part Six

Research Methodology for the Future

Michael Von Korff
Gregory E. Simon

18

Methodologic Perspective: Getting Answers to the Most Important Questions

Research methods are a means of getting valid, or meaningful, answers to important questions. A seemingly elegant study design, state-of-the-art measurement methods, and sophisticated methods of data analysis are worthless if they do not contribute in some way to answering an important question. Research on the psychological illnesses of primary care patients generally seeks to answer one or more of the following kinds of questions:

1. Which forms of psychological illness are common in primary care?
2. Which common forms of psychological illness are most significant?
3. To what extent is psychological illness recognized and treated in accordance with normative standards of patient care?
4. What mental health interventions are effective under ideal conditions?

Note: This work was supported by National Institute of Mental Health grants R01 MH41739 and R01 MH47765.

5. What mental health interventions are cost effective within the context of primary care?
6. What are more efficient and effective ways of training providers and delivering care?

Other chapters summarize the state of the art with respect to these important questions. This chapter presents methodological perspectives on efforts to get the right answers to these questions. An underlying theme of the chapter is that knowledge concerning psychological illness among primary care patients has progressed to a point where experimental and quasi-experimental designs are needed to answer the most critical research questions facing the field today. Throughout this chapter, research on depressive illness is used to exemplify methodological perspectives.

Methodologic Perspectives on Key Questions

We will consider the six questions listed above in turn.

Which forms of psychological illness are common in primary care? Answering this question requires reliable and valid approaches to case definition that can be applied in epidemiologic studies. For some time, assessment technologies have been available with acceptable reliability and convergent validity. In the case of depression, measurement properties have been assessed for a number of widely used self-rating scales (Derogatis, 1977; Weissman, Sholomskas, Pottenger, Prusoff, & Locke, 1977; Beck, Ward, Mendelson, Mock, & Erbaugh, 1961; Goldberg & Williams, 1988), clinician-rating scales (Hamilton, 1960; Rush et al., 1986), and diagnostic instruments (Robins, Helzer, Ratcliff, & Seyfried, 1982; Robins et al., 1988). Research comparing self-rating, clinician-rating, and diagnostic instruments has shown that they are strongly correlated when the item content is standardized (Tondo, Burrai, Scamonatti, Weissenburger, & Rush, 1988; Feinberg, Carroll, Smouse, & Rawson, 1981; Ancill, Rogers, & Carr, 1985), but that self-rating scales identify more patients as cases than diagnostic instruments do (Von Korff et al., 1987). Clinician-rating scales tend to show higher agreement with diagnostic instruments than self-rating scales (Tondo et al., 1988).

The construct validity of assessment methods is not as well established as reliability and convergent validity. Two key questions are: (1) At what threshold of severity are cases distinguished from noncases? (2) What distinct forms of illness can be differentiated among persons with clinically significant illness?

Threshold questions are especially critical in primary care, where many patients present with illness near or below conventional severity thresholds. While use of a diagnostic instrument to define case thresholds is now widely accepted, the shortcomings of simple dichotomous classifications have also become more apparent. Contrary to the dictum that a diagnosis should "carve nature at its joints," the validity of the thresholds differentiating subclinical and clinical illness remain ambiguous. Many primary care patients show a relapsing-remitting course of illness in which they meet diagnostic criteria at some points in time and show subthreshold illness at other points in time (Katon & Von Korff, 1990). Little attention has been paid to the implications of this within-subject variability for diagnostic and therapeutic decisions. The threshold at which depressive illness responds to pharmacological intervention does seem to be near the conventional diagnostic threshold for major depression (Paykel, Hollerman, Freeling, & Sedgewick, 1988), but important features of subclinical depression (for example, insomnia, pain) respond to pharmacological intervention among patients not meeting criteria for major depression (Egbunike & Chaffee, 1990; Stimmel & Escobar, 1986). Severity thresholds that predict therapeutic response have been identified using clinical rating scales that do not necessarily coincide with the severity thresholds used in diagnostic criteria. For these and other reasons, the validity of severity thresholds remains open to question.

The problems in differentiating distinct forms of psychological illness are more significant than the problems in establishing severity thresholds. In terms of ability to differentiate distinct forms of psychological illness, it has been shown repeatedly that depression and anxiety are highly correlated when assessed by self-rating scales (Eaton & Ritter, 1988; Breslau, 1985a, 1985b). The correlation of somatoform symptoms with depression and anxiety is somewhat lower, but in our own research has typically fallen between .40 and .60. Diagnostic assessments also find considerable overlap among depressive disorders, anxiety disorders, and somatoform disorders (Simon & Von Korff, 1991b; Boyd et al., 1984). Although major depression and panic disorder have been conceived and described as distinct (American Psychiatric Association, 1987), the two syndromes overlap considerably (Noyes et al., 1990; Lesser et al., 1988). Epidemiologic data now suggest that risk of suicide attempts may be as high for panic disorder as for depression (Weissman, Klerman, Markowitz, & Ouellette, 1989). Anxiety disorders respond to pharmacological and behavioral interventions that are also used to treat depression (Sheehan, Ballenger, & Jacobsen, 1980). Thus, the extent to which assessment methods are able to differentiate clearly distinct forms of psychological illness remains uncertain (Tyrer, 1985).

These problems and ambiguities in case definition suggest that classification criteria for psychological disorders in primary care should be viewed as conventions for classifying patients into clinically meaningful groups, rather than as syndromal or disease entities that differentiate clearly pathological states from clearly normal states. This situation is analogous to hypertension, which is diagnosed in terms of severity thresholds superimposed on dimensions (systolic and diastolic blood pressure). Approaches to superimposing psychiatric diagnoses on symptom dimensions are receiving increased theoretical and empirical attention (Clark & Watson, 1991), but it is unclear whether methods of practical value will emerge.

What approaches might help resolve the current deficiencies in methods of assessing and classifying psychological illness in primary care patients? A possible approach is to revise diagnostic criteria based on meta-analyses of existing studies and expert judgment of persons familiar with the special needs of assessment and classification in primary care. Such efforts are currently underway and can be expected to yield diagnostic criteria more suitable for application in primary care. Such an approach is, of course, limited by the existing state of knowledge and expertise.

A second approach is to apply advanced psychometric or pattern recognition methods to clinical data to identify measurement models and classification criteria that more adequately describe the psychological illnesses of primary care patients (Eaton & Bornstedt, 1989). While these methods may yield new insights into patterns in symptom data, they may also overestimate the ability of statistical methods to identify meaningful syndromes and underestimate the ambiguity of the underlying illnesses.

A third approach takes a different tack. This approach, most closely identified with the field of clinical epidemiology (Fletcher, Fletcher, & Wagner, 1982), regard diagnostic criteria as a tool of clinical decision making whose utility should be evaluated in terms of its contribution to patient management and outcomes. From this perspective, a diagnosis is useful to the extent that it increases the ability of the provider to accurately assess prognosis and to prescribe effective treatments. In the case of hypertension, diagnostic criteria have been strongly influenced by the results of longitudinal studies assessing the predictive value of blood pressure levels for adverse outcomes and by randomized controlled trials identifying blood pressure levels at which therapeutic intervention makes a difference in outcomes (Veterans Administration Cooperative Study on Hypertensive Agents, 1967). If treatment response is the ultimate test of the validity of a diagnosis *within the context of primary care,* classifications used in primary care should be developed in light of the treatments that are feasible and effective in that setting. For example, the ideal diagnostic thresholds for depression would predict which patients would benefit from recognition and intervention by the primary care physician. Similarly, distinctions between different disorders would be most useful if they corresponded to differences in appropriate treatment (Lewis, 1976). If, within the range of treatments used in primary care practice, two conditions respond to the same interventions, the differential diagnosis becomes less significant. This clinical epidemiologic approach to case definition forges a link between diagnostic criteria and the clinical decisions of primary care providers.

It is of more than passing interest that hypertension research has shown that valid assessment requires measurement of blood pressure on multiple occasions (Llabre et al., 1988). In contrast, it has generally been assumed that data collected at a single point in time will yield a valid classification of mental disorder status if the assessment method and diagnostic criteria are reliable. New approaches in measurement theory (Shavelson & Webb, 1991) provide theoretical and methodological bases for evaluating how many times a patient needs to be assessed in order to obtain an assessment generalizable across time. This approach, referred to as *generalizability theory,* also provides approaches for evaluating the impact of such factors as instrumentation, setting, and subject characteristics on the generalizability of an assessment.

When applying data from longitudinal and experimental studies to the task of improving the assessment and classification of depressive illness in primary care, several strategies are germane. First, research is needed estimating the severity thresholds at which risks of chronic psychological illness, disability, suicide, and other deleterious outcomes become appreciably greater than normal. Second, randomized controlled trials are needed that establish severity thresholds and diagnostic criteria predicting differential treatment response. Ideally, diagnostic criteria employed in primary care practice should be closely tied to provider needs to provide a prognosis, to decide whether and when to initiate active treatment, and to choose an effective form of treatment.

Which common forms of psychological illness are most significant? As summarized in other chapters, epidemiologic, health services, and clinical research has now convincingly demonstrated the public health significance of the psychological illnesses that are common among primary care patients. This research has shown that common forms of psychological illness, like depression, panic disorder, and substance abuse, are associated with increased use of health care services, functional disability, and increased risk of suicide.

This research has begun to fundamentally change public perceptions of the significance of mental disorders. When the results of the ECA surveys were first reported, a well-known commentator wrote, "Saying one in every five people has a mental disorder is like saying the average person is crazy. The average person isn't crazy. He or she may act crazy sometimes but that's all part of being normal. The average person is average. If being a little crazy is part of that, so be it" (Rooney, 1984, p. 49). Research showing that common psychological illnesses have significant social costs in terms of impaired work performance, family dysfunction, increased use of health care, risks of self injury, and other deleterious effects has since contradicted the opinion of this ill-informed vox populi.

While there is growing evidence that common mental disorders are associated with disability, excess health care costs, and increased mortality, the implications of these findings for intervention are ambiguous. Recent research concerning disability among depressed patients exemplifies this point. The Medical Outcomes Survey (Wells et al., 1989) has reported that general medical patients with major depression, on average, report levels of disability comparable to patients with heart disease. Data from the Epidemiologic Catchment Area (ECA) surveys also showed significant and sustained disability among persons with depressive illness (Wells, Golding, & Burnam, 1988; Broadhead, Blazer, George, & Tse, 1990). More recently, it has been shown among depressed high utilizers of health care (Von Korff, Ormel, Katon, & Lin, 1992), and among consecutive primary care patients with psychological illness (Ormel et al., 1993), that disability levels remain elevated over long-term follow-up periods if the depressive illness does not improve, but that disability improves substantially among patients whose depression does improve. These findings are ambiguous, because none of these studies establish the extent to which disability is *controlled* by depression. Specifically, one would like to know the extent to which effective treatment of depression reduces disability among depressed primary care patients. Randomized controlled trials have not routinely assessed the effects of treatment on behavioral outcomes like disability and health care use, so experimental data are generally lacking.

Is it possible to determine whether depression controls disability (or other deleterious behavioral correlates of depression) using observational data alone? Some have advocated applying structural equation models to multiwave survey data to address this type of question. For example, LISREL has been used to study the relationship between depression and disability using data from a longitudinal survey (Aneshensel, Frerichs, & Huba, 1984). In this work, the objective was to develop a causal model of the relationship between physical illness and depression that assessed "reciprocal causal effects" within time and across lags of four, eight, and twelve months. The results were interesting. Increased illness (a latent variable measured by disability days and number of illness episodes) was associated with moderate *concurrent* increases in depression. Increased depression was associated with a modest increase in illness four months later. It was concluded that a considerable amount of the concurrent association between depression and illness was causal in nature, but that this causal effect was attenuated over longer periods of time. It was inferred that physical illness and associated restriction of activities generated depressive symptoms within a short period of time and that this impact continued over time if illness and disability persisted. It was also inferred that elevated levels of depressive symptomatology increased the risk of physical disorder over a period of time, but not immediately. While these results are consistent with synchronous change of depression and disability, it is unclear why concurrent and longitudinal correlations permit such strong, complex, and directional causal inference. Relatively weak time-lagged effects can be difficult to replicate. Synchronous change of two variables may occur if *either* variable is influencing the other, if there is an unmeasured variable influencing both variables in a similar fashion, if both variables are affected by a common measurement bias, or if the two variables are overlapping constructs. In addition, applying structural equation models to longitudinal data introduces significant logical and statistical difficulties that arise when "causal" effects are estimated in a nonequivalent group design (Rogosa, Brandt, & Zimowski, 1982). In this regard, Rogosa (1987, pp. 193–194) states, "I've come to view the phrases causal inference, explanatory research, and so forth, as often deceptive and polarizing ways of thinking. My view is that investigators set out to address research questions, and not all important research questions are explanatory in the sense of seeking as-if-by-experiment inferences. Attempts to answer experimental (i.e., causal, explanatory, etc.) research questions with nonexperimental data seem fundamentally askew. And it seems this mismatch generates some adversarial feelings between statisticians and social scientists."

Whether disability, use of health care, or other possible behavioral correlates of depression can be reduced by mental health intervention is properly addressed by experimental or quasi-experimental designs. However, it is sometimes not recognized that showing that reductions in disability, health care use, or other behavioral variables occur after treatment of depression is not equivalent to showing that depression is an initiating cause of the behavioral effect. Longitudinal data gathered in a nonexperimental design can play an important role in improving understanding of the longitudinal relationship between depression, disability, and other behavioral variables. For example, if an observational study found that disability and depression did not show synchronous change, it would reduce the plausibility of depression having a controlling effect on disability (or disability having a controlling effect on depression). On the other hand, showing that change in depression and disability is synchronous does not usually provide a much stronger basis for an inference that depression has a controlling effect on disability (or vice versa) than observing a cross-sectional association. Appropriate uses of longitudinal data not collected in an experimental or quasi-experimental design include the following: identifying typical individual-level trajectories of depression and disability, assessing the extent of stability and change of depressive illness and disability across time, determining whether depression and disability show synchronous change, estimating the magnitude of change in disability among patients whose depression does or does not improve, using fine-grained measurements to identify time lags between changes in depression and changes in disability levels and vice versa, and identifying prognostic factors for improvement in depression and disability. This kind of information strengthens the empirical footing of theory without necessarily permitting strong causal inference. Such information is also useful in the design of experimental studies. A risk of the application of complex causal models to longitudinal data is that presentation of the parameter estimates of the model take precedence over presentation of important descriptive data regarding the natural history.

Fortunately, it is becoming commonplace for primary care researchers to use experimental methods in which strong causal inferences may be possible. The value of experimental interventions for inference about the role of depression in causing behavioral dysfunction might be enhanced if the studies were designed in light of an explicit statement of the sequence of events believed to be necessary for intervention effects to occur—what has been called *a small theory of treatment effects* (Lipsey, 1990). For example, in experimental studies concerning depressive illness underway at the

Center for Health Studies, we view depression, physical symptoms, and dysfunctional illness behaviors as a dynamically interrelated *system* of variables (Von Korff, Katon, & Lin, 1990). An intervention that alters any single variable can be expected to have corresponding effects on other biological, psychological, and behavioral components of the illness. In the context of an experimental intervention to reduce depression, an experiment might be designed to assess whether the following sequence of events occurred in the intervention group relative to the controls: (1) assignment to the intervention group increases exposure to pharmacological and behavioral interventions; (2) adherence to the interventions reduces levels of depressive symptoms, increases activity levels, and reduces dysphoric physical symptoms; (3) a reduction in symptoms (psychological and physical) increases activity levels, increases social role performance, and cuts down on functional disability; (4) reduced symptoms and disability decrease motivation for seeking health care services; and (5) reduced contact with health care providers and reduced disability decrease the risks of entering a chronic sick role characterized by dependence on family members, health care providers, co-workers, and/or the social welfare system. While the primary research question of a study might be whether exposure of the patient to the experimental intervention had a positive effect on depression, selected secondary questions concerning effects of the intervention on physical symptoms, disability, health care use, or social role performance can be addressed by the same study without substantially increasing its cost or complexity. This may be true even if the sample size required to detect effects on behavioral outcomes is greater than required to detect effects on depressive illness.

An explicit model of the process and outcomes of an experimental intervention can guide development of experimental interventions and the identification of measures needed to test critical links between process and outcomes. Such a model might be elaborated by specifying the magnitude, variability, and expected time course of hypothesized changes to guide the specification of sample size and the timing of measurement. This sort of statement, if made before data are analyzed, provides protection against opportunistic interpretation of results of studies with multiple process and outcome variables. For example, if a mental health intervention produced an effect on health care use without affecting the patient's depression, physical symptoms, or disability, one would wonder whether the result was robust, or if substitution of one form of care for another was a better explanation than an effect of treatment on the patient's illness.

To what extent is psychological illness recognized and treated in accordance with normative standards of patient care? A long series of studies have shown that primary care providers often do not recognize psychological distress (Knights & Folstein, 1977; Zung, Magill, Moore, & George, 1983; Goldberg, Steele, Johnson, & Smith, 1982). Research has also shown that depressed patients who are recognized often receive inadequate pharmacological treatment (Johnson, 1974; Katon, Von Korff, Lin, Bush, & Ormel, 1992; Simon & Von Korff, 1991a). When normative standards of psychiatric practice are applied, primary care is often characterized as deficient. But applying normative standards of psychiatric practice without considering the differences between specialty practice and primary care may not be appropriate.

Recognition studies, for example, have generally not considered such as the following: the feasibility of assessing and treating depression at the index visit in light of the patient's presenting problem, the relationship between depression and the patient's presenting physical illness, whether the depression is sufficiently severe and acute to warrant active treatment, whether the patient has received prior treatment for depression from the primary care provider or is currently receiving treatment from some other provider, whether the provider is the patient's usual source of care or is seeing the patient on a one-time basis, whether the provider would be capable of effectively treating depression if it were recognized, and the patient's receptiveness and motivation to carry out mental health treatment if it was offered. By studying recognition out of its clinical context, the significance of low recognition is difficult to evaluate, and how to improve recognition is often unclear. A result of inadequate understanding of low recognition is that studies attempting to increase recognition by providing screening scale results have sometimes not achieved expected results (Hoeper, Nycz, Cleary, Regier, & Goldberg, 1979; Shapiro et al., 1987), perhaps because the major barrier to effective treatment of psychological illness is not recognition failure but rather the lack of skills, time, and resources to implement treatments effectively.

Normative studies of pharmacological management of depression have reported less-than-optimal selection of medications, inadequate dose and duration of pharmacological treatment, infrequent follow-up relative to psychiatric standards, and poor adherence to prescribed medication regimens by patients (Katon et al., 1992; Simon & Von Korff, 1991a). While this kind of study can provide a basis for improving the process of care, little research has tried to identify the specific barriers to improving the process of treating depression in primary care. Even fewer studies have tried to experimentally alter the primary care of psychological illness in a way that might improve the process and outcomes of care. Research currently underway at several centers is evaluating the effectiveness of integrating mental health care into primary care. This research may provide more meaningful information on how to improve the process and outcomes of psychological illness in primary care and on whether such efforts can be cost effective.

What mental health interventions are effective under ideal conditions? It has long been recognized that the randomized controlled trial is the most reliable means of assessing the efficacy of medical and psychological treatments. As a result of experimental studies conducted in mental health specialty settings, a wide range of mental health interventions now exist whose efficacy has been demonstrated in reasonably well-designed and executed clinical trials. However, these studies have significant shortcomings in guiding primary care practice.

The *intensity or mode of specialty mental health interventions* is often difficult to replicate within the context of primary care. Randomized controlled trials conducted in specialty settings typically establish a clinical protocol for study purposes that is more highly structured than usual care in that setting. Study protocols are probably more likely to provide optimal treatment conditions than usual care even in a specialty setting. In primary care research, it is often necessary to integrate the experimental intervention with the regular delivery of primary care, making it substantially more difficult to provide optimal therapeutic conditions. As a result, the effectiveness of a treatment evaluated under optimal conditions in a specialty setting may not be generalizable to primary care. For example, randomized controlled trials of antidepressant medications often employ protocols requiring weekly follow-up of patients. Frequent follow-up tends to increase adherence and the likelihood of achieving therapeutic dosage levels, while regular follow-up of patients being treated with antidepressants in primary care is the exception rather than the rule.

Another limitation of some randomized controlled trials of mental health interventions is that *they report data on the basis of treatments provided rather than intention to treat.* It is widely accepted among methodologists that intention to treat (that is, randomization group) is the soundest basis for analysis of results of a controlled trial, whether the treatment was actually delivered or not (Meinert, 1986). When patients assigned to an intervention group do not receive the intended pharmacological or psychological treatment, clinical researchers may feel the patient does not provide a fair test of the treatment. Such beliefs lead some to exclude treatment dropouts from the study. The biases potentially introduced by analysis on the basis of treatment received rather than intention to treat have been reviewed elsewhere (Lee, Ellenberg, Hirtz, & Nelson, 1991). This dilemma can be avoided by keeping dropout rates as low as possible.

When there are enough dropouts to make a difference in inference, the investigator should obtain outcome data on treatment dropouts whenever possible, examine results with dropouts included and excluded, and report whether or not analysis by treatment received or intention to treat made a difference. To the extent that outcome data are not obtained on treatment dropouts, studies should routinely report rates at which patients were lost to follow-up in the intervention and control groups separately. Because nonadherence rates are generally high for health care interventions (Haynes, Taylor, & Sackett, 1979), reporting the extent to which patients drop out of intervention and control arms of an experiment separately is highly pertinent to assessing the feasibility of the intervention.

A further problem exists. *Generalizability from specialty patients enrolled in clinical trials to primary care patients is uncertain.* Subjects who are not highly motivated, with concurrent chronic disease, with a chronic form of psychological illness, who may believe their illness is physical rather than psychological, or who have a second concurrent psychological illness are unlikely to be enrolled in clinical trials conducted in specialty settings. Several of these characteristics are associated with poor prognosis. Excluding these kinds of patients limits the extent to which results of controlled trials with specialty mental health patients can be generalized to primary care patients.

An additional limitation of many controlled trials conducted in specialty settings is that *a limited range of outcome variables are assessed for a limited period of time.* Controlled trials showing that intervention group patients, relative to control group patients, have lower levels of symptoms over a six-month period leave important questions unanswered that may be critical for assessing cost-effectiveness. Did the intervention improve overall quality of life, from the patient's perspective? To what extent did the intervention increase or reduce total health care costs? To what extent did the intervention improve the patient's performance at work, or reduce the likelihood of the patient becoming work disabled, thereby offsetting disability costs to an employer? Over what time horizon were benefits of the intervention realized? Over what time horizon, and at what costs, do patients continue to receive services? These are critical questions rarely addressed by randomized controlled trials of mental health interventions in specialty settings.

What mental health interventions are cost effective within the context of primary care? It is becoming apparent that the disproportionate share of the gross domestic product spent on health care and national defense is having a deleterious effect on economic vitality in the private sector. It is also undermining the ability of state and federal governments to pursue critical social goals, such as education and housing. Within this context, the social value of health care services whose cost-effectiveness is unknown can reasonably be questioned when services are purchased with public funds or tax-exempt insurance benefits.

Mental health services provided either in primary care or in specialty settings should not be exempt from this kind of scrutiny. For example, in the Group Health Cooperative of Puget Sound, Washington, a health maintenance organization (HMO) providing services to 370,000 enrollees, the annual budget for a single newly released antidepressant medication quickly reached $1 million a year—the fastest-increasing pharmaceutical cost experienced by the HMO at that time. Observational data suggested that adherence and therapeutic dosage levels were more likely to be achieved with this medication than with older and less expensive antidepressants (Simon & Von Korff, 1991a). However, these observational data did not answer the fundamental question of whether the benefits of the antidepressant justified its greater costs. To put the costs of this medication in perspective, if its added costs had been available for other uses within Group Health's mental health service, at least ten professional staff positions could have been added to the mental health service. If its added costs had been available for general medical services, it might have been used to double the number of women screened—from 8,000 to over 16,000 per year—in Group Health's population-based breast cancer screening program. Comparable resources, if diverted by employers to employee benefits other than health care, could have fully supported the annual budget of a high-quality preschool serving 200 children. The methodological challenge facing mental health researchers is to develop data that provide a more rational basis for explicit and implicit resource allocation decisions of individuals, health care providers, insurers, employers, and government.

A series of methodological challenges exist that must be faced in carrying out a cost-effectiveness trial in primary care. Fielding an intervention whose *efficacy is plausible* and *selecting patients who might benefit* from the intervention are both critical difficulties in primary care research. In a specialty setting, it is easier to identify homogeneous patient groups, to enroll those patients in an acute phase of their illness, and to expose those patients to a strong intervention. In primary care research, identifying a patient sample with the same disorder is time consuming and difficult, identifying patients at an acute phase of their illness can be problematic, and fielding an intervention whose efficacy is credible can be especially difficult. These difficulties may explain, in part, the high rate of negative results of randomized controlled trials conducted among primary care patients.

An important methodological issue in conducting randomized controlled trials that evaluate cost-effectiveness in primary care is the identification of an appropriate control group. Typically, primary care researchers are interested in the effectiveness of an intervention relative to services currently provided. Outside of the mental health field, employing a usual care control group is a widely accepted methodological strategy. From a practical standpoint, it would often be unethical to withhold usual care from a patient entered into a cost-effectiveness trial if the patient was assigned to the control group. The issue in a cost-effectiveness study is typically whether adding a service changes the cost-effectiveness of care relative to current practice. A usual care control group is an appropriate comparison to address this type of question.

What are more efficient and effective ways of training providers and delivering care? In addition to research testing particular interventions for specific mental disorders, a need exists for services research that seeks to understand how to improve the skills of providers, the organization of services, and the processes of care delivery. Researchers who wish to study these issues using experimental methods are faced with inducing planned change in how providers deliver care. Strategies for changing how providers deliver care are, in fact, critical methods in the design of experimental research testing the effects of innovations in patient care.

Persons wishing to alter patterns of care of primary care providers need to be aware of the difficulties in changing provider behavior and of the results of research assessing the potency of different forms of intervention. There is now substantial evidence that traditional educational approaches, typically employed in continuing medical education (CME) programs, are ineffective in producing meaningful change in practice patterns. Recent research on modification of provider behavior has identified more effective techniques than old-style CME. Key principles emerging from this research are: (1) Change strategies should begin with identification of barriers to change, involve providers as active participants to the extent possible, and concentrate on a limited number of points presented multiple times via multiple modalities (Eisenberg, 1985; Heyssel, Gainter, Kues, Jones, & Lipstein, 1984; Thompson, Kirz, & Gold, 1983). (2) Brief one-on-one education is more effective than written materials or seminar-type sessions (Avorn & Soumerai,

1983). (3) Health care practices are influenced by communication networks of providers practicing in proximity to each other (Coleman, Katz, & Menzel, 1966). (4) Modeling of desired treatment practices by clinical leaders with opportunities for practice is important in producing change (Geertsma, Parker, & Whitbourne, 1982). (5) Educational interventions delivered through identified clinical opinion leaders can be more effective than standard audit and feedback systems in changing patterns of care (Lomas et al., 1991). (6) Interventions directed at the patient, particularly those that increase doctor-patient communication and the level of participation of the patient in care, can improve both the process and the outcomes of care (Greenfield, Kaplan, Ware, Yano, & Frank, 1988; Greenfield, Kaplan, & Ware, 1985; Uhlmann, Inui, Pecoraro, & Carter, 1988). (7) Reminder systems (McDonald et al., 1984; McDonald, 1976) and ongoing surveillance systems with feedback to provider and patients (Barnett, Winikoff, Dorsey, Morgan, & Lurie, 1978; Winikoff, Coltin, Morgan, Buxbaum, & Barnett, 1984) can improve patient adherence to prescribed treatments. And (8) carefully designed training sessions, with clear-cut behavioral goals and structured training, can change how providers deliver care (Roter & Hall, 1991).

The complexity of producing important changes in how care is provided, and the necessity of integrating a study with the delivery of care in a study clinic, leads many researchers to favor observational studies over experimental interventions or to attempt interventions only in residency clinics. If mental health treatment is to be fundamentally improved in primary care, it will be important for primary care researchers to find ways of conducting experimental research with experienced providers in settings other than residency training programs. A major obstacle to such research is the sheer volume of patient care that occurs in most primary care settings. Interventions need to fit into the schedules of busy doctors and nurses and to be consistent with existing methods of patient care.

Experimental interventions to improve care must direct the design, the intervention, and the analysis of data at the appropriate system level (that is, the patient, the provider, the clinic or the delivery system). Attempts to change the process of care may sometimes require interventions applied across an entire clinic or physician group. A true experiment to evaluate such an intervention might require randomization of clinics. Since changing provider practice patterns may require working with all physicians in a clinic, randomization of providers within a single clinic is sometimes not a feasible study design. Analysis of data from a study in which either a physician or a clinic is the intervention target, but in which intervention effects are measured at the level of the patient, may require inference and statistical techniques appropriate for multilevel data (Von Korff, Koepsell, Curry, & Diehr, 1992; Haney, 1980).

Mental health researchers have not fully recognized that major issues in improving care for psychological illness in primary care are similar to problems in the care of other common chronic conditions. For example, improving adherence to an antidepressant medication regimen is likely to require techniques and systems similar to those used in improving adherence to antihypertensive medications. Because research tends to be divided along specialty lines, there has been a failure to identify common methods and systems of patient care that have utility across multiple conditions. As a result, researchers trying to improve the management of a single condition have no *infrastructure of patient care* to call on. Infrastructure of patient care includes standard systems supporting patient care and techniques of patient management shared by different members of the provider team. When behavioral techniques, information systems, and routinized methods of patient care are developed to deal with generic difficulties in problem recognition, patient education, behavioral change, and adherence, it may become less difficult to induce and evaluate the effectiveness of innovations in patient care for psychological illness. Because the infrastructure of primary care is grossly deficient, a researcher must invent methods of trying to change patient care and must contend with the limited ability of health care systems to change what they are doing in a meaningful way.

Conclusion

Mental health research in primary care has succeeded in developing meaningful morbidity statistics on what mental disorders are common in primary care. There are also excellent data demonstrating the public health significance of these conditions. A major shortcoming of existing research is that diagnostic criteria and morbidity statistics are not closely linked to the clinical decisions of primary care providers. Thus, the relationship between diagnosis and management is weak from the perspective of the primary care physician. Properly designed randomized controlled trials could help rectify this situation by identifying the level of severity at which treatment is preferred over watchful waiting and by identifying criteria for conditions that show differential response to different forms of treatment.

While experimental data have been produced that evaluate the efficacy of pharmacological and behavioral interventions for specific mental disorders in specialty settings, the generalizability of this research to primary care practice is uncertain. The interventions are usually more intensive than is practical in primary care and often exclude many patients similar to those seen in primary care. As a result, the efficacy of widely used mental health interventions is largely unknown when they are applied in primary care.

Even less is known about the cost-effectiveness of mental health interventions in primary care than is known about their efficacy. Implicit or explicit claims that mental health intervention is cost effective because it controls health care costs or reduces disability are plausible, but these claims are largely unsupported by experimental data. Showing that mental disorders are associated with significant health care and disability costs is not equivalent to showing that intervention is effective in reducing those costs. For already-overburdened primary health care providers to become enthusiastic about aggressively improving care of mental disorders, researchers will probably have to produce credible evidence that the work required is justified by improved patient outcomes or reduced health care costs.

Approaches to improving management of mental disorders in primary care will need to be consistent with other innovations taking place in health care delivery, or they will be less likely to be widely adopted. A major barrier to improving care of both physical and psychological conditions in primary care is the lack of infrastructure for key elements of patient care—problem recognition, patient education, behavioral change, adherence, and relapse prevention. Mental health researchers might look to research currently being carried out for other common chronic conditions to identify strategies for improving patient care that may have general applicability, rather than viewing mental health care as having problems and solutions that are completely unique to mental disorders.

Finally, we need to begin to routinely measure how mental health interventions affect the patient's quality of life, use of health care, and functional disability. The ultimate value of mental health interventions to society should be judged by their ability to produce significant and enduring benefits in terms of improved quality of life, reduced health care costs, and enhanced social role performance. Primary care research on mental disorders has shown that the burden of mental disorders in these areas is great, but research has yet to demonstrate that widely used interventions are either effective or cost efficient when delivered in primary care.

References

American Psychiatric Association. (1987). *Diagnostic and statistical manual of mental disorders* (3rd ed., rev.). Washington, DC: Author.

Ancill, R. J., Rogers, D., & Carr, A. C. (1985). Comparison of computerized self-rating scales for depression with conventional observer ratings. *Acta Psychiatrica Scandinavica, 71,* 315–317.

Aneshensel, C. S., Frerichs, R. R., & Huba, G. J. (1984). Depression and physical illness: A multiwave, nonrecursive causal model. *Journal of Health and Social Behavior, 25,* 350–371.

Avorn, J., & Soumerai, S. B. (1983). Improving drug-therapy decisions through educational outreach: A randomized controlled trial of academically based "detailing." *New England Journal of Medicine, 308,* 1457–1463.

Barnett, G. O., Winikoff, R., Dorsey, J. L., Morgan, M. M., & Lurie, R. S. (1978). Quality assurance through automated monitoring and concurrent feedback using a computer-based medical information system. *Medical Care, 16,* 962–970.

Beck, A. T., Ward, C. H., Mendelson, M., Mock, J. E., & Erbaugh,

J. K. (1961). An inventory for measuring depression. *Archives of General Psychiatry, 4,* 561–571.

Boyd, J. H., Burke, J. D., Gruenberg, E., Holzer, C. E., Rae, D. S., George, L. K., Karno, M., Stoltzman, R., McEvoy, L., & Nestadt, (1984). Exclusion criteria of DSM-III: A study of co-occurrence of hierarchy-free syndromes. *Archives of General Psychiatry, 41,* 983–989.

Breslau, N. (1985a). Depressive symptoms, major depression, and generalized anxiety: A comparison of self-reports on CES-D and results from diagnostic interviews. *Psychiatry Research, 15,* 219–229.

Breslau, N. (1985b). Further evidence. *Psychiatry Research, 16,* 177–179.

Broadhead, W. E., Blazer, D. G., George, L. K., & Tse, C. K. (1990). Depression, disability days, and days lost from work in a prospective epidemiologic study. *Journal of the American Medical Association, 264,* 2524–2528.

Clark, L. A., & Watson, D. (1991). Tripartite model of anxiety and depression: Psychometric evidence and taxonomic implications. *Journal of Abnormal Psychology, 100,* 316–336.

Coleman, J. S., Katz, E., & Menzel, H. (1966). *Medical innovation: A diffusion study.* New York: Bobbs-Merrill.

Derogatis, L. R. (1977). *Symptom Checklist-90: Administration, scoring, and procedures manual for the Revised Version.* Baltimore, MD: Clinical Psychometric Research.

Eaton, W. W., & Bornstedt, G. (1989). Latent variable models for dichotomous outcomes: Analysis of data from the Epidemiologic Catchment Area program. *Sociological Research and Methods, 18,* 1–183.

Eaton, W. W., & Ritter, C. (1988). Distinguishing anxiety and depression with field survey data. *Psychological Medicine, 18,* 155–166.

Egbunike, I. G., & Chaffee, B. J. (1990). Antidepressants in the management of chronic pain syndromes. *Pharmacotherapy, 10,* 262–270.

Eisenberg, J. M. (1985). Physician utilization: The state of research about physicians' practice patterns. *Medical Care, 23,* 461–483.

Feinberg, M., Carroll, B. J., Smouse, P. E., & Rawson, S. G. (1981).

The Carroll Rating Scale for Depression: 3. Comparison with other rating instruments. *British Journal of Psychiatry, 138,* 205-209.

Fletcher, R. H., Fletcher, S. W., & Wagner, E. H. (1982). *Clinical epidemiology: The essentials.* Baltimore, MD: Williams & Wilkins.

Geertsma, R. H., Parker, R. C., & Whitbourne, S. K. (1982). How physicians view the process of change in their practice behavior. *Journal of Medical Education, 57,* 752-761.

Goldberg, D., Steele, J. J., Johnson, A., & Smith, C. (1982). Ability of primary care physicians to make accurate ratings of psychiatric symptoms. *Archives of General Psychiatry, 39,* 829-833.

Goldberg, D., & Williams, P. (1988). A user's guide to the General Health Questionnaire. Windsor, Berkshire, England: NFER-Nelson.

Greenfield, S., Kaplan, S., & Ware, J. E. (1985). Expanding patient involvement in care: Effects on patient outcomes. *Annals of Internal Medicine, 102,* 520-528.

Greenfield, S., Kaplan, S. H., Ware, J. E., Yano, E. M., & Frank, H. J. L. (1988). Patients' participation in medical care: Effects on blood sugar and quality of life in diabetes. *Journal of General Internal Medicine, 3,* 448-457.

Hamilton, M. (1960). A rating scale for depression. *Journal of Neurology, Neurosurgery, and Psychiatry, 12,* 56-62.

Haney, W. (1980). Units and levels of analysis in large-scale evaluation, in *Issues in Aggregation.* New Directions for Methodology of Social and Behavioral Science. San Francisco: Jossey-Bass.

Haynes, R. B., Taylor, D. W., & Sackett, D. L. (1979). *Compliance in health care.* Baltimore, MD: Johns Hopkins University Press.

Heyssel, R. M., Gainter, J. R., Kues, I. W., Jones, A. A., & Lipstein, S. H. (1984). Decentralized management in a teaching hospital. *New England Journal of Medicine, 310,* 1477-1480.

Hoeper, E. W., Nycz, G. R., Cleary, P. D., Regier, D. A., & Goldberg, I. D. (1979). Estimated prevalence of rdc mental disorder in primary medical care. *International Journal of Mental Health, 8,* 6-15.

Johnson, D. A. W. (1974). A study of the use of antidepressant medication in general practice. *British Journal of Psychiatry, 125,* 186-192.

Katon, W., & Von Korff, M. (1990). Caseness criteria for major depression: The primary care clinician and the psychiatric epidemiologist. In C. C. Attkisson & J. M. Zich (Eds.), *Depression in primary care: Screening and detection*. New York: Routledge, 41-62.

Katon, W., Von Korff, M., Lin, E., Bush, T., & Ormel, J. (1992). Adequacy and duration of antidepressant treatment in primary care. *Medical Care, 30,* 67-76.

Knights, E. B., & Folstein, M. F. (1977). Unsuspected emotional and cognitive disturbance in medical patients. *Annals of Internal Medicine, 87,* 723-724.

Lee, Y. J., Ellenberg, J. H., Hirtz, D. G., & Nelson, K. B. (1991). Analysis of clinical trials by treatment actually received: Is it really an option? *Statistics in Medicine, 10,* 1595-1605.

Lesser, I. M., Rubin, R. T., Pecknold, J. C., Rifkin, A., Swinson, R. P., Lydiard, R. B., Burrows, G. D., Noyes, R., Jr., & Dupont, R. L., Jr. (1988). Secondary depression in panic disorder and agoraphobia. *Archives of General Psychiatry, 45,* 437-443.

Lewis, A. (1976). A note on classifying phobia. *Psychological Medicine, 6,* 21-22.

Lipsey, M. W. (1990). Theory as method: Small theories of treatment. In L. Sechrest, E. Perrin, & J. Bunker (Eds.), *AHCPR conference proceedings: Research methodology: Strengthening causal interpretations in community intervention of nonexperimental data* (DHHS Publication No. (PHS) 90-3453). Washington, DC: U.S. Government Printing Office.

Llabre, M. M., Ironson, G. H., Spitzer, S. B., Gelllman, M. D., Weidler, D. J., & Schneiderman, N. (1988). How many blood pressure measurements are enough?: An application of Generalizability Theory to the study of blood pressure measurement. *Psychophysiology, 25,* 97-106.

Lomas, J. L., Enkin, M., Anderson, G. M., Hannah, W. J., Vayda, E., & Singer, J. (1991). Opinion leaders vs audit and feedback to implement practice guidelines: Delivery after previous cesarean section. *Journal of the American Medical Association, 265,* 2202-2207.

McDonald, C. J. (1976). Protocol-based computer reminders, the quality of care, and the nonperfectability of man. *New England Journal of Medicine, 295,* 1351–1355.

McDonald, C. J., Hui, S. L., Smith, D. M., Tierney, W. M., Cohen, S. J., Weinberger, M., & McCabe, G. P. (1984). Reminders to physicians from an introspective computer medical record: A two-year randomized trial. *Annals of Internal Medicine, 100,* 130–138.

Meinert, C. L. (1986). *Clinical trials: Design, conduct, and analysis.* New York: Oxford University Press.

Noyes, R., Reich, J., Christiansen, J., Suelzer, M., Pfohl, B., & Coryell, W. A. (1990). Outcome of panic disorder: Relationship to diagnostic subtypes and comorbidity. *Archives of General Psychiatry, 47,* 809–818.

Ormel, J., Von Korff, M., van den Brink, W., Katon, W., Brilman, W., & Oldehinkel, T. (1993). Depression, anxiety, and social disability show synchrony of change: A 3½ year longitudinal study in primary care. *American Journal of Public Health, 83,* 385–390.

Paykel, E. S., Hollerman, J. A., Freeling, P., & Sedgewick, P. (1988). Predictors of therapeutic benefit from amitriptyline in mild depression: A general practice placebo-controlled trial. *Journal of Affective Disorders, 14,* 83–95.

Robins, L. N., Helzer, J. E., Ratcliff, K. S., & Seyfried, W. (1982). Validity for the Diagnostic Interview Schedule, Version II: DSM-III diagnoses. *Psychological Medicine, 12,* 855–870.

Robins, L. N., Wing, J., Wittchen, H.-U., Helzer, J. E., Babor, T. F., Burke, J., Farmer, A., Jablensky, A., Pickens, R., Regier, D. A., Sartorius, N., & Towle, L. H. (1988). The Composite International Diagnostic Interview: An epidemiologic instrument suitable for use in conjunction with different diagnostic systems and in different cultures. *Archives of General Psychiatry, 45,* 1069–1076.

Rogosa, D. (1987). Casual models do not support scientific conclusions: A comment in support of Freedman. *Journal of Educational Statistics, 12,* 185–195.

Rogosa, D., Brandt, D., & Zimowski, M. (1982). A growth curve approach to measurement of change. *Psychological Bulletin, 92,* 726–748.

Rooney, A. (1984, October 7). Off center: Statistics show one out of five are mentally ill. *Seattle Times and Post Intelligencer.*

Roter, D., & Hall, J. (1991, September). *Recruitment and training of primary care physicians in interviewing skills to identify and address patients' psychosocial distress.* Paper presented at the fifth annual NIMH International Research Conference on the Classification, Recognition, and Treatment of Mental Disorders in General Medical Settings, Bethesda, MD.

Rush, A. J., Giles, D. E., Schlesser, M. A., Fulton, C. L., Weissenburger, J., & Burns, C. (1986). The Inventory for Depressive Symptomatology (IDS): Preliminary findings. *Psychiatry Research, 18,* 65–87.

Shapiro, S., German, P. S., Skinner, E. A., Von Korff, M., Turner, R. W., Klein, L. E., Teitelbaum, M. L., Kramer, M., Burke, J. D., & Burns, B. J. (1987). An experiment to change detection and management of mental morbidity in primary care. *Medical Care, 25,* 327–339.

Shavelson, R. J., & Webb, N. M. (1991). *Generalizability Theory: A primer.* Newbury Park, CA: Sage.

Sheehan, D. V., Ballenger, J., & Jacobsen, G. (1980). Treatment of endogenous anxiety with phobic, hysterical, and hypochondriacal symptoms. *Archives of General Psychiatry, 37,* 51–59.

Simon, G., & Von Korff, M. (1991a, September). *Antidepressant prescribing patterns in primary care: Factors influencing effectiveness.* Paper presented at the fifth annual NIMH International Research Conference on the Classification, Recognition, and Treatment of Mental Disorders in General Medical Settings, Bethesda, MD.

Simon, G., & Von Korff, M. (1991b). Somatization and psychiatric disorder in the NIMH Epidemiologic Catchment Area study. *American Journal of Psychiatry, 148,* 1494–1500.

Stimmel, G. L., & Escobar, J. I. (1986). Antidepressants in chronic pain: A review of efficacy. *Pharmacotherapy, 6,* 262–267.

Thompson, R. S., Kirz, H. L., & Gold, R. A. (1983). Changes in physician behavior and cost savings associated with organizational recommendations on the use of "routine" chest X-rays and multichannel blood tests. *Preventive Medicine, 12,* 385–396.

Tondo, L., Burrai, C., Scamonatti, L., Weissenburger, J., & Rush,

J. (1988). Comparison between clinician-rated and self-reported depressive symptoms in Italian psychiatric patients. *Neuropsychobiology, 19,* 1–5.

Tyrer, P. (1985, March 23). Classification of mental disorders: Neurosis divisible? *Lancet, 1,* 685–688.

Uhlmann, R. F., Inui, T. S., Pecoraro, R. E., & Carter, W. B. (1988). Relationship of patient request fulfillment to compliance, glycemic control, and other health care outcomes in insulin-dependent diabetes. *General Internal Medicine, 3,* 458–463.

Veterans Administration Cooperative Study on Antihypertensive Agents. (1967). Effects on morbidity in hypertension: 1. Results with patients with diastolic blood pressure averaging 115 through 129 mm Hg. *Journal of the American Medical Association, 202,* 1028–1034.

Von Korff, M., Katon, W., & Lin, E. (1990). Psychological distress, physical symptoms, utilization, and the cost off-set effect. In N. Sartorius (Ed.), *Psychological disorders in general medical settings.* Bern: Huber.

Von Korff, M., Koepsell, T., Curry, S., & Diehr, P. (1992). Multilevel analysis in epidemiologic research on health behaviors and outcomes. *American Journal of Epidemiology, 135,* 1077–1082.

Von Korff, M., Ormel, J., Katon, W., & Lin, E. (1992). Disability and depression among high utilizers of health care: A longitudinal analysis. *Archives of General Psychiatry, 49,* 91–100.

Von Korff, M., Shapiro, S., Burke, J. D., Teitelbaum, M., Skinner, E. A., German, P., Turner, R. W., Klein, L., & Burns, B. (1987). Anxiety and depression in a primary care clinic: Comparison of the DIS, GHQ, and practitioner assessments. *Archives of General Psychiatry, 44,* 152–156.

Weissman, M. M., Klerman, G. L., Markowitz, J. S., & Ouellette, R. (1989). Suicidal ideation and suicide attempts in panic disorder attacks. *New England Journal of Medicine, 321,* 1209–1214.

Weissman, M. M., Sholomskas, D., Pottenger, M., Prusoff, B. A., & Locke, B. Z. (1977). Assessing depressive symptoms in five psychiatric populations: A validation study. *American Journal of Epidemiology, 106,* 203–214.

Wells, K. B., Golding, J. M., & Burnam, M. A. (1988). Psychiatric disorders and limitations in physical functioning in a sample of the Los Angeles general population. *American Journal of Psychiatry, 145,* 712–717.

Wells, K. B., Stewart, A., Hays, R. D., Burnham, A., Rogers, W. Daniels, M., Berry, S., Greenfield, S., & Ware, J. (1989). The functioning and well-being of depressed patients: Results from the Medical Outcomes Study. *Journal of the American Medical Association, 262,* 914–919.

Winikoff, R. N., Coltin, K. L., Morgan, M. M., Buxbaum, R. C., & Barnett, G. O. (1984). Improving physician performance through peer comparison feedback. *Medical Care, 22,* 527–534.

Zung, W. W. K., Magill, M., Moore, J. T., & George, D. T. (1983). Recognition and treatment of depression in a family medicine practice. *Journal of Clinical Psychiatry, 44,* 3–6.

Name Index

C

D

G

H

I

J

K

L

Subject Index

E

F

G

H

I

J

L

M

Q

R

S